BONE TUMORS

BONE TUMORS

General Aspects and Data on 6,221 Cases

(Third Edition)

by

DAVID C. DAHLIN, M.D.

Consultant

Section of Surgical Pathology, Mayo Clinic

Professor of Pathology

Mayo Medical School

University of Minnesota

Rochester, Minnesota

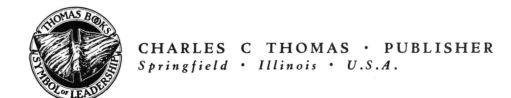

CHARLES C THOMAS · PUBLISHER
Springfield · Illinois · U.S.A.

Published and Distributed Throughout the World by
CHARLES C THOMAS • PUBLISHER
BANNERSTONE HOUSE
301-327 East Lawrence Avenue, Springfield, Illinois, U.S.A.

© *1957, 1967, and 1978 by* CHARLES C THOMAS • PUBLISHER
ISBN-0-398-03692-6
Library of Congress Catalog Card Number: 77-24333

First Edition, 1957
Second Edition, First Printing, 1967
Second Edition, Second Printing, 1970
Second Edition, Third Printing, 1973
Third Edition, 1978

With THOMAS BOOKS *careful attention is given to all details of manufacturing and design. It is the Publisher's desire to present books that are satisfactory as to their physical qualities and artistic possibilities and appropriate for their particular use.* THOMAS BOOKS *will be true to those laws of quality that assure a good name and good will.*

Library of Congress Cataloging in Publication Data

Dahlin, David C.
  Bone tumors. Third Edition.

  Includes bibliographies and index.
    1. Bones—Tumors. I. Title. [DNLM: 1. Bone
neoplasms. WE258 D131b]
  RC280.B6D33 1977   616.9'92'71   77-24333
  ISBN 0-398-03692-6

Printed in the United States of America
C-1

Preface to Third Edition

THE BASIC CLASSIFICATION (modified from Lichtenstein's) employed in the first two editions has gained wide acceptance, does not vary in significant degree from the classifications used by other authors, and is used again in this book. The entities recognized have characteristic roentgenographic patterns, and their usefulness demands that they have significant clinical and therapeutic implications.

The eleven years ending December 31, 1975, have provided 2,234 additional tumors in patients who have been seen in consultation at the Mayo Clinic. Their tumors, all studied pathologically, have been incorporated into the total. The overall group has provided new studies of many types of tumor in collaboration with colleagues in pathology, roentgenology, and the therapeutic fields. The continuing cooperation of the Department of Medical Statistics and Epidemiology has provided us with follow-up data on 97 to 100 percent of the various categories of malignant bone tumor. Such continuing studies are essential to learning the biology of and therapeutic results for any series of tumors. Those myelomas diagnosed by marrow aspiration have not been studied in detail by me, but the 398 myelomas diagnosed from surgical material and all of the remainder of the bone tumors have been.

The institution of a section of Orthopedic Oncology has aided in standardizing management of these tumors. Doctor J. C. Ivins, Chairman of that section, has edited the short comments on therapy in this book. They are obviously not comprehensive since it is not my purpose to afford the reader with details in this area. Doctor J. W. Beabout and Doctor R. A. McLeod of our Department of Diagnostic Roentgenology have cooperated on the procurement of suitable roentgenograms for illustration of the various lesions and have edited the remarks concerning them.

The new data have necessitated increasing the size of most of the chapters. Concepts gained from the study of our own cases amplified by about 5,000 sent in for consultation have been incorporated when indicated. Notable additions are the new chapters on benign and malignant (fibrous) histiocytomas. Recognizable subtypes of osteosarcoma and chondrosarcoma are described and illustrated. Several new examples of bone tumor simulators are illustrated and briefly described in Chapter 28. Pertinent new references are included in the bibliography for each chapter.

Members of the Section of Photography and the Section of Medical Graphics have made indispensable contributions to this work. Doctor Marc A. Shampo of our Editorial staff has gone over this work in detail with me.

D. C. DAHLIN, M.D.

Preface to Second Edition

THE BASIC CLASSIFICATION (modified from Lichtenstein's) employed in the first edition, with tumors comprising histologically distinctive types that have significant clinical and therapeutic implications, has stood the test of time and has gained wide acceptance. Nevertheless, some minor but useful modifications and additions have been developed and are incorporated in this volume. A few of the tumors in the earlier series have been reclassified in the light of recent knowledge.

The nine years ending December 31, 1964, have provided more than 1,700 additional tumors, all in patients who consulted the Mayo Clinic and all studied pathologically, to augment the original series. These new cases have been incorporated into the total. The combined material has been reviewed pathologically and clinically in continuing studies in collaboration with my colleagues in the Section of Orthopedics and the Section of Diagnostic Roentgenology. It has provided significantly more follow-up information, which is critical to advancement of knowledge concerning each type of tumor. The continuing cooperation of our Section of Medical Statistics, Epidemiology, and Population Genetics has provided us with follow-up data on from 97 to 100 percent of the various categories of malignant bone tumor. The only group I have not studied in detail is the series of 1,044 myelomas that have been diagnosed on material obtained by aspiration of bone marrow. Patients in this group are examined and treated in the Special Hematology Laboratory, the Section of Therapeutic Radiology, and the Section of Clinical Oncology.

The new data have necessitated amplification of most of the chapters. Illustrations have been increased in order to document many of the concepts gained from study of our own material and of material sent in from elsewhere on some 1,200 problem cases in the past few years. Notable additions include comments on desmoplastic fibroma, mesenchymal chondrosarcoma, postirradiation sarcomas, and sarcomas secondary to chondromatosis and to multiple exostoses. A new chapter deals with odontogenic tumors. The bibliography for each chapter has been increased. Many of the articles that cover general aspects of diagnosis and treatment of bone tumors and several of the more comprehensive texts available are listed at the end of Chapter 1.

Members of the Section of Publications, the Section of Photography, and the Section of Medical Illustrations and Scientific Exhibits have made indispensable contributions to this work.

D. C. D.

vii

Preface to First Edition

MANY OF THE MAJOR ADVANCES in present-day understanding of neoplastic and nonneoplastic diseases of bone have been made in the last two decades. In the light of current concepts, I have reviewed systematically all the bone tumors in the files of the Mayo Clinic prior to 1956. I began this review nine years ago, and have had the help of several of my colleagues who have collaborated in the study of various facets of the overall problem, as is indicated in the bibliography. The study has embraced more than 2,000 consecutive, unselected bone tumors. Correlation of the clinical features with the gross and microscopic features has been possible because both the case records and the gross and microscopic specimens have been available for study. Complete follow-up studies were available in almost 100 percent of cases largely because of the work of Doctor Henry W. Meyerding, emeritus member, Section of Orthopedic Surgery, Mayo Clinic, and emeritus professor of orthopedic surgery, Mayo Foundation, Graduate School, University of Minnesota, whose active interest in bone tumors covered a span of nearly forty years.

Data derived from this study were first presented in the form of an exhibit at the annual meeting of the American Medical Association held in Chicago in June, 1956. Information on skeletal localization and on age and sex distribution, as well as roentgenograms, photomicrographs, and illustrative moulages of gross specimens, was included. As a result of this exhibit, a number of orthopedic surgeons, roentgenologists, and pathologists asked me to make the accumulated data available for reference. This I have attempted to do in this small volume, which is an amplification of the material presented in the exhibit.

Because proper understanding of the neoplasms of bone demands correlation of their roentgenologic, gross and microscopic features, these features are liberally illustrated. Textual material has been kept to a minimum and theoretical considerations have been almost completely avoided. The bibliography has been restricted to a few of the pertinent contributions on each subject.

In the final chapter I have discussed briefly several nonneoplastic diseases of bone because they are among those that may be confused clinically and roentgenologically with neoplasms of bone. Odontogenic tumors, because of the special problems they pose, have not been included in the series.

I am indebted to Doctor David G. Pugh, of the Section of Roentgenology of the Mayo Clinic, for his review of the illustrative roentgenograms and of the comments on the roentgenologic features of bone tumors. From Doctor Einer W. Johnson, Jr., and Doctor William H. Bickel of the Section of Orthopedic Surgery, I have received invaluable aid in preparation of the comments on therapy. I am also indebted to the entire staff of the Section of Orthopedic Surgery for their cooperation in this project. To Doctor Carl M. Gambill, of the Section of Publications, and to the Section of Photography, the Section of Biometry and Medical Statistics and the Art Studio I am grateful for their contributions to this book. Doctor Arthur H. Bulbulian, of the Mayo Foundation Museum of Hygiene and Medicine, did much of the work on the original exhibit of bone tumors.

D. C. D.

Contents

xi

BONE TUMORS

Chapter 1

Introduction and Scope of Study

THE TABULATED STATISTICS included in this book are those of an unselected series of bone tumors except for the following factors. A case was included only if a complete surgical specimen or adequate material for biopsy had been obtained. No case was included in which histologic verification of the diagnosis according to modern pathologic concepts was impossible. The pathologic features were currently reviewed in every case. The patients had all come to the Mayo Clinic for care, thus introducing a possible selection factor of questionable significance.

Accurate analysis of many of the tumors from the earlier years embraced by this study would have been impossible but for the fact that the entire gross specimen, preserved in 10% formalin solution, was available for review in practically every case. A sufficient number of new microscopic sections were made to assure that the various gross features of each lesion could be studied histologically. Such new sections were essential for the correct interpretation of certain lesions. In the average aneurysmal bone cyst, for example, the microscopic section on file was often from a nonspecific solid portion, and it was necessary to embed the curetted fragments from the specimen bottle in paraffin to obtain a preparation that reconstructed the true pathologic appearance to a degree sufficient for correct diagnosis.

Roentgenograms or the interpretation of them were correlated with the gross and histopathologic features. Although roentgenographic shadows do not supplant microscopic sections in the final diagnosis, they frequently afford practically conclusive evidence of the malignant or benign nature of bony lesions and often indicate the histologic type. The roentgenogram may be considered part of the gross pathologic findings, delimiting as it does the part of the bone affected and, in large measure, the extent of the disease. The pathologist responsible for the diagnosis of osseous lesions handicaps himself immeasurably if he ignores their roentgenographic features. These features provide a useful guide for proper biopsy. Anyone can determine, for instance, the inadequacy of an inconclusive needle biopsy specimen or a gram of necrotic tissue excised from a tumor that gives the roentgenologic appearance of having destroyed half of a femur. A recognized limitation is that rather gross destruction, especially of cancellous bone, is necessary for a lesion to be reflected in the roentgenogram. This is well illustrated in Figures 27-4 and 27-5, pages 349 and 350.

In rare instances, as with every diagnostic modality, the roentgenogram provides misleading information. A pertinent case is illustrated on page 417.

In most bone tumors, the patient's local symptoms and the results of physical examination are relatively nonspecific. The usual symptoms, pain or swelling or both of these, serve mainly as a guide to the correct site for roentgenographic studies and for biopsy. Accordingly, clinical features of bone tumors have been relegated to a relatively minor place in the discussions to follow. Occasionally, however, as with osteoid osteoma that may give referred pain at a site well away from the lesion, clinical judgment is all-important.

Laboratory studies are of little aid in the diagnosis of the average bone tumor. Myeloma, with its sometimes practically pathognomonic alteration of proteins in serum or urine, is a notable exception. Alkaline phosphatase levels may be elevated in osteoid-producing neoplasms, either primary or metastatic. Elevated levels of acid phosphatase are suggestive of metastatic prostatic carcinoma. The ominous nature of rapidly growing sarcomas such as Ewing's tumor may be suggested by systemic evidences that include fever, anemia, and rapid sedimentation rate of erythrocytes.

Physiologists, chemists, and electron microscopists are attempting to clarify some of the basic problems relative to the diagnosis and nature of neoplasms, including those in bone. Some day a simpler method may be found for indicating the biologic capability of each bone tumor that presents a problem. As of now, however, the diagnosis on which therapy must be predicated and prognosis estimated depends upon correct interpretation of material removed for biopsy and stained by techniques that have been known for decades, sometimes augmented significantly by gross pathologic alterations including those reflected in the roentgenogram.

In the interest of brevity, a somewhat dogmatic stand will be presented in the chapters to follow. This will be based on the study of Mayo Clinic cases and a review of the literature. When significant differences of opinion exist, these will be indicated in the text or in the bibliography.

Practical Approach to Rapid Histologic Diagnosis

Successful therapy of malignant disease depends upon the institution of treatment before systemic dissemination has occurred. It is axiomatic, therefore, that when the treatment of choice is ablative surgery it should be instituted at the earliest practicable moment in an attempt to remove the tumor before the neoplastic embolization that leads to death of the patient has occurred.

At least 90 percent of bone tumors have soft portions that can be sectioned and examined for immediate diagnosis. In most cases, these soft portions afford the best material for diagnosis. For example, in sclerosing osteosarcoma there are almost invariably such noncalcified zones at the periphery of the tumor. Study of the roentgenogram will guide the surgeon to these zones from which to obtain biopsy specimens for early diagnosis. Pathologists are becoming increasingly aware that they can, after examination of the roentgenograms, give the surgeon valuable counsel regarding the biopsy procedure. Protracted decalcification of densely sclerotic portions of the tumor or adjacent cortical bone only delays the institution of therapy.

Fresh-frozen sections allow an immediate, accurate, definitive diagnosis in more than 90 percent of the cases of bone tumor. There should be no problem in recognizing the rare lesion that is too difficult or too ossified for rapid interpretation. As with fixed sections of various types, good histologic preparations and sound basic understanding of the pathologic features are requisites for successful interpretation of fresh-frozen sections. Deficiency in either requisite will tend to make one deprecate this diagnostic medium. Actually the fresh-frozen technique has several advantages over conventional permanent-section techniques. First, it allows immediate appraisal of the adequacy of the specimen for biopsy. Edematous tissue around the tumor, necrotic neoplastic tissue, or benign portions of the lesion with frankly malignant foci may otherwise be considered representative of the pathologic process. Second, if the lesion proves to be inflammatory, the pathologist is guided to proper bacteriologic techniques. Third, it allows immediate appraisal of the adequacy of attempted total resection or the adequacy of level of amputation. Finally, and most important, in malignant tumors that are best treated by ablative surgery, definitive therapy can be carried out immediately. Dockerty, in 1953, detailed the technique that has been employed successfully in our laboratory, with minor variations, for more than sixty years.

The pathologist who is averse to making a definitive diagnosis on fresh-frozen sections should have permanent sections ready for diagnosis generally within twenty-four hours, provided the surgeon has procured the most suitable tissue for biopsy.

Ultrastructural studies and staining techniques other than the ordinary technique with hematoxylin and eosin are rarely necessary because they are of insignificant value in most cases. On some occasions, a stain for mucus helps in the differentiation of metastatic carcinoma from primary neoplasm of bone. A stain for reticulin in examples of reticulum cell sarcoma has questionable value because atypical tumors often show equivocal amounts of stainable reticulin. Even techniques for the demonstration of alkaline phosphatase in fresh material are of no value in classification, this enzyme appearing in such cells as those of a pure chondrosarcoma and the endothelial cells intermixed in typical reticulum cell sarcoma. The demonstration of glycogen within the cytoplasm of malignant "small round cell" tumors of bone is outlined by Schajowicz in his study of Ewing's sarcoma. Fixation in 80% ethanol is recommended. Glycogen is usually absent in the cells of malignant lymphoma and present in those of Ewing's tumor.

The procurement of material for biopsy of bone tumors by aspiration through a needle or trochar has become increasingly advocated. Positive results obtained by this technique are dependable and of value, and at the Mayo Clinic, its greatest usefulness has been in lesions of the vertebrae where it can supplant an extensive operation for surgical removal of tissue. The use of this technique is limited, however, since a negative result has little value if there is clinical and roentgenologic evidence of significant disease. Also, in some tumors such as low-grade, well-differentiated chondrosarcomas, a large sample may be necessary to provide adequate evidence of malignant disease or to find the highly malignant areas that may be present in an otherwise low-grade tumor.

When decalcification is necessary, a number of satisfactory techniques are available. Detailed considerations of them were published by Morris and Benton in 1956. A good principle is to avoid the dense bone that requires severe measures for

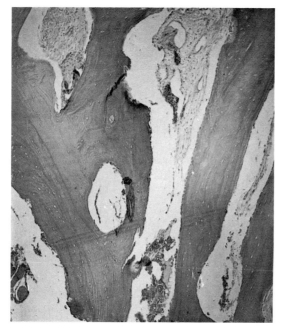

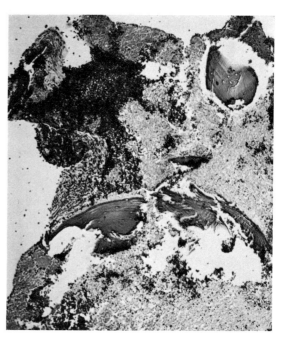

Figure 1-1. Lymphoma permeating dense bone, a poor place for biopsy. Decalcification has ruined cytologic features. (×50)

Figure 1-2. Nondiagnostic, necrotic tissue. Frozen sections could have provided guidance to adequate tissue. (×75)

decalcification. Careful selection of the abnormal material minimizes the decalcification of immaterial and sometimes voluminous adjacent bone. Relatively thin and small blocks should be prepared. Coarse and slow-moving saw teeth increase artifact produced by the forcing of bone fragments into soft tissue areas, especially in very thin blocks. We have employed 20% formic acid successfully, and it works relatively rapidly. Ethylenediaminetetraacetic acid (EDTA) provides adequate decalcification of small, not heavily calcified fragments such as those from cancellous bone. This ion-exchange material has the advantage that its basic solution is 10% formalin to which, in the ratio of 4 g to 80 ml, the EDTA has been added.

In the laboratory, we use a butcher's meat saw with a disposable blade 65 cm long for cutting large bone specimens and an X-acto® saw, which contains a fine-toothed, disposable blade 11.4 cm long, for producing small blocks that are to be decalcified and processed into microscopic sections. Band saws and other related units with external power sources are large, somewhat dangerous, and generally unnecessary.

Literature

Numerous articles and books concerned with bone tumors have appeared in recent years. Most authors now recognize that a useful classification must comprise entities that are pathologically distinct and have significant clinical, therapeutic, and prognostic implications. Nearly everyone has accepted the several entities that have

---

* Throughout this book, hematoxylin-eosin stain has been used in tissue samples unless legend states otherwise.

been clarified by the works and writings of Jaffe and Lichtenstein. There are still some differences of opinion regarding exact definitions of some tumors. Accordingly, at the end of this chapter, I have provided the interested reader with a bibliography that includes the major texts that have been written in English. The list also includes many of the classic articles related to diagnostic techniques, therapy, and etiology of tumors, as well as some of the comprehensive studies of bone tumors in general and of those in special locations.

Classification

The classification used in this book (Table I) is similar to that advocated by Lichtenstein. One of the significant differences is that there has been little attempt to draw a relationship between the benign and the malignant tumors because so few of the latter take origin from the former. The classification is based on the cytology or the recognizable products of the proliferating cells. In most instances, the tumors

TABLE 1

CLASSIFICATION OF 6,221 PRIMARY TUMORS OF BONE*

(All were Mayo Clinic Patients)

Histologic type	Benign	Cases	Malignant	Cases
Hematopoietic 2,572 cases (41.4%)			Myeloma Reticulum cell sarcoma	2,245 327
Chondrogenic 1,300 cases (20.9%)	Osteochondroma Chondroma Chondroblastoma Chondromyxoid fibroma	579 162 44 30	Primary chondrosarcoma Secondary chondrosarcoma Dedifferentiated chondrosarcoma Mesenchymal chondrosarcoma	367 52 51 15
Osteogenic 1,199 cases (19.3%)	Osteoid osteoma Benign osteoblastoma	158 43	Osteosarcoma Parosteal osteogenic sarcoma	962 36
Unknown origin 607 cases (9.8%)	Giant cell tumor (Fibrous) histiocytoma	264 7	Ewing's tumor Malignant giant cell tumor Adamantinoma (Fibrous) histiocytoma	299 20 17 (35)[+]
Fibrogenic 234 cases (3.8%)	Fibroma Desmoplastic fibroma	72 4	Fibrosarcoma	158
Notochordal 195 cases (3.1%)			Chordoma	195
Vascular 99 cases (1.6%)	Hemangioma	69	Hemangioendothelioma Hemangiopericytoma	25 5
Lipogenic 5 cases	Lipoma	5		
Neurogenic 10 cases	Neurilemmoma	10		
	Total benign	1,447	Total malignant	4,774

* Classification based on that advocated by Louis Lichtenstein. Classification of Primary Tumors of Bone, *Cancer* 4: 335–341, 1951.

+ Numbers in parentheses not in data totals.

apparently arise from the type of tissue they produce, but such an assumption cannot be proved correct. For example, most chondrosarcomas begin in portions of bone that normally contain no obvious benign cartilaginous zones. In any event, basing a classification on what is actually seen histologically allows reduplication of results on subsequent analysis. Some of the lesions in the general classification are probably not neoplasms in the strict sense.

Myxomas of the jaws are probably of odontogenic derivation. Myxomas are practically never seen elsewhere in the skeleton. One myxosarcoma that I have seen in the humerus was metastatic from a similar tumor of the uterus. I have seen two periosteal myxomas that have eroded nearby bone. I have seen in consultation three large expansile tumors of the ends of femurs of elderly patients that appeared to be myxoma alone. Chondrosarcomas, fibrosarcomas, chondromyxoid fibromas, and portions of fibrous dysplasia may have prominent myxoid features.*

HEMATOPOIETIC TUMORS: The hematopoietic tumors, numbering 2,572, were the most prevalent tumors of bone in the files of the Mayo Clinic. These included 2,245 cases of myeloma. Malignant lymphomas of bone, which ordinarily contain a predominance of reticulum cells and are generally referred to as reticulum cell sarcomas, contributed 327 cases. Leukemic tumor nodules in bone, while commonly found in the terminal phases of leukemia, rarely masquerade clinically as primary malignant disease of bone, although osteoarticular symptoms and signs may be prominent in acute leukemia.

CHONDROGENIC TUMORS: The second largest group consisted of chondrogenic tumors. The tumors in this group were placed there because their histologic appearance proved or suggested a relationship to hyaline cartilage. More than one fifth of the total series were in this group, and the osteochondromas (osteocartilaginous exostoses) constituted 45 percent of the chondrogenic group. Osteochondromas result from growth of their cartilaginous caps, making them basically chondrogenic. Chondromas, whether they be centrally or subperiosteally located, are tumors of hyaline cartilage which may show variable amounts of calcification and ossification within their substance. Benign chondroblastomas have been separated from the "wastebasket" of giant cell tumors of bone because their proliferating cells produce foci of a matrix substance quite like that of hyaline cartilage. Although chondromyxoid fibromas have a variegated histologic appearance, large or small zones ordinarily bear a striking resemblance to hyaline cartilage. Both primary and secondary chondrosarcomas occur. Approximately 10 percent of either type dedifferentiate into highly malignant neoplasms. Mesenchymal chondrosarcoma is recognized as a distinctive lesion.

OSTEOGENIC TUMORS: In the osteogenic group of tumors, the 998 sarcomas dominated the group. For a tumor to qualify for this group, the malignant neoplastic cells of the given tumor must, in at least some portions, produce recognizable osteoid substance. With this basic qualification the osteosarcomas logically fall into three classes, namely osteoblastic, chondroblastic, and fibroblastic, depending upon the dominant histologic structure. The basic biologic behaviors of these three tumor

---

* All data in this book pertain to Mayo Clinic patients unless otherwise indicated.

subtypes, however, are similar, as will be shown in the chapter devoted to osteosarcoma.

Periosteal osteosarcoma is now recognizable as a separate entity, and its features will be illustrated. The twenty-five tumors that we have segregated as definite and recognizable "telangiectatic" osteosarcomas will be described.

The clinically indolent and pathologically slowly progressing low-grade tumors that have become generally known as parosteal or juxacortical osteosarcomas have been placed in a separate subdivision.

In the Mayo Clinic files there are 158 examples of ordinary osteoid osteoma. Without delving into the controversy as to whether this lesion represents a true neoplasm or some peculiar reaction in bone, we have arbitrarily classed it with the bone tumors. The forty-three tumors that we previously called "giant osteoid osteomas" represent an unusually controversial group of cases. Lesions of this type have been called "osteogenic fibromas," "ossifying fibromas," and more recently "osteoblastomas." We employed the term "giant osteoid osteoma" because this tumor bears such a close histologic resemblance to ordinary osteoid osteoma. The prefix "giant" was meant to indicate a different biologic behavior, since tumors of this type do not share the strictly limited growth potential of the average osteoid osteoma. Benign osteoblastoma is now the generally accepted name for this tumor. Larger size is its greatest difference from osteoid osteoma.

TUMORS OF UNKNOWN ORIGIN: The most common tumor of unknown origin was Ewing's tumor, constituting 299 cases. Benign giant cell tumor, with 264 cases, was almost as prevalent. The giant cells of the benign giant cell tumor appear to arise from the stromal cells, the exact origin of which is unknown. It has been suggested that they arise from undifferentiated mesenchymal cells of bone. The diagnosis of malignant giant cell tumor cannot be substantiated unless one can demonstrate typical zones of benign giant cell tumor in the current or previous tissue from the same case. We had only twenty bona fide malignant giant cell tumors. Adamantinoma of long bones is of unknown origin and only seventeen examples were present in this series. Fibrous histiocytomas, both benign and malignant, are now included in the discussion. The exceptionally controversial status of lesions that appear to belong in these two categories will be amplified.

FIBROGENIC TUMORS: The pathologic entity called "fibromas of bone," although quite likely not neoplastic, has been included among the bone tumors because of common usage. The files contained seventy-two examples. Only 158 pure fibrosarcomas of bone were encountered. It should be stressed, however, that multiple sections of all of the tumors were made, and osteoid production in any portion of a predominantly fibroblastic tumor relegated it to the osteosarcoma group. The four desmoplastic fibromas encountered, although histologically benign, will be discussed in relation to fibrosarcomas.

NOTOCHORDAL TUMORS: This series included 195 chordomas. Metastasis is somewhat unusual, but this tumor commonly produces death of its host by local recurrence and extension, and hence it has been placed in the category of malignant tumors.

TUMORS OF VASCULAR ORIGIN: Although the angiomatous tumors are relatively commonly manifested in roentgenograms, only 1.6 percent of the histologically verified neoplasms in this series were in this group. Sixty-nine of these were hemangiomas, five were hemangiopericytomas, and twenty-five were malignant blood vascular tumors.

LIPOGENIC TUMORS: Five lipomas of bone were found. In no case did it seem possible to substantiate the unequivocal diagnosis of liposarcoma of bone. The occasional tumor with multinucleated malignant cells, possessing foamy cytoplasm and suggesting the possibility of an origin from adipose connective tissue, was classed with the osteosarcomas or with the (fibrous) histiocytomas. This decision was based on the observation that a similar histologic appearance was present in other tumors which contained zones of obvious osteosarcoma or qualified as (fibrous) histiocytomas.

NEUROGENIC TUMORS: Four of the ten neurilemmomas of bone in the present series involved the mandible. No malignant neurogenic tumors originating in bone were recognized.

UNCLASSIFIED TUMORS: A few tumors had to be discarded from the total series because there was insufficient tissue for accurate classification. Another group, constituting approximately 1 percent of the total, did not fall into a niche in the classification. These neoplasms form a heterogeneous group that, for the time being, must be called "unclassified."

Skeletal and Age Distribution

The skeletal distribution of the various types of tumors is shown in Table 2. It affords the reader a convenient guide for comparative incidence whether he is interested in a specific neoplasm or an affected bone. The knowledge that certain bones are practically immune to some tumors and have a marked predilection to be the site of development of other neoplasms often assists one in arriving at a correct diagnosis. It is noteworthy, for instance, that only 3 of 962 osteosarcomas affected bones of the hands and wrists and that all but 2 of the 34 tumors of the sternum were malignant.

Some tumors have a decided predilection for patients in certain age groups. Knowledge of this predilection is often useful in arriving at a preoperative diagnosis. The succeeding chapters indicate, with bar graphs, the age distribution for each neoplasm. For specific figures, the reader is referred to Table 3.

TABLE 2

LOCALIZATION DATA ON BONE TUMORS

(Exclusive of 1,847 Patients with Multiple Myelomas, 63 with Multiple Exostoses, and 26 with Multiple Chondromas)

	Femur	Tibia	Fibula	Tarsals	Foot	Patella	Humerus	Radius	Ulna
Osteochondroma	185	83	24	4	1		99	8	3
Chondroma	27	2	4		9	1	18	2	1
Chondroblastoma	11	7		1			6		
Chondromyxoid fibroma	6	9		1	6			2	1
Osteoid osteoma	59	41	2	6	2		13	2	4
Benign osteoblastoma	3	5	1	1		1	3		
Giant cell tumor	79	69	7	3			16	27	8
Fibrous histiocytoma	2	1					1		
Fibroma	27	31	8				4	2	
Desmoplastic fibroma				1			1	1	
Hemangioma	5	1	1			1	2		
Lipoma	1								1
Neurilemmoma	2								
Total benign	407	249	47	17	18	3	163	44	18
Myeloma	26	4					20		1
Malignant lymphoma	78	22	1	3		1	26	1	3
Primary chondrosarcoma	89	15	2	2	4		36	2	1
Secondary chondrosarcoma	5	4	4				4		
Mesenchymal chondrosarcoma	1				1				
Osteosarcoma	405	178	30	8	1		100	7	5
Parosteal Osteosarcoma	28	5					2		1
Ewing's tumor	66	26	20	9	7		33	4	4
Malignant giant cell tumor	11	2					3		
Adamantinoma	1	13	1						2
(Fibrous) histiocytoma	(15)	(4)	(1)				(3)		(1)
Fibrosarcoma	43	26	2	2			12	2	1
Chordoma									
Hemangioendothelioma	1	3	1	1		1	3		
Hemangiopericytoma									
Total malignant	754	298	61	25	13	2	239	16	18
Total series	1,161	547	108	42	31	5	402	60	36

* Includes 2 multi(bi)focal giant cell tumors and 1 multifocal fibroma.

+ Excludes 4 myelomas diagnosed on basis of lymph nodes, 4 other soft-tissue sites, and 1,847 on marrow.

‡ Primary chondrosarcoma includes 51 dedifferentiated tumors. Excludes 3 chondrosarcomas of hyoid and 1 of knee joint.

TABLE 2 *(Continued)*

Carpals	Hand	Scapula	Clavicle	Ribs	Sternum	Vertebra	Sacrum	Innominate	Skull	Mandible	Maxilla and nasal cavity	Total
1	9	26	3	15		14	3	39				517
1	55	2		4	1	5	1	3				136
		4		3		1		8	2	1		44
							1	4				30
2	8	4				9		5		1		158
1				1		16	3		1	7		43
	1			3	1	9	23	17	3			266*
							2	1				7
			1									73
										1		4
				1		17		1	29	4	7	69
				1					2			5
		1		1			1		1	4		10
5	73	37	4	29	2	71	34	78	38	18	7	1,362
		9	17	65	10	135	16	46	13	8	20	390+
	1	20		29	7	29	17	46	21	22		327
1	7	20	2	60	11	28	9	104	2	1	18	414‡
		4	1	1		3	2	24				52
		1		3		1		2	1	2	3	15
	3	13	5	12	3	17	11	81	17	30	36	962
												36
	1	16	7	23	1	7	15	53	4	3		299
							2	2				20
												17
	(1)							(4)	(4)	(1)	(1)	(35)
		5		3		6	9	21	6	17	3	158
						28	96		71			195
	1			3		5		5	1			25
				1		1		2			1	5
1	13	88	32	200	32	260	177	386	136	83	81	2,915
6	86	125	36	229	34	331	211	464	174	101	88	4,277

TABLE 3

DISTRIBUTION OF TUMORS BY HISTOLOGIC TYPE AND BY AGE OF PATIENTS

Histologic type	Age distribution by decades									Total patients
	1	*2*	*3*	*4*	*5*	*6*	*7*	*8*	*9*	
Benign										
Hematopoietic										None
Chondrogenic										
Osteochondroma	54	279	115	62	36	24	7	2		579
Chondroma	15	40	29	27	29	11	10	1		162
Chondroblastoma	1	24	6	4	3	6				44
Chondromyxoid fibroma	5	6	10	3	3	3				30
Osteogenic										
Osteoid osteoma	22	80	39	11	3	2	1			158
Benign osteoblastoma	2	20	14	4	1	1	1			43
Unknown origin										
Giant cell tumor	2	37	99	66	36	14	7	3		264
(Fibrous) histocytoma			2		3	1	1			7
Fibrogenic										
Fibroma	17	44	10	1						72
Desmoplastic fibroma		2	2							4
Notochordal										None
Vascular										
Hemangioma	2	3	10	13	22	11	7	1		69
Lipogenic										
Lipoma				1	2		1	1		5
Neurogenic										
Neurilemmoma		4	2		1		2	1		10
Total benign	120	539	338	192	139	73	37	9		1,447

TABLE 3 *(Continued)*

Histologic type	Age distribution by decades									Total patients
	1	*2*	*3*	*4*	*5*	*6*	*7*	*8*	*9*	
Malignant										
Hematopoietic										
Myeloma			5	20	77	124	115	53	3	398*
Malignant lymphoma	11	36	37	35	52	80	55	17	4	327
Chondrogenic										
Chondrosarcoma										
Primary	3	15	38	64	76	96	56	16	3	367
Secondary		2	18	16	11	4	1			52
Mesenchymal chondrosarcoma		2	5	4	3	1				15
Dedifferentiated chondrosarcoma		1		5	10	24	5	5	1	51
Osteogenic										
Osteosarcoma	46	472	168	74	80	54	47	20	1	962
Parosteal osteosarcoma		7	12	10	6	1				36
Unknown origin										
Ewing's tumor	59	171	46	14	6	3				299
Malignant giant cell tumor			3	7	3	6	1			20
Adamantinoma	1	5	8	1		2				17
Malignant (fibrous) histiocytoma	(1)	(7)	(3)	(7)	(6)	(2)	(8)	(1)		(35)+
Fibrogenic										
Fibrosarcoma	1	23	18	38	25	28	16	6	3	158
Notochordal										
Chordoma	1	6	12	32	41	53	35	13	2	195
Vascular										
Hemangioendothelioma	1	4	4	5	6	2	3			25
Hemangiopericytoma				2	1		1	1		5
Lipogenic										None
Neurogenic										None
Total malignant	123	745	374	327	397	478	335	131	17	2,927

* Exclusive of 1,847 tumors diagnosed only by marrow aspiration.
+ Numbers in parentheses not in data totals.

Bibliography

1948   Guri, J. P.: Tumors of the Vertebral Column. *Surg Gynecol Obstet, 87:*583-598.
1948   Hatcher, C. H.: The Diagnosis of Bone Sarcoma. *Rocky Mt Med J, 45:*968-978 (Nov.)
1949   Geschickter, C. F., and Copeland, M.M.: *Tumors of Bone,* ed. 3. Philadelphia, Lippincott, 810 pp.
1951   Pugh, D. G.: *Roentgenologic Diagnosis of Diseases of Bones.* Baltimore, Williams & Wilkins, pp. 352-568.
1951   Lichtenstein, L.: Classification of Primary Tumors of Bone. *Cancer, 4:*335-341.
1953   Dockerty, M. B.: Rapid Frozen Sections—Technique of Their Preparation and Staining. *Surg Gynecol Obstet, 97:*113-120.
1953   Johnson, L. C.: A General Theory of Bone Tumors. *Bull N Y Acad Med, 29:*164-171.
1955   Schajowicz, F.: Aspiration Biopsy in Bone Lesions. Cytological and Histological Techniques. *J Bone Joint Surg, 77A:*465-471.

1955 Lichtenstein, L.: Tumors of Periosteal Origin. *Cancer, 8:*1060-1069.

1955 Barrett, N. R.: Primary Tumors of Rib. *Br J Surg, 43:*113-132.

1955 Thomson, A. D., and Turner-Warwick, R. T.: Skeletal Sarcomata and Giant-Cell Tumour. *J Bone Joint Surg, 37B:*266-303.

1956 Morris, R. E., Jr., and Benton, R. S.: Studies on Demineralization of Bone: I. The Basic Factors of Demineralization. II. The Effect of Electrolytic Technics in Demineralization. III. The Effect of Ion Exchange Resins and Versenate in Demineralization. IV. Evaluation of Morphology and Staining Characteristics of Tissues After Demineralization. *Am J Clin Path, 26:*579-595, 596-603, 771-777, 882-898.

1956 Sirsat, M. V.: Sarcoma of Bone: Observations on 150 Cases, With Special Reference to Incidence, Location and Pathology. *Indian J Surg, 18:*1-30.

1957 Schobinger, R., and Stoll, H. C.: The Arteriographic Picture of Benign Bone Lesions Containing Giant Cells. *J Bone Joint Surg, 39A:*953-960.

1957 Bickel, W. H., and Lewis, R. C., Jr.: Hemipelvectomy for Malignant Disease. *JAMA, 165:*8-12.

1957 Tracey, J. F., Brindley, H. H., and Murray, R. A.: Primary Malignant Tumors of Bone. *J Bone Joint Surg, 39A:*554-560.

1958 Jaffe, H. L.: *Tumors and Tumorous Conditions of the Bones and Joints.* Philadelphia, Lea & Febiger, 629 pp.

1959 Bucalossi, P., Di Pietro, S., and Rock, T.: Tumori della Gabbia Toracica. *Tumori, 45:*695-750.

1959 Strickland, B.: The Value of Arteriography in the Diagnosis of Bone Tumours. *Br J Radiol, 32:*705-713.

1962 Vittali, Horst-Peter: Zur Diagnose der Bösartigen "Zystischen" Knochentumoren. *Munch Med Wochenschr, 104:*2494-2497; 2511-2512.

1963 Gilmer, W. S., Higley, G. B. Jr., and Kilgore, W. E.: *Atlas of Bone Tumors: Including Tumorlike Lesions.* Saint Louis, Mosby, 165 pp.

1964 Gabrielsen, T. O., and Kingman, A. F., Jr.: Osteocartilaginous Tumors of the Base of the Skull. Report of a Unique Case and Review of the Literature. *Am J Roentgenol, 91:*1016-1023.

1964 Cohen, D. M., Dahlin, D. C., and MacCarty, C. S.: Apparently Solitary Tumors of the Vertebral Column. *Mayo Clin Proc, 39:*509-528.

1969 Boyd, J. T., Doll, R., Hill, G. B., and Sissons, H. A.: Mortality From Primary Tumors of Bone in England and Wales, 1961-63. *Br J Prev Soc Med, 23:*12-22 (February).

1971 Murray, R. O., and Jacobson, H. G.: *The Radiology of Skeletal Disorders: Exercises in Diagnosis.* Baltimore, Williams & Wilkins, 1320 pp.

1971 Spjut, H. J., Dorfman, H. D., Fechner, R. E., and Ackerman, L. V.: Tumors of Bone and Cartilage. In *Atlas of Tumor Pathology,* Fascicle 5. Washington, D.C., Armed Forces Institute of Pathology, 454 pp.

1972 Lichtenstein, L.: *Bone Tumors,* ed. 4. Saint Louis, Mosby, 441 pp.

1972 Schajowicz, F., Ackerman, L. V., and Sissons, H. A.: Histologic Typing of Bone Tumours. In *International Histological Classification of Tumours No. 6.* Geneva, World Health Organization, 59 pp.

1972 Volkov, M. V.: *Childhood Osteology: Bone Tumors and Dysplasias.* Moscow, Mir Publishers, 466 pp.

1973 Dorfman, H. D.: Malignant Transformation of Benign Bone Lesions. In *Proceedings of the Seventh National Cancer Conference.* Philadelphia, Lippincott, pp. 901-913.

1973 Edeiken, J., and Hodes, P. J.: *Roentgen Diagnosis of Diseases of Bone,* ed. 2, vols. 1 and 2. Baltimore, Williams & Wilkins, 1156 pp.

1973 The Netherlands Committee on Bone Tumours: *Radiological Atlas of Bone Tumours,* vols. 1 and 2. Baltimore, Williams & Wilkins, 600 pp.

1973 Uehlinger, E.: Pathologische Anatomie der Knochengeschwülste. *Helv Chir Acta, 40:*5-27 (March).

1974 Adler, C. P.: Klinische und Morphologische Aspekte Maligner Knochentumoren. *Dtsch Med Wochenschr, 1, No. 14:*665-671 (April).

1974 Larsson, S.-E., and Lorentzon, R.: The Geographic Variation of the Incidence of Malignant Primary Bone Tumors in Sweden. *J Bone Joint Surg, 56A:*592-600 (April).

1974 Larsson, S.-E., and Lorentzon, R.: The Incidence of Malignant Primary Bone Tumors in Relation to Age, Sex, and Site: A Study of Osteogenic Sarcoma, Chondrosarcoma and Ewing's Sarcoma Diagnosed in Sweden From 1958 to 1968. *J Bone Joint Surg, 56B*:534-540 (August).

1974 Weinert, C. R., Jr., McMaster, J. H., and Ferguson, R. J.: Immune Response to Sarcomas: A Review. *Clin Orthop, 102*:207-216 (July-August).

1975 Aegerter, E. E., and Kirkpatrick, J. A., Jr.: *Orthopedic Diseases: Physiology, Pathology, Radiology,* ed. 4. Philadelphia, Saunders, 792 pp.

1975 Finkel, M. P., Reilley, C. A., Jr., and Biskis, B. O.: Viral Etiology of Bone Cancer. *Front Radiat Ther Oncol, 10*:28-39.

Chapter 2

Osteochondroma (Osteocartilaginous Exostosis)

T HIS MOST COMMON of the benign bone tumors logically belongs in the chondrogenic group. Although the average osteochondroma is predominantly osseous, the bony mass is produced by progressive enchondral ossification of its growing cartilaginous cap. Growth of these tumors usually parallels that of the patient, and the lesions often become quiescent when the epiphyses have closed.

One may question whether osteochondromas are correctly classed with the neoplasms of bone, but their clinical features and their rare malignant transformation make it reasonable to include them among the tumors. Their pathologic features make it apparent that the tumors are produced by growth of aberrant foci of cartilage on the surface of bone. Hence, one could consider these tumors among the congenital anomalies.

A few of the reported lesions have arisen after radiation that involved a bone. Bony spurs that result from such things as trauma and degenerative joint disease are not truly osteochondromas.

Multiple Osteochondromas

A much smaller group of patients has numerous osteochondromas affecting many bones. In this condition, which has a strong familial tendency, each individual tumor has the characteristics that will be described for the solitary form. The incidence of development of secondary chondrosarcoma in patients with multiple osteochondromas is probably more than 10 percent. The exact risk of sarcomatous change is unknown because of selection factors related to indications for surgery in individual cases with benign or suspected malignant tumors and the lack of follow-up from birth to death in a large unselected group of patients with multiple osteochondromas. The same criticisms apply with regard to the risk for patients with multiple chondromas. Osteochondromas result from a distinctive form of dysplasia that should not be confused with enchondromatosis. Most patients with multiple exostoses have many, sometimes innumerable, lesions that may be grossly deforming. An occasional patient has only two or three. One patient in our study had polyposis of the colon.

Subungual Exostoses

These peculiar projections from the distal portion of a terminal phalanx, usually of the first toe, are almost certainly the result of trauma with or without superimposed infection. They are not included in the data on osteochondromas although they possess many of the roentgenologic and pathologic features of them.

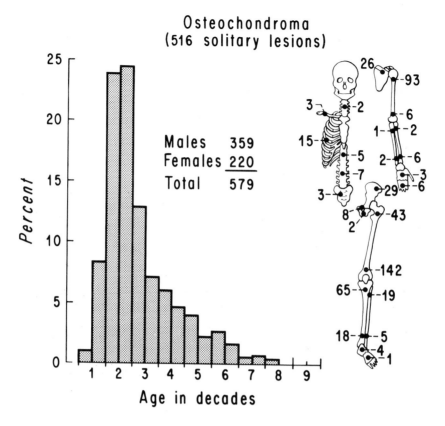

Figure 2-1. Skeletal, age, and sex distribution of osteochondromas.

Incidence

Osteochondromas comprised 40 percent of the benign bone tumors and 9.3 percent of the total in this series. Many of these tumors are asymptomatic and never found, and many of those discovered are never excised, so their actual incidence is much greater than these figures for surgical cases indicate. Nearly 90 percent (516) of the patients had solitary lesions. None could be related to prior radiation therapy.

Sex

A trifle more than 60 percent of patients in both the solitary and multiple exostoses groups were males. The literature indicates little sex predilection.

Age

Approximately 57 percent of the patients were less than twenty years of age at the time of excision of their osteochondromas, and 48.2 percent were in the second decade of life. The age at the time of first operation for those with multiple exostoses was used in the illustration above and paralleled closely the age of patients with single exostoses who required surgical treatment.

Localization

Osteochondromas may occur on any bone that develops by enchondral ossification. They usually occur in the metaphyseal region of the long bones of the limbs; rarely they are near or in the middle third of such bones. Nearly half in this series involved the femur and humerus. The ilium contributed twenty-nine of the thirty-nine arising from innominate bones. Nine of fifteen in ribs involved the first four ribs.

Symptoms

The patient's complaints are related to the size of the tumor; the complaint of a hard swelling, usually of long duration, is the most common. The presence of the mass may induce the patient, because of fear or vanity, to seek medical care. Pain may result from the tumor's impinging on neighboring structures, from weight-bearing or other activity, or be caused by an overlying bursa. Pain was due to fracture of the tumor's stalk in four patients in this series.

Physical Findings

Palpable mass is ordinarily the only finding. Secondary effects may occur, especially when the tumor infringes upon the spinal canal.

Roentgenologic Features

The characteristic appearance is that of a projection composed of a cortex continuous with that of the underlying bone and a spongiosa, similarly continuous. The adjacent cortex often flares to become the base of the tumor. The projection may have a broad base or be distinctly pedunculated. Irregular zones of calcification may be present, especially in the cartilaginous cap, but extensive calcification with consequent irregularities of the cap should arouse the suspicion of malignant

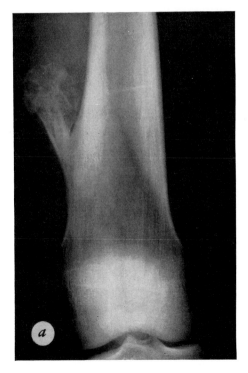

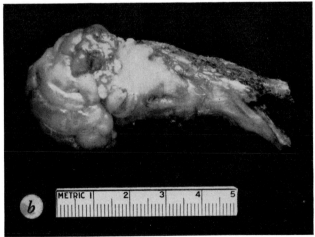

Figure 2-2. *a.* Pedunculated osteochondroma of medial aspect of femur. *b.* Gross specimen in same case showing regular, smooth cartilaginous cap.

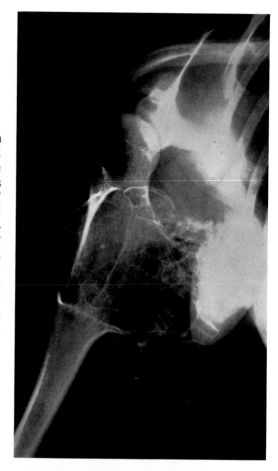

Figure 2-3. *Right.* Osteochondroma of nineteen years' known duration in twenty-four-year-old woman. Mass had been partially excised at the age of eleven years. This roentgenogram shows flaring of bony cortex as it becomes the base of the tumor. *Below.* Excised tumor is composed chiefly of fatty, cancellous bone. Cortex is markedly attenuated where it covers the broad stalk of tumor. Most of cartilaginous cap has undergone involution. Excised segment of humerus was replaced by bone graft. Similar block excisions were employed for two other humeral osteochondromas and one femoral osteochondroma because size and roentgenographic appearance suggested the possibility of chondrosarcoma.

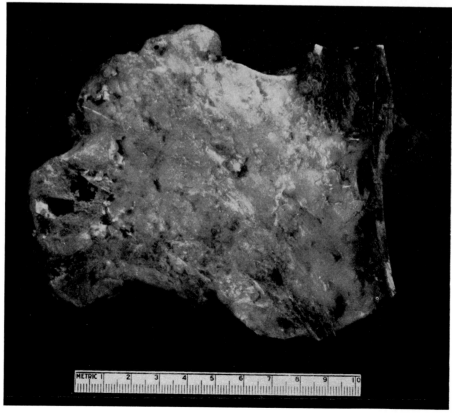

change. Osteochondromas commonly arise at the site of tendon insertions, and the direction of their growth is often along the line of the tendon's pull. The affected bone is often abnormally wide at the level of an osteochondroma owing to failure of normal tubulation. Such widening is especially likely to be seen in patients with multiple exostoses. The bone harboring the tumor may be shortened.

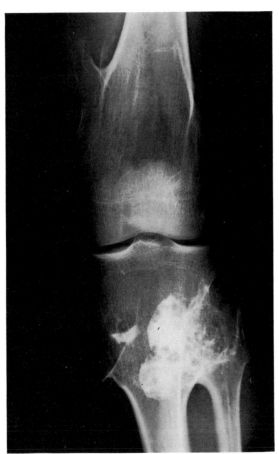

Figure 2-4. Hereditary multiple osteochondromas about the knee.

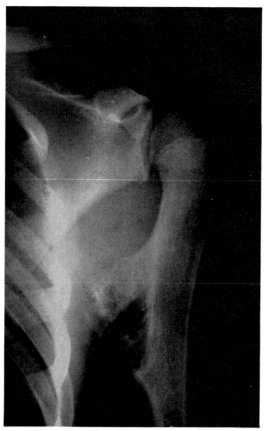

Figure 2-5. Sessile exostosis in one of more common sites. Gross specimen is shown in Figure 2-8.

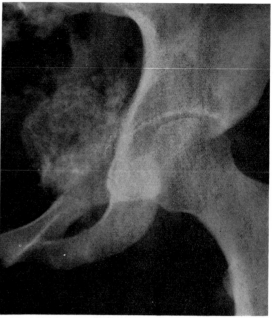

Figure 2-6. Osteochondroma proved to be benign but with roentgenologic features suggestive of chondrosarcoma.

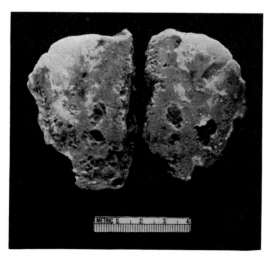

Figure 2-7. Osteocartilaginous exostosis with prominent irregular cartilaginous cap. Such lesions require careful sampling to exclude secondary chondrosarcomatous change. Note cyst formation secondary to degeneration.

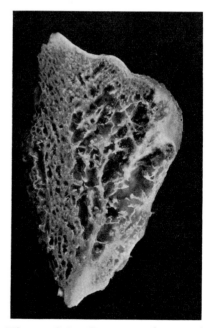

Figure 2-8. Gross specimen of lesion illustrated in Figure 2-5. There is prominent cancellous core and thin cartilaginous cap.

Gross Pathology

The gross pathologic features confirm the roentgenologic pattern. Sessile exostoses may be flat, whereas pedunculated ones are sometimes long and slender, and all gradations between these exist. Many are cauliflower-shaped with or without a stalk.

The tumor's cortex and its periosteal covering are continuous with those of the underlying bone. A bursa often develops over the exostosis. The marrow of the tumor may be fatty or hematopoietic, often mirroring the status of the spongiosa of the underlying bone with which it merges.

The hyaline cartilage of the tumor's cap is ordinarily 2 to 3 mm thick. This cap may cover the entire external surface of a sessile tumor, whereas it covers only the rounded end of a stalked exostosis. The cartilage may be 1 cm or more thick in the actively growing benign exostosis of adolescence. Irregularity and thickening of the cap, especially when the patient is adult, demand careful histologic study because of the likelihood of secondary chondrosarcoma. If the cartilaginous rim is thin and regular and the underlying spongiosa appears to be normal, the tumor is always benign. If this exostosis is arrested, there may be practically no cartilaginous cap.

The bursa overlying an exostosis may be the site of ossified or calcified cartilaginous loose bodies. In this series, there were three lesions with numerous and two with single such loose bodies. There may be hemorrhage into the bursa, or the exostosis may traumatize nearby arteries, especially the distal femoral or the popliteal, and it may even produce false aneurysms.

Histopathology

Microscopic study confirms the gross appearance of regular cortical and underlying medullary bone with its fatty or hematopoietic component. Sections not taken at right angle to the periphery may give an erroneous impression of the thickness of the cartilage. The chondrocytes of the cartilaginous cap are often arranged in clusters in parallel, oblong lacunar spaces, reminiscent of normal epiphyseal cartilage. This histologic orientation strongly suggests that the lesion is benign. The typical benign chondrocyte has a single small nucleus. During the age of active bone growth, binucleate cartilage cells may be seen fairly frequently in benign exostoses. Malignant transformation of an exostosis is nearly always in the form of chondrosarcoma, the histologic features of which are described in a later chapter. Other sarcomas in osteochondromas are rare and, hence, medical curiosities. Islands of cartilage are sometimes imbedded in the underlying cancellous bone, and these may undergo degeneration with irregular calcification, which is sometimes demonstrable on the roentgenograms. The exostosis is covered by periosteum which is continuous with that of the adjacent bone. As indicated by the gross appearance, the cartilaginous cap involutes after growth of the osteochondroma ceases, and it may even disappear entirely.

Trauma may produce fibroblastic proliferation and even new bone formation, especially in the peripheral portions of an osteochondroma. Those few osteochon-

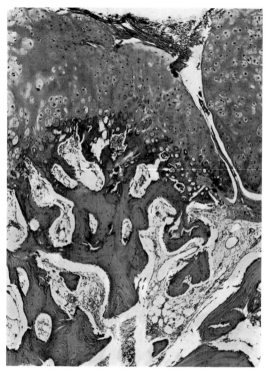

Figure 2-9. Slightly lobulated cartilaginous cap of benign osteochondroma. Enchondral ossification is producing regular bony trabeculae separated by fatty marrow. Strip of periosteum overlies tumor. (×30)

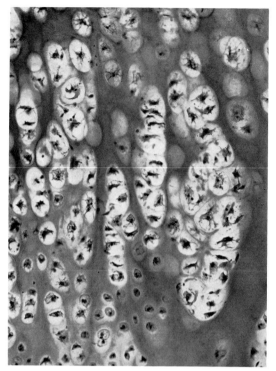

Figure 2-10. Linear clusters of chondrocytes mimicking normal epiphysis. Individual nuclei are small, and multinucleated chondrocytes are rare in the average benign osteochondroma. (×110)

dromas of the hands and feet not in the subungual zones tended to have more admixed fibroblastic tissue and less regularity of their cartilaginous and bony components, suggesting that they may have resulted from prior trauma; many are probably related to the non-neoplastic proliferation seen in subungual exostoses.

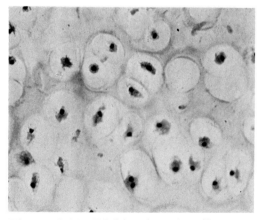

Figure 2-11. Multinucleated cells occur frequently in some of benign exostoses of childhood. (×210)

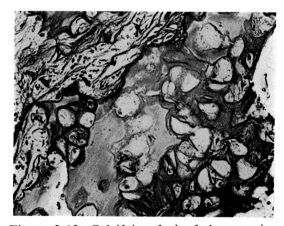

Figure 2-12. Calcifying foci of degenerating cartilage in stalk of osteochondroma. (×170)

Treatment

The presence of an osteocartilaginous exostosis is, in itself, insufficient reason for surgical extirpation since malignant transformation occurs in only about 1 percent of clinically recognized osteochondromas. Removal is indicated if the tumor is unsightly, is producing pain or disability, has roentgenologic features suggestive of malignancy, or shows abnormal increase in size.

Removal of the tumor flush with the bone of origin is the treatment when surgical intervention is indicated. The entire cartilaginous cap should be removed. In some locations, such as a rib, block excision of the affected bone is best, especially if the diagnosis is uncertain.

Although chondrosarcoma will develop in approximately 10 percent of patients with multiple osteocartilaginous exostoses, the precursor tumors are too numerous to allow prophylactic removal. The same general principles should govern removal of a tumor in this condition as in the solitary form of the disease.

Prognosis

Osteochondromas, if benign, are practically always cured by complete excision. Approximately 2 percent of the tumors were recurrent when the patients came to our clinic or recurred after excision here. These recurrent lesions made a second operation necessary at intervals that varied from one year to twenty-six years, although all were benign. Second operations in these cases proved to be curative. Failure to remove the entire cartilaginous cap or even its overlying periosteum probably explains most recurrences. Sometimes a nearby similar cartilaginous focus is unwittingly left behind and produces a second tumor.

Recurrence suggests the possibility that the original tumor was a chondrosarcoma. Such was the case in some of the earlier tumors erroneously misclassified as osteochondroma in our series.

Subungual Exostoses

Forty-four exostoses removed from the distal portions of the distal phalanges were not included in the data on tumors. Patients with these lesions frequently give such a convincing history of trauma and repeated or continuous infection at the site of the lump that these seem likely to have a part in its genesis. The proliferating fibrocartilaginous tissue capping a growing subungual exostosis resembles callus in its morphologic gradations to mature bony trabeculae, further supporting the likelihood of the tumor's being a response to injury. Sometimes the advancing margin of these lesions is so actively growing as to mimic sarcoma much the way that a march fracture may. Attention to the lack of true anaplasia and to the orderly progression to mature bone provides the clues of benignity.

These frequently painful projections from the distal phalanges are usually under the nail and are rarely more than 1 cm in diameter. Pain and swelling are the result. Ulceration and infection may be present and make subungual melanoma a consideration clinically. Of the forty-four tumors, thirty-three affected the first toe; six,

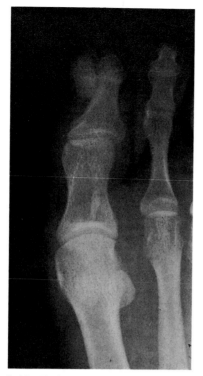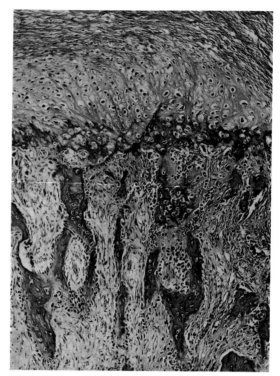

Figure 2-13. *Left.* Exostosis protruding dorsomedially from distal phalanx of first toe. *Right.* Relatively early stage in development of subungual exostosis with proliferating cartilage maturing into bone. Orderly progression to bone is evident, although the process is earlier than that depicted in accompanying roentgenogram. (×50)

the other toes; four, the thumb; and one, the index finger. The ages of the affected patients ranged from eight to sixty-five years, but 45 percent were in the second and 27 percent in the third decade of life. Despite occasional recurrence, surgical removal effects cure of these exostoses, and they have no premalignant potential. Similar non-neoplastic projections are seen on other surfaces of the small bones of the hands and feet.

Sarcomas in Solitary Osteochondroma

Twenty-two exostoses, not included in the foregoing data on osteochrondromas, gave rise to chondrosarcomas. The features of these tumors will be further elaborated in the chapter on chondrosarcoma. Roentgenologic, gross, and microscopic evidence indicated the relationship of these malignant tumors to the benign precursor. These twenty-two tumors comprised 4.1 percent of all solitary exostoses treated surgically, but this figure does not represent accurately the incidence of malignant change since so many benign ones are not treated surgically. Furthermore, it is likely that patients with sarcomatous change are seen in medical centers.

Two osteosarcomas arose in a parosteal or juxtacortical location but within lesions that bore stigmata of preexisting osteochondroma. One lesion was on the medial aspect and one on the posteromedial aspect of the distal portion of the shaft of the femur, but neither was characteristic of ordinary parosteal (juxtacortical) osteosarcoma.

Sarcoma in Multiple Exostoses

None of the sixty-three patients with multiple exostoses included in Figure 2-1 had sarcomas, but an additional twenty-four with multiple exostoses have been treated for secondary chondrosarcomas at the Mayo Clinic. Although this represents a 27.6 percent incidence of malignant change, the selection factors again make firm conclusions unwise. A single osteosarcoma complicated multiple exostoses; it occurred in an osteochondroma of the temporal bone.

Bibliography

1943   Jaffe, H. L.: Hereditary Multiple Exostosis. *Arch Pathol, 36:*335-357.

1954   Harsha, W. N.: The Natural History of Osteocartilaginous Exostoses (Osteochrondroma) *Am Surg, 20:*65-72.

1962   Murphy, F. D., Jr., and Blount, W. P.: Cartilaginous Exostoses Following Irradiation. *J Bone Joint Surg, 44A:*662-668 (June).

1963   Bethge, J. F. J.: Hereditäre, Multiple Exostosen und Ihre Pathogenetische Deutung. *Arch Orthop Unfallchir, 54:*667-696.

1963   Anastasi, G. W., Wertheimer, H. M., and Brown, J. R.: Popliteal Aneurysm with Osteochondroma of the Femur. *Arch Surg, 87:*636-639.

1964   Solomon, L.: Hereditary Multiple Exostosis. *Am J Hum Genet, 16:*351-363.

1964   Morton, K. S.: On the Question of Recurrence of Osteochondroma. *J Bone Joint Surg, 46B:*723-725.

1966   Evison, G., and Price, C. H. G.: Subungual Exostosis. *Br J Radiol, 39:*451-455 (June).

1971   Schweitzer, G., and Pirie, D.: Osteosarcoma Arising in a Solitary Osteochondroma. *S Afr Med J, 45:*810-811 (July).

1972   Lénárt, G., and Szepesi, D.: Eigenartiger Knorpeliger Tumor am Finger. *Arch Orthop Unfallchir, 73:*7-10.

1972   Hershey, S. L., and Lansden, F. T.: Osteochondromas As a Cause of False Popliteal Aneurysms. Review of the Literature and Report of Two Cases. *J Bone Joint Surg, 54A:*1765-1768 (December).

Chapter 3

Chondroma

THIS BENIGN TUMOR is composed of mature hyaline cartilage. Most commonly, chondromas are centrally located in bone, and such tumors are called "enchondromas." Less often they are distinctly eccentric and bulge the overlying periosteum; this type has been called "periosteal chondroma." In thin or flat bones such as the ribs, scapula, or innominate bone, the exact origin of chondromas, that is, whether central or subperiosteal, often cannot be determined because of destruction of landmarks by the tumor.

Multiple Chondroma

This dysplasia of bone is characterized by failure of normal enchondral ossification with the production of tumefactive cartilaginous masses in the epiphyseal and adjacent regions of the shaft. A few or many bones may be affected. With widespread involvement and a tendency to unilaterality, this condition is often called "Ollier's disease." In addition to tumefaction, there are concomitant bowing and shortening of bones as a result of this disease. In fact, multiple chondroma and fibrous dysplasia both result from disordered ossification, and this relationship is emphasized by lesions containing histopathologic features of both. Patients with multiple chondroma should be sharply differentiated from those with skeletal osteochondromatosis (multiple osteochondromas). Skeletal chondromatosis when associated with angiomas of the soft tissues is called Maffucci's syndrome. Other rarer syndromes associated with skeletal chondromas have been recognized. Completely reliable figures are not available, but approximately one third of the cases of multiple chondroma are complicated by chondrosarcoma.

Extraosseous Cartilaginous Tumors

Not included in this series are cartilaginous tumors arising in unusual sites such as the larynx and the synovial membranes. These have unusual characteristics, the most significant of which is that their clinical behavior is less aggressive than that suggested by their histology. The same applies to the not uncommon extraosseous cartilaginous tumors of the hands and feet, most of which are small and many of which probably derive from synovium. Frankly malignant extraosseous definitely cartilaginous neoplasms are rare.

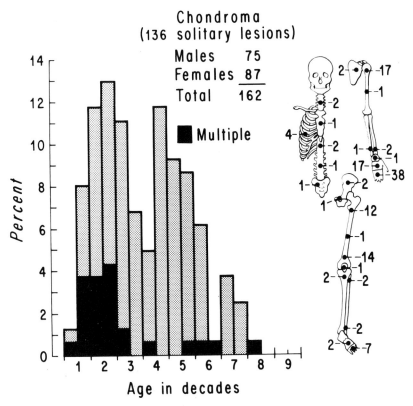

Figure 3-1. Skeletal, age, and sex distribution of chondromas.

Incidence

Chondromas comprised only 11.2 percent of the benign tumors of the present series and 2.6 percent of the entire series.

Sex

Experience in the present series of cases bears out recorded data which indicate no significant sex predilection. Sixteen of the twenty-six with multiple chondromas were males.

Age

Cases were fairly evenly distributed throughout life, but 59 percent were in the ten– to thirty-nine-year age-group. Patients with multiple lesions required operation at an average younger age.

Localization

More than 40 percent of the tumors were in the hands and feet, chiefly in the phalanges, and 86 percent of these were in the hands. Chondroma is by far the commonest tumor of the small bones of the hand. One of the three lesions of the innominate bone involved the pubis and two the ilium. The bones most commonly affected by chondrosarcoma are relatively immune to chondroma. None of the rare chondromatous tumors at the base of the skull were encountered in this series, and some of those reported are probably chordomas or related to them. Two intra-cranial chondromas of meningeal origin were excluded. The 9 by 8 by 6 cm patellar chondroma was on its surface and may have been an example of para-articular chondrome.

Symptoms

Many chondromas are asymptomatic, which can be attributed to their extremely slow rate of growth. Some are discovered accidentally on roentgenographic examination. Pathologic fracture often ushers in the symptoms of the commonly seen chondroma of the distal portions of the extremities. Notable swelling is rarely produced. Pain unassociated with pathologic fracture should arouse the suspicion of malignancy because it suggests that the tumor is invasive.

Physical Findings

Physical examination contributes little to the diagnosis of chondroma of bone. Tumefaction is rarely produced except by lesions of the small bones of the hands and feet. Large tumors at such sites may be malignant. The occurrence of pain or pathologic fracture merely directs one's attention to the appropriate region for roentgenographic study.

Roentgenologic Features

The average chondroma produces a localized central region of rarefaction. Any portion of the small tubular bones of the hands and feet may be affected, but the tumor is ordinarily diaphyseal in location. From slight to very prominent stippled or mottled calcification of the tumor is frequently seen, especially in those chondromas occurring in the large tubular bones. Ossification within the lesion may contribute radiopacity. The cortex overlying a chondroma of small bones is often expanded, and the expansion may be eccentric. The presence of calcification within a well-circumscribed rarefying tumor affords strong evidence that the lesion contains hyaline cartilage that is undergoing degenerative change. Periosteal chondromas lie eccentrically, beneath the periosteum, in a well-demarcated cortical defect. Thirty-one of the solitary chondromas in this series were so located.

Chondromas may be solitary or multiple. Especially in younger persons, there may be stigmata indicating they are an expression of skeletal dysplasia, as in Figures 3-2 and 3-7. Chondrodysplasia is often associated with large chondromas that are benign.

Many of the small asymptomatic central lesions that are obviously cartilaginous because of their areas of radiodensity are not operated upon if their small size and lack of endosteal erosion indicative of aggressiveness suggest that they are benign. Large size and invasiveness indicated by endosteal erosion produce the suspicion of malignancy.

Bone infarcts resemble calcifying cartilaginous neoplasms, but infarcts typically contain central rarefactions and are well separated from surrounding normal bone by a zone of calcification or even ossification at their peripheries.

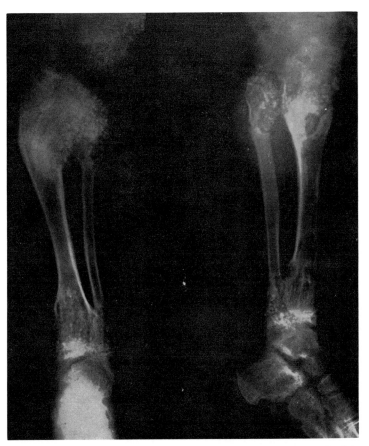

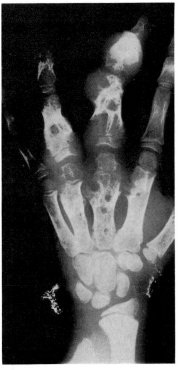

Figure 3-2. Enchondromatosis (Ollier's dyschondroplasia) in a ten-year-old boy with multiple deforming cartilaginous tumors with punctate calcification in lesional tissue. (Reproduced with permission from: Pugh, D. G.: *Roentgenologic Diagnosis of Diseases of Bones.* Baltimore, Williams & Wilkins, 1954, pp. 438-442.)

Figure 3-3. Multiple deforming enchondromas in ten-year-old boy.

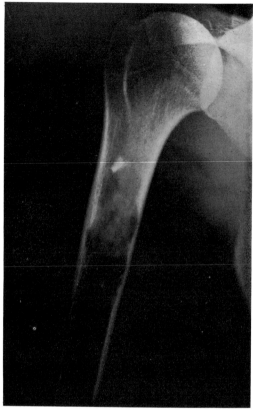

Figure 3-4. Chondroma of humerus in thirty-two-year-old woman. Despite endosteal erosion and occasional binucleated cells, patient was well fourteen years after thorough curettage.

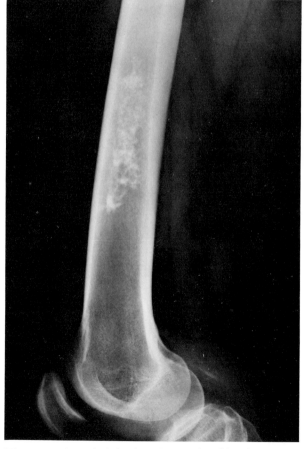

Figure 3-5. Painful chondroma in fifty-four-year-old man. Patient was well ten years after curettage.

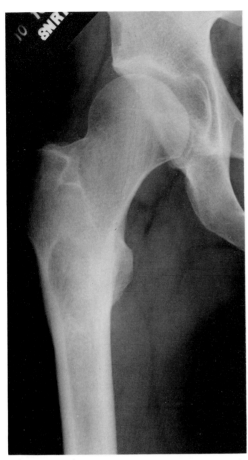

Figure 3-6. "Cellular" chondroma in thirty-nine-year-old man. Curettage was followed by small grade 1 chondrosarcoma eighteen years later. Grade 2 chondrosarcoma involved entire femur and produced pulmonary metastasis twenty-five years after first treatment.

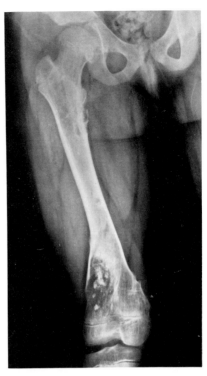

Figure 3-7. Chondromas of Ollier's disease in nine-year-old girl. Tissue from largest lesion, in distal part of femur, showed chondroma six years previously. Stigmata of Ollier's disease permit increased cellularity in large cartilaginous tumors that have a benign clinical course. Patient had deformity and shortening of that leg but was otherwise well nineteen years after biopsy at age of three years.

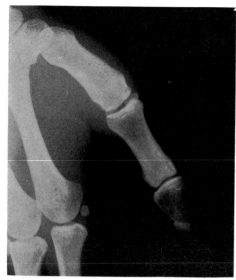

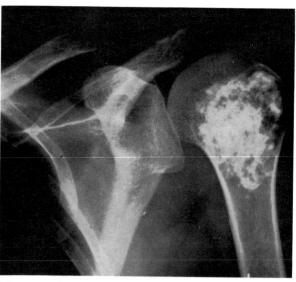

Figure 3-8. Typical central chondroma of small bone, in this case affecting distal phalanx of thumb. Many of these small chondromas show stippled calcification.

Figure 3-9. Heavily calcified chondroma. Such density is ordinarily the result of calcification secondary to necrosis. Such lesions resemble infarcts.

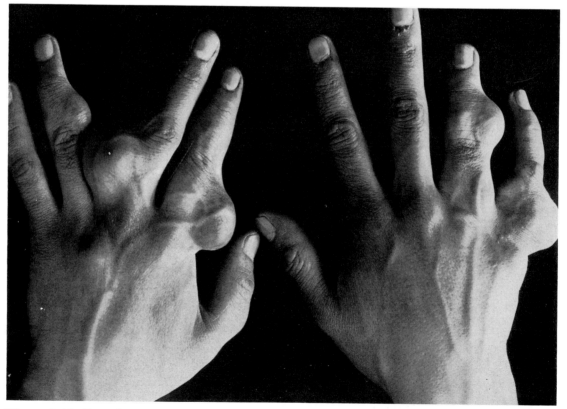

Figure 3-10. Rare but markedly deforming multiple chondromas, in this case affecting only the hands. This may be mild manifestation of Ollier's dyschondroplasia. Enchondromas of hands usually produce no visible swelling. (Reproduced with permission from: Shellito, J. G., and Dockerty, M. B.: *Surg Gynecol Obstet, 86*:465-472, 1948.)

Gross Pathology

The characteristic chondroma is composed of confluent masses of bluish, semitranslucent, hyaline cartilage with a distinctly lobular arrangement. The lobules vary from a few millimeters to a centimeter or more in diameter. The periphery of the lesion may be somewhat indistinct, because ramifications of the cartilaginous tumor sometimes penetrate into adjacent marrow spaces. Some of the tumors are very soft and mucinous. Those characterized by x-ray evidence of punctate areas of calcification have calcified masses scattered throughout the tumor, and occasional lesions are heavily calcified and ossified. The gross characteristics of the solitary tumor and of the individual tumors of the multiple variety are similar.

As previously indicated, most chondromas are central in location, but some of them are under the periosteum and produce a well-marginated defect in the underlying cortex and a bulge in the contour of the bone. These subperiosteal chondromas lie in an excavation in the bone, and their internal limits are marked by a thin sclerotic zone. The upper part of the shaft of the humerus is a favorite site for periosteal chondromas, which may be up to approximately 5 cm in greatest dimension.

Chondromas are characteristically small tumors, and when one encounters a tumor of hyaline cartilage that is several centimeters in diameter, one should check carefully for evidence of malignancy. Lysis of cortex over a central chondroma, especially if associated with extraosseous extension, is an ominous sign and is often indicated on the roentgenogram.

Chondroid lesions that are difficult to diagnose are often located at the neck of the femur. Periosteal chondroma, synovial chondromatosis, para-articular chon-

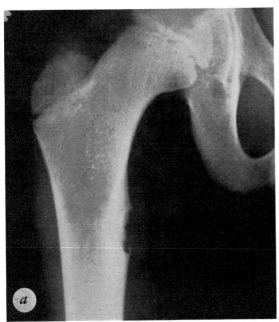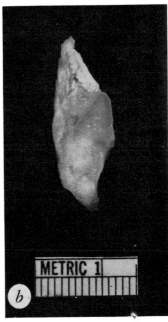

Figure 3-11. *a.* Typical subperiosteal chondroma lying in slightly sclerotized concavity in cortex. *b.* Gross specimen from same case. Semitranslucent nature of hyaline cartilage is apparent.

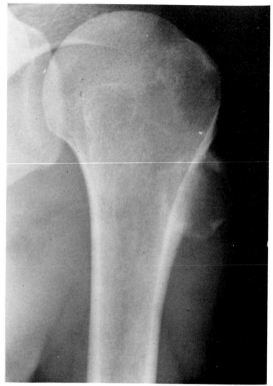

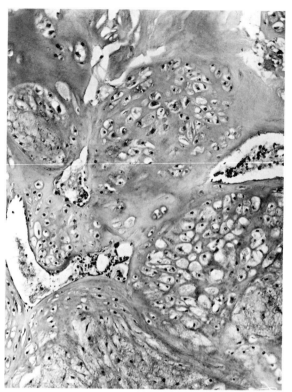

Figure 3-12. Cellular "active" periosteal chondroma in twenty-three-year-old man who had had pain and swelling for two years.

Figure 3-13. Chondroma, 8 by 5 by 3 cm, in upper part of humeral shaft in patient with dyschondroplasia. (×160)

droma with osseous erosion, and non-neoplastic entities such as predominantly chondroid fibrocartilaginous dysplasia must be considered.

Histopathology

The chondrocytes that make up the cellular component of a chondroma are small cells that lie in lacunar spaces and have a round, regular nucleus similar to that of the chondrocyte seen in non-neoplastic hyaline cartilage. The degree of cellularity varies remarkably in chondromas, some of the enchondromas of the small bones being highly cellular. Hence, cellularity affords little help in differentiating chondroma from chondrosarcoma. Large, oblong lacunar spaces similar to those seen in a growing epiphyseal line and containing a cluster of chondrocytes are sometimes present, and such a finding affords strong presumptive evidence that the lesion is benign. Multinucleated chondrocytes and cells with large nuclei are uncommon and should arouse the suspicion of malignancy. A lobular arrangement is sometimes apparent microscopically. Finely granular calcific debris or prominent sheets of calcific, substance, when present, are apparently at sites of degeneration. The hyaline cartilage may contain foci of enchondral ossification in some of these neoplasms. In others, the ground substance has a myxoid or mucinous appearance.

It is necessary to examine numerous fields in these tumors to be certain that there are not areas with sufficient evidence for a diagnosis of malignancy. This is especially true if the lesions are large or if they are located in a long bone near the body, in the pelvic or shoulder girdle, or in a rib. Evidence for chondrosarcoma is sometimes found in only isolated areas within a tumor. The histologic criteria of chondrosarcoma will be detailed in the chapter dealing with that subject. Differentiation of benign from malignant chondromatous tumors of bone requires careful correlation of clinical, roentgenologic, and histopathologic features.

Periosteal chondromas often have an alarming degree of cellular atypia. They may be difficult to distinguish from periosteally located chondrosarcomas; roentgenographic alterations aid in the differentiation. Wide local resection is indicated for those with equivocal evidence for malignancy. The junction of a periosteal chondroma with underlying bony trabeculae may simulate such a junction at the cap of an osteochondroma.

Areas of definite fibrous dysplasia in a central cartilaginous lesion indicate that it is an example of fibrocartilaginous dysplasia. Such benign chondroid masses can be several centimeters in diameter. Most dysplasias of this type involve the upper part of the shaft or the neck of the femur.

Fracture or recent injury such as produced by surgery may cause active fibrocartilaginous proliferation that should not be mistaken for malignancy.

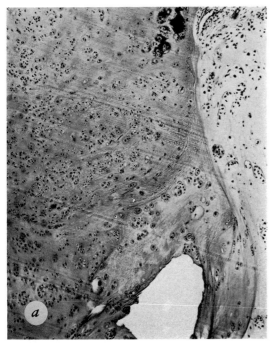 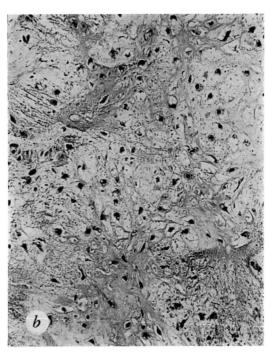

Figure 3-14. *a.* Chondroma under low magnification showing lobular pattern, clustering of cells, and small focus of calcification. (×65) *b.* Higher magnification to show that each cell has single small nucleus. (×185)

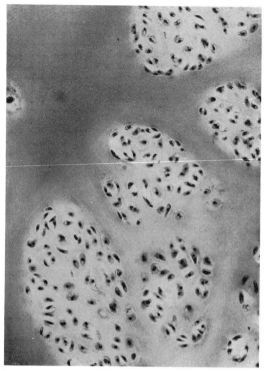

Figure 3-15. Small, usually single, nuclei are typical of benign chondroma. Cells often occur in clusters. (×140)

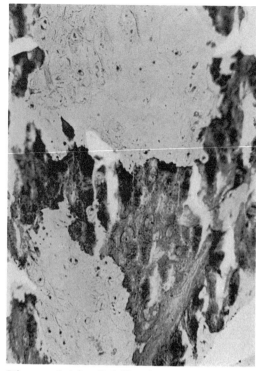

Figure 3-16. Calcification secondary to degeneration. This is lesion illustrated in Figure 3-9. (×160)

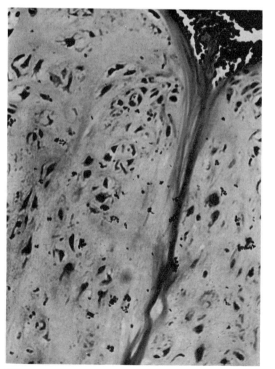

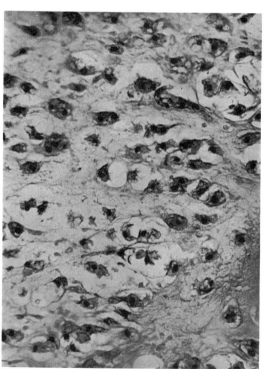

Figure 3-17. *Left.* Periosteal chondroma. Fair numbers of binucleate cells and considerable cytologic atypia have less significance in chondromas lying in cortical defect, as in Figure 3-11 *a.* (×175) *Right.* Binucleate cells and cellularity are likewise less ominous in roentgenologically benign-appearing chondromas of the hand such as this one. (×350)

Treatment

Curettage, filling the defect with bone chips if necessary, is the usual treatment. After curettage, some recommend chemical cauterization of the cavity and collapse of the cortical bone over the defect. If the tumor is in a small bone such as a rib that can be sacrificed or is in the subperiosteal region of a large bone and it can be excised en bloc with a surrounding portion of normal bone, that is the proper treatment. Such total excision is especially desirable when the possibility of malignancy cannot be excluded preoperatively. Curettage is likely to leave fragments of a lobulated tumor behind so that the tumor can recur even if it is benign.

Central tumors of major bones that are "active" or borderline for malignancy histologically have been treated successfully by widely exposing the lesion and removing it meticulously at surgery. Cautery of the tumor base is probably important in prevention of recurrence. This approach permits preservation of functional integrity of the bone. Long-term follow-up observation is necessary in such cases. There appears to be no justification for partial removal of such "worrisome" lesions with the view of assessing their nature histologically. Such assessment is notoriously difficult.

Prognosis

With the treatment outlined, the prognosis in chondroma is good and recurrence is unusual even after curettage. Occasionally, however, a tumor that seemed to be completely benign recurs, and the recurrent tumor is characterized, in rare instances, by increased anaplasia with obvious evidence of malignancy. Frequently, this apparent increase in cellular activity is actually the result of failure of correct interpretation of the original specimen; sometimes the apparent discrepancy is accounted for by the fact that insufficient microscopic sections were made to evaluate completely the original specimen. Actually in chondroma of the hand, the average lesion is so innocuous that curettage is usually curative. With larger lesions, resection that includes the surrounding shell of bone and grafting may be necessary.

Multiple Chondroma

Not included in the localization data in Figure 3-1 were twenty-six patients with benign but multiple chondromas. These patients required operation for various reasons. In nine, tissue was removed from a lesion for diagnosis. Deforming tumors were locally excised from the hand in eight patients and from the foot in one. A toe of one patient was amputated, and three others had one or more fingers amputated. One of these latter three patients required disarticulation at the shoulder later for a huge tumor of the humerus, from which tissue was not available for study. One patient required amputation through the femur because of severe and disabling tibial deformity. The final patient required amputation of an affected arm for an associated angiosarcoma of the soft tissues which complicated chronic lymphedema and caused death within a year.

The severity of skeletal chondromatosis varied markedly in this group. Six pa-

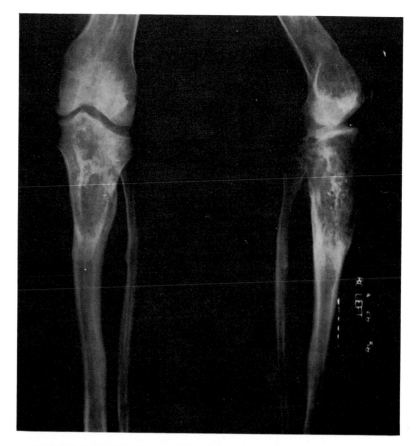

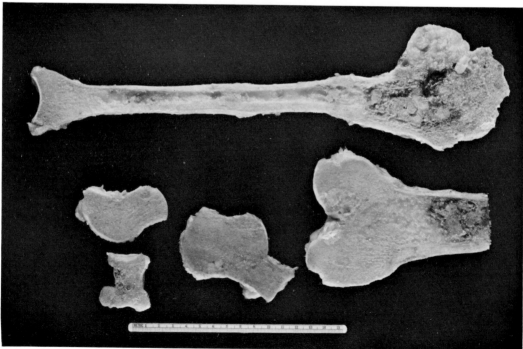

Figure 3-18. *Top.* The forty-seven-year-old man in this case had chondromas in left femur, tibia, and bones of foot. Chondrosarcoma had developed in tibia. *Bottom.* Sarcoma had perforated tibial cortex posteriorly. Chondromas were found at amputation level, in distal end of femur, and in several bones of the foot. This chondrosarcoma had dedifferentiated, and all of numerous metastatic lesions seen at autopsy fifty-eight months after amputation were grade 3 fibrosarcoma, as seen in Figure 17-24.

tients had the bones of only one hand involved, and two others had the bones of but one foot involved. One of the latter patients had only two tumors. In the hands and feet, nearly all the chondromas were in phalanges, metacarpals, and metatarsals. One patient had chondromas distributed throughout three extremities, and four others had two limbs similarly affected. The remainder had diffuse involvement of one extremity, often with involvement of the bones of the ipsilateral shoulder or pelvic girdle. Ribs were involved in one case.

Sarcomas in Multiple Chondroma

In addition to the previously mentioned twenty-six patients with skeletal chondromatosis, there were eight with the same disease complicated by chondrosarcoma. They are included in the data on malignant tumors. Four extremities were involved by chondromas in one case, three in one case, and two in one case; the remainder had monomelic disease. Three of the chondrosarcomas occurred in the upper part of the tibia, two in the distal part of the femur, and one each in the ilium, the upper part of the humerus, and a metatarsal. The patients' ages at the time of diagnosis of sarcoma ranged from twenty-three to fifty-five years. An additional patient developed osteosarcoma of the upper part of the femur and multiple chondromas of the bones of the same leg.

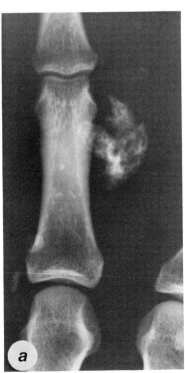
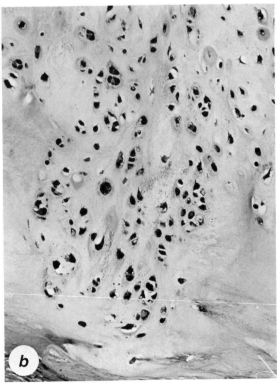

Figure 3-19. *Left.* Chondroma (synovial) in soft tissue of phalanx. Although tumor is heavily mineralized, bone is not primarily involved. *Right.* Cellularity and cellular atypia as shown is present in many of these benign lesions. (×250)

Cartilaginous Tumors of the Soft Tissues of the Hands and Feet

Chondrosarcoma of the classic type is seen in very rare instances in various soft tissues, including the breast. In addition to such malignant tumors of distinctly hyaline-cartilage type, there are a number of "chondroid" neoplasms, as described by Lichtenstein and Bernstein, that are not definitely cartilaginous. The latter are often of debatable histologic type and clinical capability.

Among tumors of soft tissue that are unequivocally cartilaginous, the vast majority are seen in the hands and feet and are benign. Twelve of seventy tumors that we reported in 1974 produced local recurrence, but none metastasized. The ages of affected patients ranged from ten to eighty-four years. The seventy tumors of the soft tissues of the hands and feet included nine with xanthomalike zones that provided further evidence, besides the common juxtaposition to tendon sheaths, of a synovial origin. Only six of the seventy tumors were larger than 5 cm in greatest dimension. Somewhat more than half of the tumors contained calcific material or bone that usually produced radiographic density. Roentgenography indicated that they were not bone tumors although bone was eroded by some. Histologic atypia suggestive of chondrosarcoma was present in most.

Bibliography

1952 Lichtenstein, L., and Hall, J. E.: Periosteal Chondroma: A Distinctive Benign Cartilage Tumor. *J Bone Joint Surg, 34A:*691-697.

1954 Pugh, D. G.: *Roentgenologic Diagnosis of Diseases of Bones.* Baltimore, Williams & Wilkins, pp. 438-442.

1958 Bean, W. B.: Dyschondroplasia and Hemangiomata (Maffucci's Syndrome). II. *AMA Arch Intern Med,* 102:544-550.

1959 Lichtenstein, L., and Bernstein, D.: Unusual Benign and Malignant Chondroid Tumors of Bone. A Survey of Some Mesenchymal Cartilage Tumors, and Malignant Chondroblastic Tumors, Including a Few Multicentric Ones, as Well as Many Atypical Benign Chondroblastomas and Chondromyxoid Fibromas. *Cancer, 12:* 1142-1157 (November-December).

1962 Murphy, F. P., Dahlin, D. C., and Sullivan, C. R.: Articular Synovial Chondromatosis. *J Bone Joint Surg, 44A:*77-86.

1963 Gilmer, W. S., Kilgore, W., and Smith, H.: Central Cartilage Tumors of Bone. *Clinical Orthopedics, No. 26.* Philadelphia, Lippencott.

1963 Goethals, P. L., Dahlin, D. C., and Devine, K. S.: Cartilaginous Tumors of the Larynx. *Surg Gynecol Obstet, 117:*77-82.

1971 Takigawa, K.: Chondroma of the Bones of the Hand. A Review of 110 Cases. *J Bone Joint Surg, 53A:*1591-1600 (December).

1972 Rockwell, M. A., Saiter, E. T., and Enneking, W. F.: Periosteal Chondroma. *J Bone Joint Surg, 54A:*102-108 (January).

1974 Dahlin, D. C., and Salvador, A. H.: Cartilaginous Tumors of the Soft Tissues of the Hands and Feet. *Mayo Clinic Proc, 49:*721-726 (October).

Chapter 4

Benign Chondroblastoma

BENIGN CHONDROBLASTOMA is one of the neoplasms of bone that has been rescued from the "wastebasket" of giant cell tumors and is now recognized as a distinct entity. The basic proliferating cells of this neoplasm are remarkably similar to those of a true giant cell tumor, but these cells have the ability to produce foci of chrondroid matrix, making it reasonable to include chondroblastoma among the tumors of cartilaginous origin. Valls and coworkers have suggested a reticulo-histiocytic origin for these tumors, but most people relate then to epiphyseal cartilage. Electron microscopic observations have supported their cartilaginous nature.

Although some of the features of this neoplasm were recognized previously, it was not until 1942 that the term "benign chondroblastoma" was introduced and its distinctive clinicopathologic features were delineated. The cellular zones of these tumors ordinarily contain at least a few mitotic figures. These, coupled with the chondroid zones, have led to the erroneous diagnosis of malignant giant cell tumor. Actually, one of the main reasons for recognizing this entity is that clinically it is relatively nonaggressive and readily curable as compared with giant cell tumor.

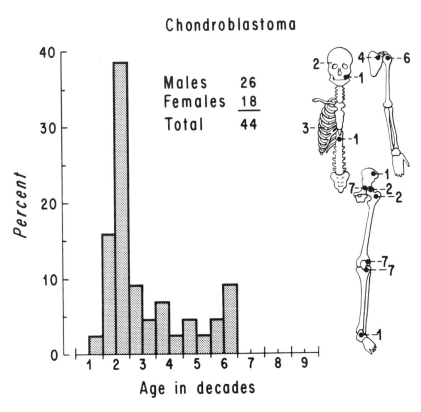

Figure 4-1. Skeletal, age, and sex distribution of benign chondroblastomas.

43

The present studies and those of others have indicated a close relationship between benign chondroblastoma and chondromyxoid fibroma. In common with most observers, my colleagues and I have recognized no malignant counterpart of benign chondroblastoma.

Several benign chondroblastomas have metastasized as benign tumors, and some, usually called "aggressive," have produced huge, occasionally lethal, local recurrence. When the component cells and overall histopathologic appearance of a lesion suggest that atypical chondroblastoma is the most likely designation, one must be sure that the actually correct diagnosis is not something else, like clear cell chondrosarcoma or even atypical fibrous histiocytoma. The roentgenographic appearance, likewise, may suggest that the diagnosis of benign chondroblastoma is erroneous.

Incidence

Less than 1 percent of this series of bone tumors were chondroblastomas, and they were one-sixth as common as were true giant cell tumors. To 1968, 182 cases were reviewed in the literature.

Sex

The Mayo Clinic series contained nearly 60 percent males. The literature as well as the nearly 150 non-Clinic cases we have seen in consultation indicate that approximately two thirds of affected patients are males.

Age

More than half of our cases and of those reported have been confirmed in the second decade of life. Six of our patients were more than fifty years old and the youngest was nine years old.

Localization

Chondroblastomas are typically centered in an epiphysis. They are seen most often in the end of a major tubular bone but can appear in any secondary center of ossification such as the greater trochanter. They have been described in a wide variety of bones including those of the hands and feet. The knee region has contributed the most examples. By contrast with the frequency of these lesions in the epiphyseal portion of a major tubular bone, of the thirteen lesions in our series that were in patients more than twenty-nine years old, only one was in a long bone. Seventeen of the lesions sent in for consultation were in patients who were in the fourth decade of life or older, and only two of those were in long bones.

Symptoms

Local pain is the most important and practically a constant symptom of benign chondroblastoma. It is often mild or moderate in degree; patients of the present series had symptoms for three months to sixteen years before they sought medical attention, and the average duration was slightly more than two years. In a reported case, the lesion was present for fifty-nine years. The complaints are ordinarily referred to the adjacent joint region. Tumefaction is usually absent because of the small size of the tumor and the presence of overlying soft tissue.

Physical Findings

Aside from local tenderness that may be present, the physical examination is of little diagnostic value. There may be wasting of the muscles in the region of the tumor owing to disuse, and limping may be observed. Some patients have increased fluid in the neighboring joint.

Roentgenologic Features

Characteristically, this neoplasm presents with a central region of bone destruction that is usually sharply delimited from the surrounding normal bone by a thin margin of increased bone density. There may or may not be mottled areas of density within the radiolucent zone, depending on the presence and degree of calcification within the tumor. Both trabeculation and active periosteal reaction are rarely seen. The tumor, when it involves the long bones, almost always affects the epiphysis and frequently the adjacent metaphysis. Large chondroblastomas cause bulging

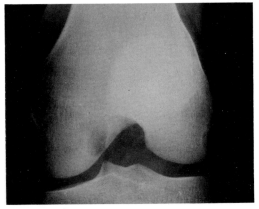

Figure 4-2. Small lytic chondroblastoma of medial condyle of femur.

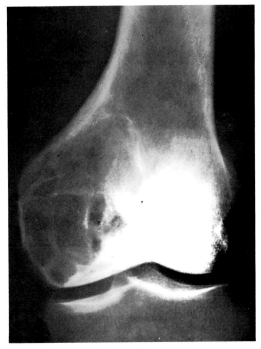

Figure 4-3. Chondroblastoma in medial condyle of femur, an asymptomatic lesion in fifty-four-year-old man found incidentally during angiography. It is well circumscribed and has a slightly sclerotic boundary. After curettage only, tumor did not progress and patient died of unrelated disease approximately ten years later.

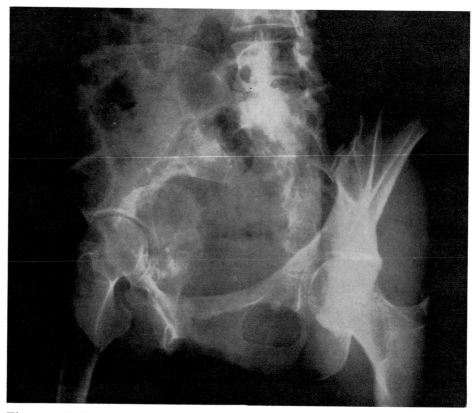

Figure 4-4. Benign chondroblastoma of right innominate bone in region of acetabulum. It has produced obvious expansion into pelvis. This tumor occurred in fifty-four-year-old woman, had produced pain for one year, and resulted in asymptomatic huge recurrence shown in Figure 4-21.

Figure 4-5. Another pertinent lesion, in this case involving the greater trochanter and adjacent neck of femur of eighteen-year-old woman who had had local pain for four months. She has remained well for thirty-six years after curettage, cautery, and radiation therapy.

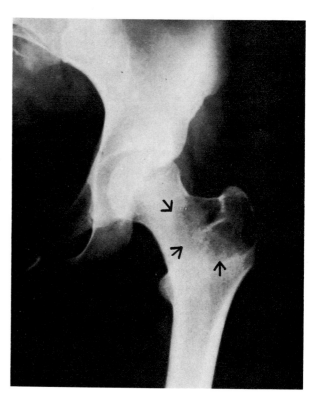

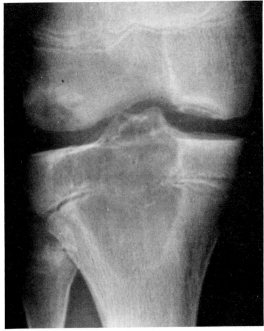

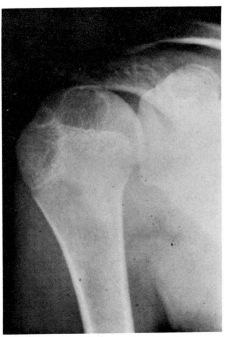

Figure 4-6. Chondroblastoma in fourteen-year-old boy has extended into metaphysis. Osteochondritis dissecans involves femoral condyles.

Figure 4-7. Classic chondroblastoma of epiphysis in sixteen-year-old boy was largely cystic, and patient was well two years after curettage.

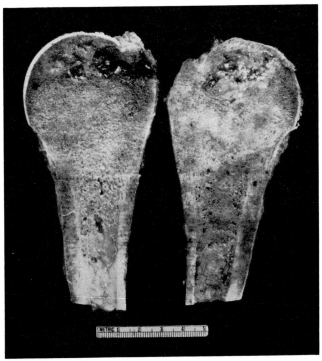

Figure 4-8. Chondroblastoma of upper 2.5 cm of humerus. Resection of specimen was performed because of erroneous diagnosis of chondrosarcoma. (Reproduced with permission from: Kunkel, M. G., Dahlin, D. C., and Young, H. H.: *J Bone Joint Surg, 38A*:817-826, 1956.)

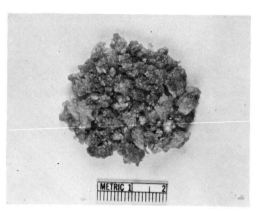

Figure 4-9. Curetted fragments of chondroblastoma of upper end of tibia. Focal chondroid appearance suggests correct diagnosis.

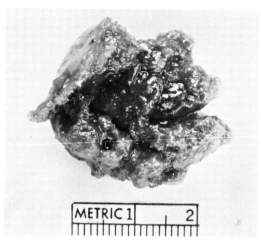

Figure 4-10. Chondroblastoma of distal end of femur. Note overlying periosteum at left and hemorrhagic soft tumor.

and thinning of the cortex of the bone. Enchondromas and chondromyxoid fibromas rarely affect the epiphysis. Chondrosarcoma and benign giant cell tumor are lesions that are likely to produce rarefaction of the end of a bone.

Chondroblastomas of pelvic bones show a remarkable tendency to originate near the triradiate cartilage. None of those in our series arose in either the periosteum or soft tissues, although no osseous abnormality was noted in a mediastinal tumor that probably arose from the first rib. In the thorough review of the roentgenographic features of seventy-two chondroblastomas, McLeod and Beabout noted that only about one fourth of the tumors had visible evidence of calcification. Some authors have suggested that the lesions may become more sclerotic in their later stages.

Gross Pathology

Chondroblastomas are ordinarily small. The primary tumors in this series varied from 1 to 7 cm in greatest diameter. There may be a thin zone of slightly sclerotic bone surrounding the tumor. The lesional tissue itself does not have pathognomonic features. It is grayish pink and may contain zones of hemorrhage or necrosis. In rare instances, the chondroid matrix is so prominent that the tumor has features similar to those of chondroma or chondrosarcoma. Although these tumors often abut on the articular cartilage of a joint, they rarely produce much destruction of this cartilage. An occasional chondroblastoma destroys the bony cortex and produces an extraosseous mass. Minute foci of calcified material may be recognized within the tumor substance. Cystic change, sometimes prominent, may occur; occasionally tumors simulate bone cysts.

Although benign chondroblastomas are usually predominantly epiphyseal in location, rare examples have been centered in the metaphyseal region with only a minimal epiphyseal component. This contrasts with the location of the closely related tumor, chondromyxoid fibroma, which almost always is at or near the end of the shaft when a long bone is affected. Both tumors are found, however, in locations consistent with the theory that they arise from cells of the epiphyseal cartilaginous plate or from "'rests" of these cells.

Histopathology

As indicated by the name of this tumor, its basic proliferating cells are considered to be chondroblasts, that is, cells related to cartilage-forming connective tissue. The round or oval nucleus of this cell is often indented, and the cell borders are ordinarily clearly defined. There is little stroma between the cells except for the zones with chondroid substance. Although mitotic figures are never numerous, they can be found in practically all chondroblastomas. Among the proliferating neoplastic cells are variable numbers of benign multinucleated cells which contain from five to forty or more nuclei. These giant cells of a chondroblastoma are, in general, smaller and less abundant than those of a genuine giant cell tumor of bone. Nuclei of the giant cells resemble closely those of the chondroblasts of the cellular portions of the tumors. These benign giant cells are often less conspicuous in tumors of older persons, as are the areas with chondroid differentiation.

Zones of a chondroid material are the distinctive feature of chondroblastomas,

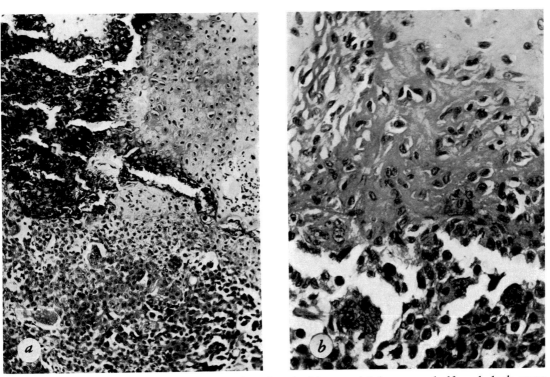

Figure 4-11. *a.* Typical chondroblasts with chondroid material in upper half and dark zone of calcification. (×130) *b.* Higher magnification to show cell detail and giant cells. (×285) (Reproduced with permission from: Kunkel, M. G., Dahlin, D. C., and Young, H. H.: *J Bone Joint Surg, 38A*:817-826, 1956.)

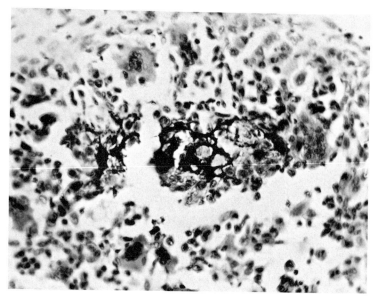

Figure 4-12. Lacelike calcification of chondroid ground substance may be seen only in small foci in benign chondroblastoma. (×285)

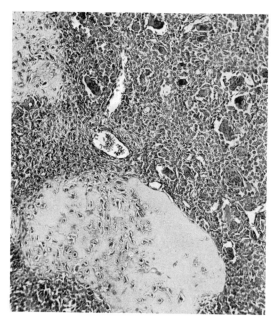

Figure 4-13. Benign chondroblastoma of head of humerus, showing again the relationship of chondroid islands to portions that mimic the appearance of genuine giant cell tumor. (×100)

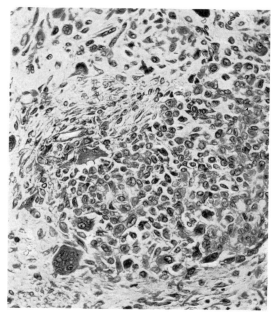

Figure 4-14. Chondroblastomatous zone in recurrence of an originally pure chondromyxoid fibroma removed by curettage twenty months previously. (×200) (Reproduced by permission from: Dahlin, D. C.: *Cancer, 9:*195-203, 1956.)

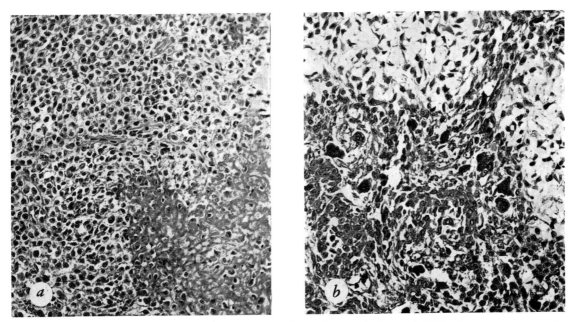

Figure 4-15. *a.* Benign chondroblastoma in region of acetabulum. (×145) Roentgenogram in this case is illustrated in Figure 4-4. *b.* Chondromyxoid fibroma of distal metaphysis of femur originally classified as chondroblastoma because of prominent zones such as those dominating this field. (×165) (Reproduced with permission from: Kunkel, M. G., Dahlin, D. C., and Young, H. H.: *J Bone Joint Surg, 38A:*817-826, 1956.)

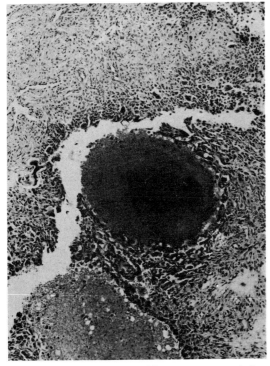

Figure 4-16. Chondroblastoma containing blood-filled spaces in central and lowest portions of photo, producing a resemblance to aneurysmal bone cyst. (×60)

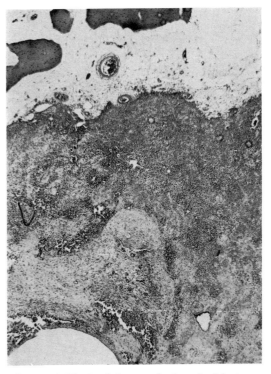

Figure 4-17. Periphery of chondroblastoma well demarcated from adjacent bone. A cyst is present in lower left corner. (×20)

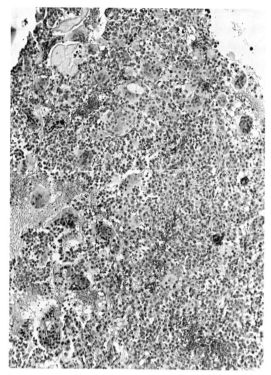

Figure 4-18. As depicted here, some chondroblastomas contain zones markedly similar to giant cell tumor. (×125)

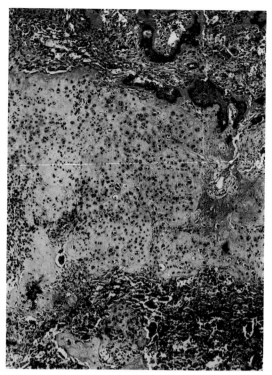

Figure 4-19. Benign chondroblastoma of phalanx. Some of its abundant cartilage is differentiating into bone, as seen especially in the peripheral portions of some of these tumors. (×50)

although these zones may be abundant or rare. In two cases of the present series, the chondroid zones overshadowed the cellular zones. Some have likened this ground substance to the chondroid material found in mixed tumors of the salivary glands, but sometimes it closely resembles mature hyaline cartilage. In most chondroblastomas, some islands of this interstitial substance undergo degeneration and subsequent calcification. These calcified portions are characteristically lacelike with residual lacunae where the degenerated chondroblasts had been. In rare cases, the calcified material is so abundant as to overshadow the diagnostic cellular foci. Recent evidence has been accumulated which indicates a strong histologic relationship between benign chondroblastoma and chondromyxoid fibroma of bone. Some tumors exhibit zones that are characteristic of each of these neoplasms.

Rare tumors contain typical zones of chondroblastoma and other regions with blood-filled spaces reminiscent of aneurysmal bone cyst; such lesions indicate that the latter process represents secondary change in a preexisting disease. Some have suggested that chondroblastomas with an aneurysmal bone cystlike component have greater than usual tendency to recur, but this has not been our experience. Occasionally, the chondroid areas show metaplasia to osteoid and bone, sometimes obscuring the separation of the lesion from adjacent bone.

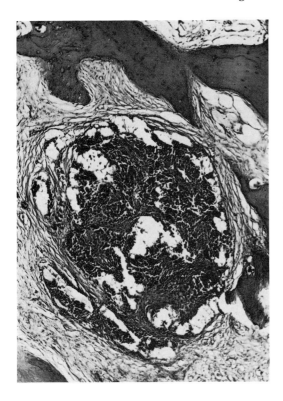

Figure 4-20. One of several foci in recurrent chondroblastoma of the tibia. Such recurrences are unusual and probably result from lobules of tumor that escape the curette. (×65)

There is a tendency to diagnose as chondroblastoma the tumors that contain atypically large nuclei or have merely a chondroid aura in zones. Some have even tried to recognize fully malignant sarcomas as related to chondroblastoma; such attempts have been unsuccessful. If atypicality is suggested by the microscopic or roentgenographic appearance, the lesion actually may be some other disease such as osteosarcoma, atypical fibrous histiocytoma, or the newly recognized clear cell chondrosarcoma.

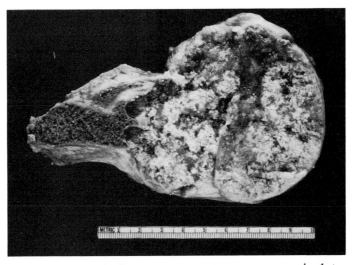

Figure 4-21. This huge recurrent tumor was excised ten years after incomplete removal of benign chondroblastoma seen in Figure 4-4. Patient died of "football-sized" intrapelvic recurrence of similar tumor fourteen years after this second operation.

Treatment

Because chondroblastomas are so benign and nonaggressive, the main danger is that too radical treatment may be instituted, sometimes because of an erroneous diagnosis. The pathologist who is not conversant with the features of this tumor is likely to mistake it for a malignant tumor, especially for chondrosarcoma or for malignant giant cell tumor. The average tumor of this type is best treated by curettage. Bone grafting of the resultant defect may be necessary. As in the management of other cartilaginous tumors, those chondroblastomas so located that they can be excised completely with a surrounding shell of normal bone should be so treated. Such complete resection is especially apropos for tumors considered atypical histologically or for those with an aggressive quality clinically.

Radiation therapy is nearly always unnecessary, and the several reported postradiation sarcomas in cases of benign chondroblastoma underscore the potential danger. In one of our patients with tibial chondroblastoma, sarcoma of the adjacent distal part of a femur developed twenty-nine years after a large dose of radiation to the benign tumor.

Prognosis

Practically all chondroblastomas may be eradicated by the treatment outlined above. Even the rare tumor that recurs or produces implantation in nearby soft tissues should be curable by total resection. Radiation has been beneficial for tumors not surgically resectable. In two well-documented cases, sarcomas replaced the benign tumors at intervals of several years with no radiation therapy.

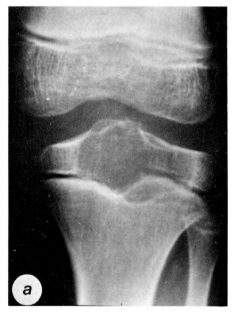 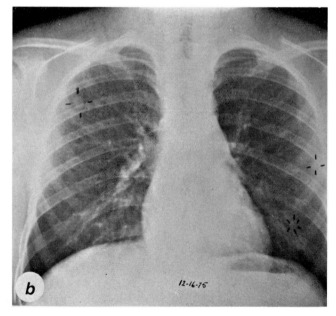

Figure 4-22. *a.* Benign chondroblastoma in nine-year-old boy. *b.* The same month, several small benign pulmonary deposits were found. (Case contributed by Doctors S. G. Parker of Decatur, Illinois, and M. Kyriakos of St. Louis, Missouri.)

Several benign chondroblastomas have metastasized to the lungs as benign tumors. These have proved to be quasi-malignant with the metastatic deposits usually nonprogressive. The need for radiation or chemotherapy for such metastasis remains debatable. Although I have seen pulmonary specimens from four such benign metastasizing tumors, none occurred in the Mayo Clinic series of forty-four cases. They must be regarded as rare.

Several "aggressive" chondroblastomas have been reported and are similar to our case shown in Figures 4-4, 4-15a, and 4-21. Although histologically similar to the remainder, those tumors have become large, usually after a prolonged course and with debatably adequate early surgery. A related problem was provided by another case in this series, a tumor of the scapula that was 18 by 14 by 12.5 cm in a forty-eight-year-old man. On two occasions, he had received radiation therapy for the lesion—at ten years and again at seven years—before its removal by forequarter amputation. Eighteen months later, local recurrence and pulmonary metastasis developed. The scapular tumor appears to be indistinguishable from the other benign chondroblastomas, except that chondroid islands are inconclusive, and so it has been included in this group of forty-four tumors.

Bibliography

1931   Codman, E. A.: Epiphyseal Chondromatous Giant Cell Tumors of the Upper End of the Humerus. *Surg Gynecol Obstet, 52:*543-548.

1942   Jaffe, H. L., and Lichtenstein, Louis: Benign Chondroblastoma of Bone: A Reinterpretation of the So-called Calcifying or Chrondromatous Giant Cell Tumor. *Am J Pathol,18:*969-992.

1949   Copeland, M. M., and Geschickter, C. F.: Chondroblastic Tumors of Bone: Benign and Malignant. *Ann Surg, 129:*724-733.

1951   Hatcher, C. H., and Campbell, J. C.: Benign Chondroblastoma of Bone: Its Histologic Variations and a Report of Late Sarcoma in the Site of One. *Bull Hosp Joint Dis, 12:*411-430.

1951   Valls, José, Ottolenghi, C. E., and Schajowicz, Fritz: Epiphyseal Chondroblastoma of Bone. *J Bone Joint Surg, 33A:*997-1009.

1956   Kunkel, M. G., Dahlin, D. C., and Young, H. H.: Benign Chondroblastoma. *J Bone Joint Surg, 38A:*817-826.

1958   Plum, G. E., and Pugh, D. G.: Roentgenologic Aspects of Benign Chondroblastoma of Bone. *Am J Roentgenol, 79:*584-591.

1964   Welsh, R. A., and Meyer, A. T.: A Histogenetic Study of Chondroblastoma. *Cancer, 17:*578-589.

1965   Steiner, G. S.: Postradiation Sarcoma of Bone. *Cancer, 18:*603-612

1968   Salzer, M., Salzer-Kuntschik, M., and Kretschmer, G.: Das Benigne Chondroblastom. *Arch Orthop Unfallchir, 64:*229-244.

1969   Kahn, L. B., Wood, F. M., and Ackerman, L. V.: Malignant Chondroblastoma: Report of Two Cases and Review of the Literature. *Arch Pathol, 88:*371-376 (October).

1970   Schajowicz, F., and Gallardo, H.: Epiphysial Chondroblastoma of Bone: A Clinicopathological Study of Sixty-nine Cases. *J Bone Joint Surg, 52B:*205-226 (May).

1970   Sirsat, M. V., and Doctor, V. M.: Benign Chondroblastoma of Bone: Report of a Case of Malignant Transformation. *J Bone Joint Surg, 52B:*741-745 (November).

1971   Gravanis, M. B., and Giansanti, J. S.: Benign Chondroblastoma: Report of Four Cases With a Discussion of the Presence of Ossification. *Am J Clin Pathol, 55:*624-631 (May).

1972   Dahlin, D. C., and Ivins, J. C.: Benign Chondroblastoma: A Study of 125 Cases. *Cancer, 30:*401-413 (August).

1972   Levine, G. D., and Bensch, K. G.: Chondroblastoma—The Nature of the Basic Cell: A Study by Means of Histochemistry, Tissue Culture, Electron Microscopy, and Autoradiography. *Cancer, 29:*1546-1562 (June).

1973   Huvos, A. G., and Marcove, R. C.: Chondroblastoma of Bone: A Critical Review. *Clin Orthop, 95:*300-312 (September).

1973   McLeod, R. A., and Beabout, J. W.: The Roentgenographic Features of Chondroblastoma. *Am J Roentgenol, 118:*464-471 (June).

1975   Green, P., and Whittaker, R. P.: Benign Chondroblastoma: Case Report with Pulmonary Metastasis. *J Bone Joint Surg, 57A:*418-420 (April).

Chapter 5

Chondromyxoid Fibroma

CHONDROMYXOID FIBROMA is a rare and peculiar benign tumor, apparently derived from cartilage-forming connective tissue. Its name, which is cumbersome, has the merit of being highly descriptive and is gaining acceptance for this distinctive tumor. It was described by Jaffe and Lichtenstein in 1948 when they presented eight cases and emphasized the danger of mistaking this benign neoplasm for a malignant lesion, especially chondrosarcoma. The relative rarity of the neoplasm should not lull one into a complacent disregard for it, because anyone dealing with bone tumors must be prepared to interpret and manage any lesion he encounters. One cannot ignore even the more complicated ramifications of a useful classification, because he cannot expect to diagnose and treat correctly a tumor with which he is unfamiliar.

Although chondromyxoid fibroma characteristically contains variable amounts of chondroid, fibromatoid, and myxoid components, certain portions within the tumor resemble hyaline cartilage and make it logical to include this neoplasm among those of cartilaginous derivation.

The rationale of this classification is enhanced by the striking histologic similarity indicated previously that chondromyxoid fibroma and benign chondroblastoma sometimes have.

Many of the tumors referred to in the literature as myxomas and fibromyxomas of bone are, no doubt, examples of chondromyxoid fibroma. The distinctive myxoma (fibromyxoma) of jawbones lacks the lobulation and varied histologic spectrum of chondromyxoid fibroma, has no exact counterpart in the remainder of the skeleton, and is apparently of odontogenic derivation.

The earlier admonition to avoid "overdiagnosing" chondromyxoid fibroma as chondrosarcoma has been taken too seriously by some pathologists. I have seen a number of instances in which errors have been made in the reverse direction, with consequent inadequate treatment of chondrosarcoma.

These tumors can be expected to behave in a benign fashion, except for the extremely rare lesion that undergoes malignant transformation spontaneously and those subjected to the slight risk of malignant alteration by radiation therapy.

Bone Tumors

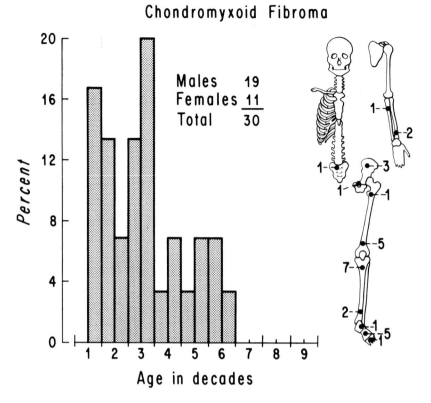

Figure 5-1. Skeletal, age, and sex distribution of chondromyxoid fibromas.

Incidence

Chondromyxoid fibroma accounted for but only half of 1 percent of bone tumors of this series. Reports in the literature indicate that it is less common than chondro-blastoma.

Sex

A definite male predilection was found in this series and has been noted in the recent literature.

Age

There is a marked predilection for patients in the second and third decades of life. The youngest in this series was six years old, and the oldest was fifty-nine years old.

Localization

The typical chondromyxoid fibroma is located in the metaphyseal region of a bone and may abut on or be a variable distance from the epiphyseal line. Occasionally, a tumor involves both the metaphysis and the epiphysis. This localization suggests that, like benign chondroblastoma, chondromyxoid fibroma possibly arises from the epiphyseal cartilaginous plate. Approximately two thirds of the recorded examples of this tumor have been in the long tubular bones, with the tibia contributing approximately one third of all cases. It occurs in other long tubular bones, in small bones of the hands and feet, and in the pelvic girdle, with sporadic examples in such bones as vertebrae, ribs, scapulae, and the skull.

Nine tumors in this series occurred in patients thirty years old or older; only three of the lesions were in the long tubular bones. Of twenty-two patients of similar age whose tumors were sent in for consultation, half had involvement of the long tubular bones.

Symptoms

Pain is by far the most common presenting symptom of patients with chondromyxoid fibroma. Occasionally, it is of several years' duration. Local swelling is occasionally a complaint of patients whose tumors are not camouflaged by a thick layer of overlying tissues. Such tumefaction has been noted by only three of the twenty patients in this series. Occasionally, these tumors are asymptomatic incidental findings on roentgenograms.

Physical Findings

Physical examination is of little diagnostic aid. Tenderness in the region of the tumor, or a tender or nontender mass, may be found and aid in exact localization.

Roentgenologic Features

The defect is characteristically an eccentric, sharply circumscribed zone of rarefaction that occasionally causes expansion of the bone. The cortical outline was partially absent over three of the tumors of the present series. A chondromyxoid fibroma, especially in a small bone, can produce fusiform expansion of its entire contour.

Trabeculae appear to traverse the defect in most cases, but these are merely the roentgenographic reflection of corrugations on the inner surface of the cavity that contains the tumor. Sometimes the bone adjacent to the tumor is characterized by a thin delimiting line of sclerosis. Although a minority of these neoplasms contain microscopic foci of calcification, these are very rarely reflected in the roentgenographic shadow.

The roentgenologic features of the tumors in this series and of those in additional cases are detailed by Turcotte and coworkers, who found that the defect uniformly looks benign.

Beabout observed that these tumors, if not round, usually have their long axis parallel to the bone; they vary from about 1 to 10 cm in greatest dimension. The tumors usually spare the epiphyseal cartilaginous plate. Pathologic fracture occurred in four of the thirty cases he studied.

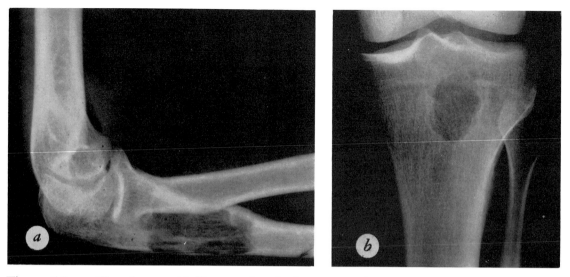

Figure 5-2. *a.* Chondromyxoid fibroma that had caused pain for eight months. There was tender swelling of upper part of ulna. *b.* This tumor occurred in twenty-eight-year-old man and had produced local pain for two years. (Reproduced with permission from: Dahlin, D. C.: *Cancer, 9:*195-203, 1956.)

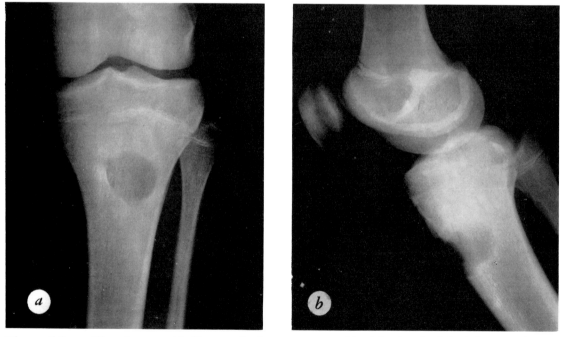

Figure 5-3. *a.* Chondromyxoid fibroma in fourteen-year-old girl who had had local pain for three months. *b.* Lateral view of same lesion. It recurred twenty months after curettage and was then treated by block excision. She was well eleven years after this wider excision. (Reproduced with permission from: Dahlin, D. C.: *Cancer, 9:*195-203, 1956.)

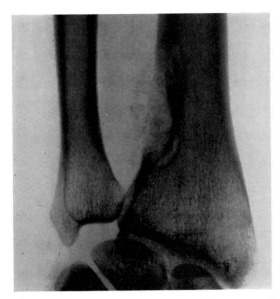

Figure 5-4. Chondromyxoid fibroma of radius showing punctate calcification. Visible mineralization in these tumors is exceedingly rare. (Case contributed by Doctors C. R. Dochat, Robert Fowler, and Charles Miller of Akron, Ohio.)

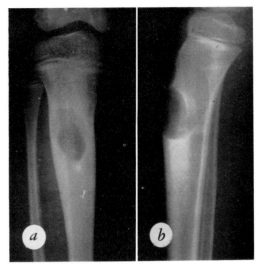

Figure 5-5. *a* and *b*. Anteroposterior and lateral views of chondromyxoid fibroma in ten-year-old boy. Foci of chondroblastoma were present in tumor. (Reproduced with permission from: Dahlin, D. C.: *Cancer, 9*:195-203, 1956.)

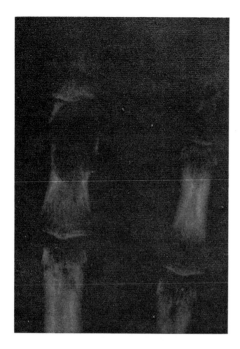
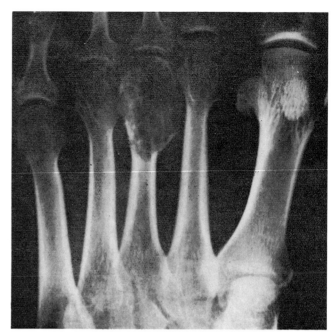
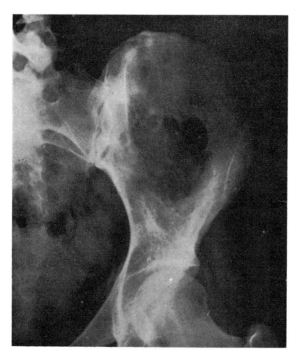
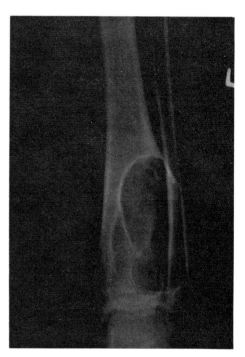

Figure 5-6. Four characteristic chondromyxoid fibromas. *Top left*. Lesion in middle phalanx of third finger with central location. (Courtesy of Doctor R. R. Williams of Middletown, Ohio.) *Top right*. Tumor in third metatarsal. *Bottom left*. Large defect in ilium, with trabeculated appearance. (Courtesy of Doctors E. H. Boyer and J. A. Finer of Youngstown, Ohio.) *Bottom right*. Large but typical tumor in tibia. (Courtesy of Doctor Lorel Stapley of Phoenix, Arizona.) (These four illustrations reproduced with permission from: Turcotte and coworkers: *Am J Roentgenol,* 87:1085-1095, 1962.)

Gross Pathology

The average tumor of this type is small, those of this series varying in size up to 5 cm in greatest diameter, although larger tumors have been reported. Grossly, the lesion may closely resemble hyaline cartilage or appear to be a somewhat translucent fibrous mass. In general, the consistency is denser than one would suspect from the histologic appearance. A striking feature is the sharp delimitation from the surrounding bone, a feature that contrasts with what one observes in chondrosarcoma. The surface of the tumor is often distinctly lobulated, and the cavity from which it is enucleated frequently is characterized by corrugations that correspond

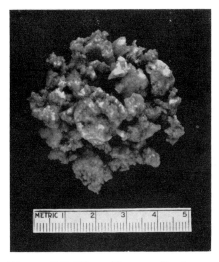

Figure 5-7. Firm, fibrocartilaginous tissue removed by curettage from lesion represented in roentgenogram shown in Figure 5-2*b*.

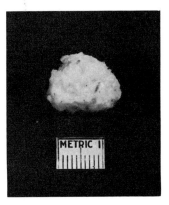

Figure 5-8. Finely lobulated tumor enucleated from defect represented in roentgenograms shown in Figure 5-3*a* and *b*. (Reproduced with permission from: Dahlin, D. C.: *Cancer, 9*:195-203, 1956.)

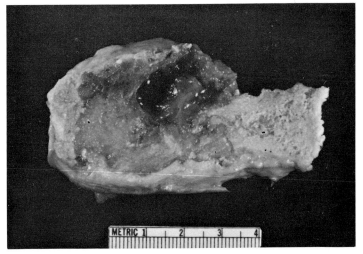

Figure 5-9. Chondromyxoid fibroma of third metatarsal of forty-three-year-old man who had noted swelling for thirty years. Dark area represents zone that simulated aneurysmal bone cyst.

with the tumor lobules. There may be a thin sclerotized zone in the bone immediately adjacent to the neoplasm.

Myxoid foci, small cysts, hemorrhagic zones, and even calcific deposits may be seen. A liquid mucinous quality strongly suggests that the tumor is a chondrosarcoma. One tumor contained a cyst with 5 ml of clear fluid.

Histopathology

The name of this tumor indicates the variation observed microscopically in different fields of a given tumor and from tumor to tumor. The gamut includes myxomatous zones, fibrous zones, and fields with a distinctly chondroid appearance. The nuclei of the cells are round, oval, crescentic, or spindle-shaped. Cytoplasmic extensions are often multipolar. The chondroid element may occupy only small foci, but it occasionally dominates the histologic pattern and introduces the hazard of mistaking the tumor for a chondrosarcoma. Chondromyxoid fibroma characteristically possesses a lobular pattern of growth, but this feature is sometimes obscured in microscopic sections prepared from curetted fragments, and the lobules are often only partially separated from each other. A highly characteristic feature is the increased concentration of nuclei observed at the periphery of the lobules and partial lobules, but this must not be confused with a similar disposition of cells in some chondrosarcomas. At the edge of the tumor, this cellular peripheral zone is sharply demarcated from the surrounding uninvolved tissues. Variable collagenization of the lobules is observed. Small amorphous foci of calcification are occasionally present, and these sometimes have the lacelike quality of the calcification seen in benign chondroblastoma.

Calcific foci were found in one fourth of the seventy-six lesions studied by Rahimi and coworkers. In some of these, however, amorphous basophilic zones were interpreted as being areas of calcification. These may be related to zones of degeneration sometimes present in the lobules. Benign giant cells and phagocytic mononuclear cells may be seen in the tissue between the lobules. As indicated in the preceding chapter, some chondromyxoid fibromas contain cellular foci indistinguishable from microscopic fields in benign chondroblastoma. Rarely one sees a tumor that is difficult to classify strictly into one category or the other.

Vascularity is seen in the connective tissue between lobules or peripheral to fused lobules. Occasionally, the vascular pattern is like that of aneurysmal bone cyst. Osteoid and newly formed bone is rare but may be seen in the interlobular connective tissue or at the periphery of lobules.

Pink staining of the cytoplasm of the stellate cells usually occurs. Jaffe has noted that the myxoid areas do not contain lipid. Alcian blue stains are positive in the chondroid areas. There is a delicate reticulin network in the myxoid zones and denser concentrations of this material at the periphery of the lobules. Mitotic figures are distinctly rare.

The most important histologic feature of chondromyxoid fibroma is that the cells in some portions of many of these tumors are large and have nuclei of irregular size and shape, and even contain multiple nuclei at times. These features, if present

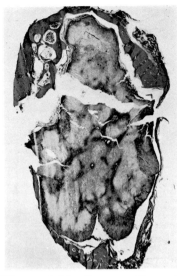

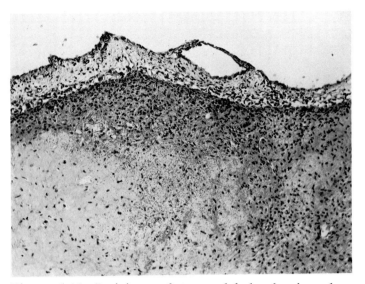

Figure 5-10. Cross-section of entire tumor that had caused some expansion of rib. (×6) (Reproduced with permission from: Dahlin, D. C.: *Cancer, 9:*195-203, 1956.)

Figure 5-11. Periphery of tumor lobule showing characteristic condensation of nuclei beneath rim of compressed adjacent tissue, here located above neoplastic tissue. (×130) (Reproduced with permission from: Dahlin, D. C., Wells, A. H., and Henderson, E. D.: *J Bone Joint Surg, 35A:*831-834, 1953.)

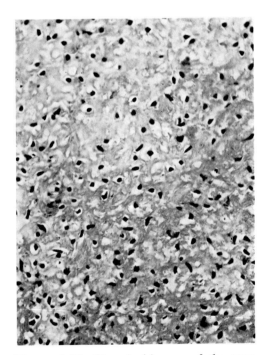

Figure 5-12. Chondroid zone of the type commonly seen in chondromyxoid fibroma. (×200) (Reproduced with permission from: Dahlin, D. C., Wells, A. H., and Henderson, E. D.: *J Bone Joint Surg, 35A:*831-834, 1953.)

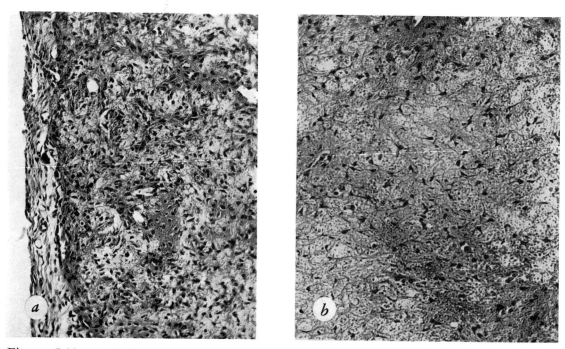

Figure 5-13. *a.* Well-demarcated periphery showing fibromatoid and chondroid features. (×180) *b.* Myxoid zone of type seen in many chondromyxoid fibromas. (×200) (Reproduced with permission from: Dahlin, D. C., Wells, A. H., and Henderson, E. D.: *J Bone Joint Surg, 35A:*831-834, 1953.)

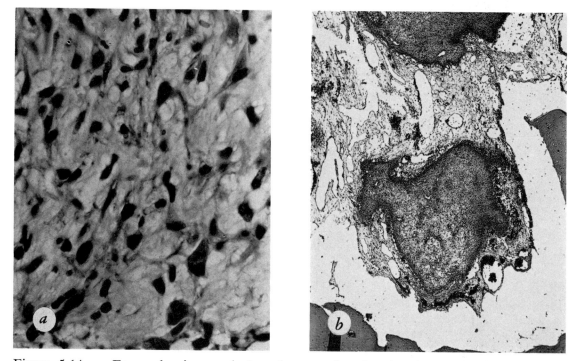

Figure 5-14. *a.* Focus showing marked nuclear atypism in chondromyxoid fibroma. Such zones have no significance in lesion that has other features of this benign tumor. (×520) *b.* Tumor lobule separated, in this plane, from main neoplasm. Such ramifications could be left behind during curettage and thus account for recurrence. (×40) (Reproduced with permission from: Dahlin, D. C.: *Cancer, 9:*195-203, 1956.)

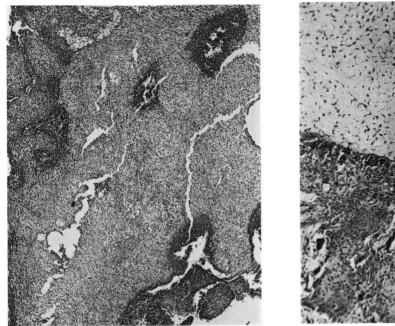
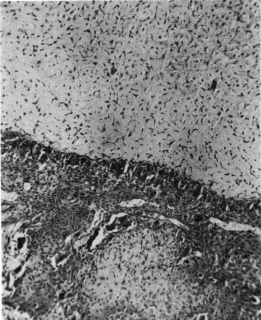

Figure 5-15. *Left.* Lobules of myxoid tissue partially separated from one another by cellular zones. One of patterns seen in chondromyxoid fibroma. (×25) *Right.* Another variation with very small multipolar cells in lobules. (×100)

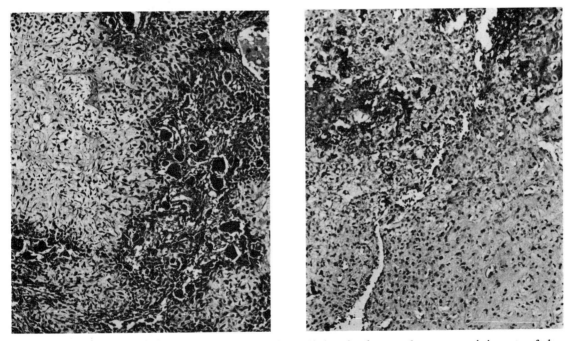

Figure 5-16. *Left.* Smaller myxoid lobules in cellular background very reminiscent of benign chondroblastoma. (×80) *Right.* Darkly staining calcific foci such as these are seen in minority of chondromyxoid fibromas. (×80)

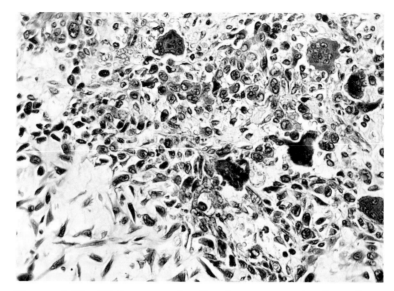

Figure 5-17. High-power detail of recurrent benign chondromyxoid fibroma containing abundant "chondroblasts." Wider local resection of recurrence resulted in cure. (×200)

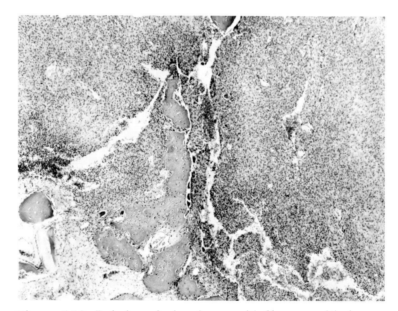

Figure 5-18. Lobules of chondromyxoid fibroma with immature bone in non-neoplastic septal area and merging with edge of tumor lobule. (×50)

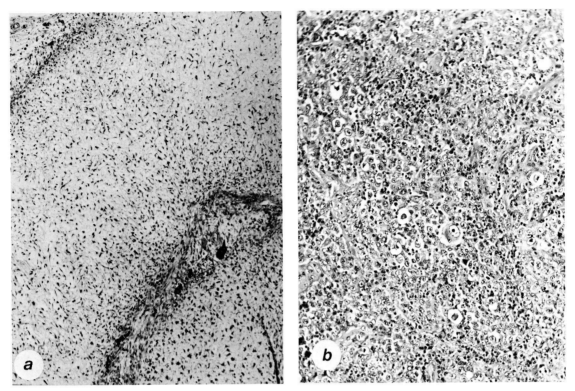

Figure 5-19. *a.* Typical chondromyxoid fibroma of pubis in forty-five-year-old man who had noted pain for one year. Note good demarcation from adjacent bone. Doctor Lent Johnson of A.F.I.P. had concurred in the diagnosis. (×100) *b.* At exploration, huge intra-abdominal extension of this benign tumor was grade 4, highly undifferentiated sarcoma. No radiation therapy had been given. Autopsy revealed no other primary lesion. Such "spontaneous" malignant transformation of chondromyxoid fibroma has not been convincingly documented previously. (×160)

in a hyaline-cartilage tumor of the chondroma-chondrosarcoma group, would be indicative of malignancy. When one recognizes, however, that these cells are only part of the overall pattern of chondromyxoid fibroma, the benign nature of the lesion is firmly established.

Treatment

Block excision of the affected area, when feasible, is the best treatment. Curettage, although ordinarily successful, imposes perhaps a 25 percent risk of recurrence. Bone grafting after excision or curettage is often necessary. Radiation therapy is not indicated except for the very rare surgically inaccessible lesion.

Three patients in this series were treated by amputation: one because of the large size of the tumor, one because of a diagnosis of sarcoma, and one because a recurrent lesion treated elsewhere was similarly misinterpreted.

Two other patients with metatarsal tumors had ray amputations.

Prognosis

Recurrent tumor developed in six patients in this series. As indicated, one patient was subjected to amputation; the remainder were successfully managed by wider excision. The lobulations on the periphery of these tumors may lead one to leave ramifications behind when treating them by curettage.

Rahimi and coworkers found that the risk of recurrence was higher in patients with tumors containing enlarged and irregular nuclei, especially if the patients were less than fifteen years old.

Malignant transformation of chondromyxoid fibroma rarely has been demonstrated convincingly in the literature, although there have been many allusions to this problem. I know of one sarcoma that developed six years after radiation to the area of chondromyxoid fibroma. One patient in this series had a lethal sarcoma develop in a classic chondromyxoid fibroma, though there had been no radiation (*see* Figure 5-19). Sarcomatous change remains a pathologic rarity in this disease.

Bibliography

1948 Jaffe, H. L., and Lichtenstein, L.: Chondromyxoid Fibroma of Bone: A Distinctive Benign Tumor Likely to Be Mistaken Especially for Chondrosarcoma. *Arch Pathol, 45:*541-551.

1953 Dahlin, D. C., Wells, A. H., and Henderson, E. D.: Chondromyxoid Fibroma of Bone: Report of Two Cases. *J Bone Joint Surg, 35A:*831-834.

1954 Wrenn, R. N., and Smith, A.G.: Chondromyxoid Fibroma. *South Med J, 47:*848-853.

1956 Dahlin, D. C.: Chondromyxoid Fibroma of Bone, With Emphasis on Its Morphological Relationship to Benign Chondroblastoma. *Cancer, 9:*195-203.

1958 Iwata, S., and Coley, B. L.: Report of Six Cases of Chondromyxoid Fibroma of Bone. *Surg Gynecol Obstet, 107:*571-576.

1961 Scaglietti, O., and Stringa, G.: Myxoma of Bone in Childhood. *J Bone Joint Surg, 43A:*67-80.

1962 Ralph, L. L.: Chondromyxoid Fibroma of Bone. *J Bone Joint Surg, 44B:*7-24.

1962 Benedetti, G. B., Canepa, G., and Garcia, M.: Il Fibroma Condromixoide dell' osso. Revisione Critica delle Letterature ed Indagini Istologiche ed Istochimiche su 8 Casi. *Arch Putti Chir Organi Mov, 17:*44-72.

1962 Turcotte, B., Pugh, D. G., and Dahlin, D. C.: The Roentgenologic Aspects of Chondromyxoid Fibroma of Bone. *Am J Roentgenol, 87:*1085-1095.

1962 Gilmer, W. S., Higley, G. B., Jr., and Kilgore, W. E.: *Atlas of Bone Tumors.* Saint Louis, Mosby, pp. 36-39.

1964 Marcove, R. C., Kambolis, C. Bullough, P. G., and Jaffe, H. L.: Fibromyxoma of Bone: A Report of 3 Cases. *Cancer, 17:*1209-1213 (September).

1965 Salzer, M., and Salzer-Kuntschik, M.: Das Chondromyxoidfibrom. *Langenbecks Arch Chir, 312:*216-231.

1970 Feldman, F., Hecht, H. L., and Johnston, A. D.: Chondromyxoid Fibroma of Bone. *Radiology, 94:*249-260 (February).

1971 Murphy, N. B., and Price, C. H. G.: The Radiological Aspects of Chrondromyxoid Fibroma of Bone. *Clin Radiol, 22:*261-269.

1971 Schajowicz, F., and Gallardo, H.: Chondromyxoid Fibroma (Fibromyxoid Chondroma) of Bone: Clinico-pathological Study of Thirty-two Cases. *J Bone Joint Surg, 53B:*198-216 (May).

1972 Rahimi, A., Beabout, J. W., Irvins, J. C., and Dahlin, D. C.: Chondromyxoid Fibroma: A Clinico-pathologic Study of 76 Cases. *Cancer, 30:*726-736 (September).

Chapter 6

Osteoma

THE ACTUAL OCCURRENCE of true osteoma is so debatable that this tumor was not included in the overall statistical data. Reactive changes from trauma, infection, or invading tumor such as meningioma can cause osseous overgrowth. Some bony outgrowths may represent ancient osteochondromas, the cartilaginous caps of which have completely involuted. Because these tumefactions produce the clinical manifestations of a neoplasm, they are often erroneously called "osteomas."

Occasional tumors of the skull, especially those involving the paranasal sinuses, are the most nearly bona fide osteomas, and yet there is room for conjecture regarding these. The gamut of fibro-osseous dysplastic lesions that affect these bones runs from soft, purely fibrous lesions to those that are heavily ossified. A few of the dense "ivory" osteomas contain softer zones of fibro-osseous dysplasia. Hence, there is no clear line of distinction between obviously dysplastic lesions and completely osseous tumors that one might wish to call "true osteomas."

Rarely, one encounters a sessile ossified neoplasm on the surface of a bone, a tumor with roentgenologic and pathologic features that relate it closely to the malignant tumor called "parosteal osteosarcoma." These benign counterparts are best regarded as parosteal osteomas.

Skeletal "osteomas" of various bones, but prominently involving the skull and jaws, are associated with intestinal polyps, fibromatous and other connective tissue lesions, and epidermal cysts in Gardner's syndrome.

The appearance of some lesions regarded as "solid" odontomas makes it possible that they are osteomas because formed elements of tooth structure cannot be absolutely identified. It seems probable that dentin can become ossified.

The dense bony overgrowths of torus palatinus and torus mandibularis are of unknown etiology but can hardly be considered neoplastic since they have very restricted growth potential. Similar reasoning applies to hyperostosis cranii.

Because of the hodgepodge of tumors included among the "osteomas," no attempt will be made to discuss their features as a group. Some of the characteristics of three pertinent types will be illustrated.

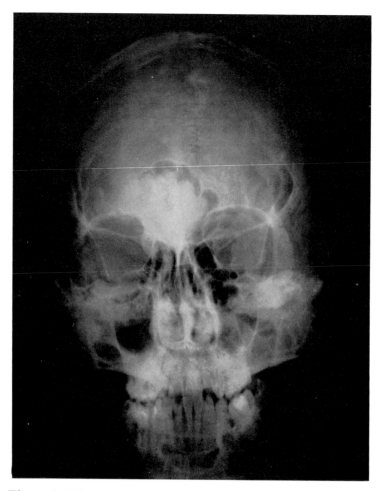

Figure 6-1. Osteoma of frontal sinus in nineteen-year-old man produced local tumefaction. Such lesions can produce symptoms by blocking drainage from the sinus or by penetrating into neighboring structures, including the cranial cavity.

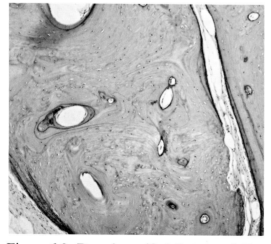

Figure 6-2. Densely ossified "osteoma." Reactive bony sclerosis can give similar appearance. (×60)

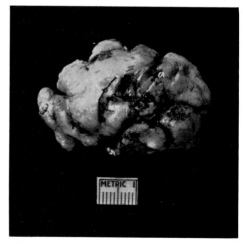

Figure 6-3. Gross specimen removed from patient whose roentgenogram is illustrated in Figure 6-1.

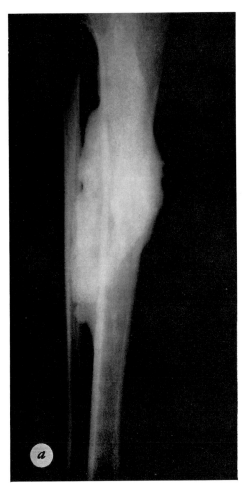 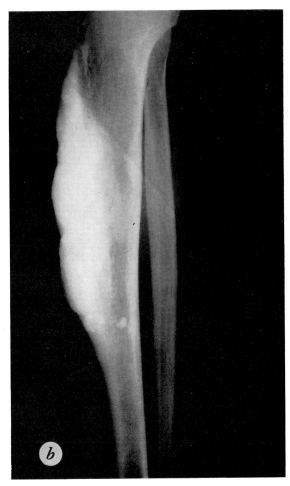

Figure 6-4. *a* and *b*. Anteroposterior and lateral views of dense parosteal osteoma of tibia of forty-three-year-old man who had noted gradually increasing swelling for thirty-one years. This tumor bears a roentgenographic resemblance to parosteal osteogenic sarcoma. Patient had no evidence of recurrence when he died with multiple myeloma fifty-eight months after resection of lesion shown in Figure 6-5.

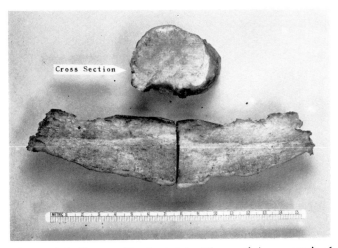

Figure 6-5. Tumor illustrated in Figure 6-4 was excised along with subjacent cortex of bone.

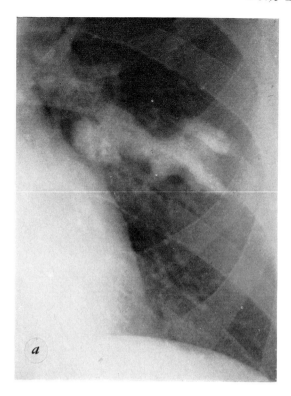 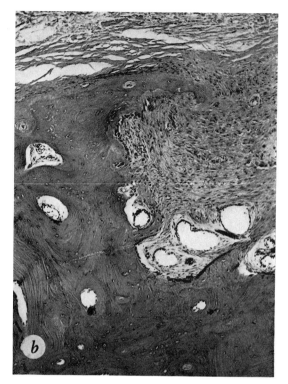

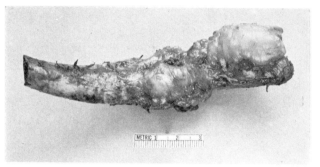

Figure 6-6. *a.* Irregular sessile osteoma of eighth rib. This was an incidental finding, having produced no signs or symptoms. *b.* Periphery of same lesion showing that osseous tissue appears to be derived from proliferating fibroblasts, apparently by a process of metaplasia. This appearance is reminiscent of what one commonly observes in parosteal osteogenic sarcoma. (×70) *Below.* Resected specimen. Patient was sixty-nine years old and well twenty years after resection.

Bibliography

1950   Hallberg, O. E., and Begley, J. W., Jr.: Origin and Treatment of Osteomas of the Paranasal Sinuses. *Arch Otolaryngol, 51:*750-760.

1958   Caughey, J. E.: The Etiology of Hyperostosis Cranii (Metabolic Craniopathy): A Clinical Study. *J Bone Joint Surg, 40B:*701-721.

1962   Gardner, E. J.: Follow-up Study of Family Group Exhibiting Dominant Inheritance for a Syndrome Including Intestinal Polyps, Osteomas, Fibromas and Epidermal Cysts. *Am J Hum Genet, 14:*376-390.

1965   Bullough, P. G.: Ivory Exostosis of the Skull. *Postgrad Med J, 41:*277-281.

1966   Colock, B. P., and Zomorodian, A. A.: Gardner's Syndrome. Multiple Polyposis of Colon, Bone Tumors and Soft-Tissue Tumors. *Postgrad Med, 40:*29-34 (July).

Chapter 7

Osteoid Osteoma

THE MAJORITY OPINION now favors the view that osteoid osteoma is a neoplasm and not the result of some obscure infection or other known specific etiologic agent. This distinctive benign osteoblastic lesion consists of a small oval or round mass, commonly called a nidus. This nidus is often associated with a surrounding zone of sclerotic bone, especially when the lesion develops in a cortical portion of bone. The nidus is the essential part of the tumor, the surrounding sclerosis being a reversible change that disappears after removal of the nidus. As will be illustrated, the major component of this tumor is a meshwork of osteoid trabeculae showing varied degrees of mineralization in a background of usually vascular fibrous connective tissue.

Certain instances of focal subacute or chronic osteomyelitis in bone produce a clinical and roentgenographic pattern that has been confused with that of osteoid osteoma, especially when these inflammatory lesions are associated with a small, discrete, central rarefied focus. Histologically, of course, the lesion produced by inflammation and that by genuine osteoid osteoma are readily distinguished when appropriate sections are made. Osteoid osteomas located immediately beneath articular cartilage have been mistaken for osteochondritis dissecans roentgenologically. Focal islands of idiopathic medullary sclerosis may be the size of a nidus of sclerotic osteoid osteoma, but they produce no clinical symptoms.

For a neoplasm, osteoid osteoma has a strangely limited growth potential, and tumors more than 1.5 cm in largest diameter are unusual. There may be remarkable histologic similarity to osteoblastoma, as described in Chapter 8. All lesions less than 1 cm in diameter McLeod and coworkers arbitrarily called "osteoid osteoma"; they called lesions more than 2 cm in diameter osteoblastoma; and they used an arbitrary dividing line of 1.5 cm for lesions indistinguishable by all other criteria.

Multiple bone involvement in this disease has not been described.

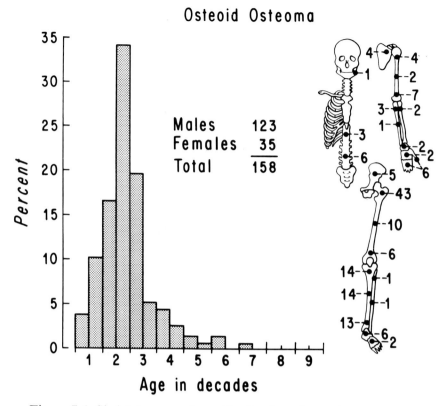

Figure 7-1. Skeletal, age, and sex distribution of osteoid osteomas.

Incidence

The 158 osteoid osteomas in the present series comprised 11 percent of the benign tumors. This is undoubtedly lower than the actual incidence, because this type of tumor was recognized only rarely before 1940.

Sex

Our series indicates a pronounced predominance of males. The females showed age and localization distributions similar to those of the total group.

Age

Paralleling the literature closely, 80 percent of the patients in this series were five through twenty-four years old. Six were less than five years old, the youngest was two years old, and the oldest was sixty-one years old.

Localization

At least half of the osteoid osteomas occur in the femur or tibia. In long bones they are usually near the end of the shaft. Other fibro-osseous processes in the mandible may simulate osteoid osteoma. In vertebrae the arch is most commonly involved. Some of the vertebral examples, as well as others, in the literature are undoubtedly benign osteoblastomas. This series contained none in the calvarium, sternum, or clavicle. Only approximately 1 percent are seen in the jaws.

Symptoms

By far the most important complaint is pain of gradually progressing severity. Its duration prior to the patient's seeking medical care may vary from weeks to several years. Many have noted that salicylates relieve the pain, which otherwise commonly interferes with sleep. The pain is often referred to the adjacent joint region, and occasionally it is referred to a site so distant from the lesion that roentgenographic studies are misdirected. In some instances, especially when the involved bone is near the skin, painful local swelling may become evident. Growth disturbances including increased bone length may occur. Scoliosis and flexion contractures have been produced by this tumor. Those near a joint may simulate arthritis.

Pain may be related to nerves, identified by special axon stains, within the nidus. Only two lesions in this series were painless.

Physical Findings

Dysfunction, often resulting in a limp, is commonly produced by an osteoid osteoma. Atrophy of some muscles of the affected extremity is common. When added to the character of the pain and the decreased muscle stretch reflexes, the atrophy may be suggestive of a neurologic disorder. In this series, two patients with a femoral osteoid osteoma and one with a tibial osteoid osteoma had been operated on mistakenly for "intervertebral disk." At least four others had symptoms that were at first believed due to protruded disk, and one had been operated on for suspected glomus tumor of soft tissues.

Roentgenologic Features

A variable, sometimes extensive, sclerotic zone ordinarily surrounds the nidus and may mask it, necessitating special roentgenographic techniques for its demonstration. Typically, the nidus appears as a small, relatively radiolucent zone. Sclerosis of the nidus adds to problems in its recognition. Osteoid ostomas without secondary sclerosis may be less dense or more dense than adjacent bone or may be practically invisible. Sometimes the reactive periosteal laminations of new bone can

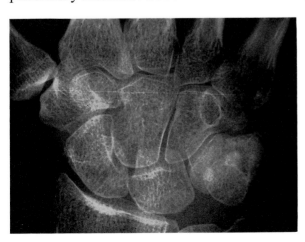

Figure 7-2. Osteoid osteoma of triangular bone. Center of nidus is denser than periphery, and there is only slight sclerosis of adjacent bone. Patient was a nineteen-year-old woman who had had pain for nineteen months. Only other carpal bone involved by osteoid osteoma in this series was the capitate.

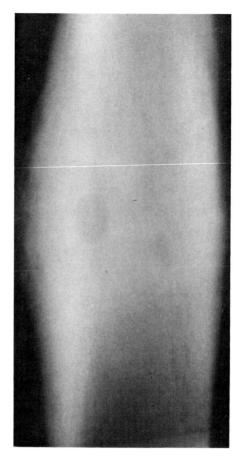

Figure 7-3. Tomogram of multifocal osteoid osteoma depicted grossly in Figure 7-4. Several relatively lucent areas are seen in a large field of sclerotic bone.

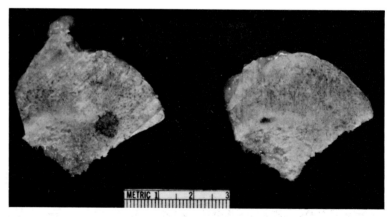

Figure 7-4. Two nidi found in osteoid osteoma illustrated in Figure 7-3. Larger and smaller dark areas represented lesions microscopically. Radiograms of excised specimen had aided in locating them. The thirty-three-year-old man had had pain for eighteen months, and operation elsewhere six months after onset of pain had failed to disclose a lesion.

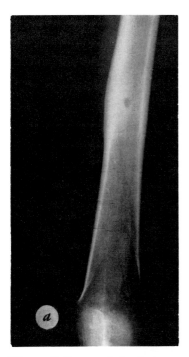
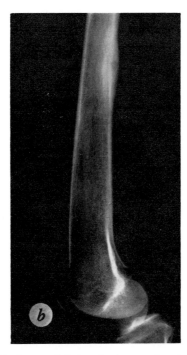
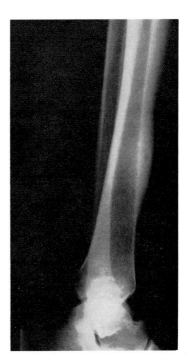

Figure 7-5. *a* and *b*. Anteroposterior and lateral views of osteoid osteoma of femur showing the typically small nidus with considerable sclerosis of adjacent bone. *Right.* Another typical osteoid osteoma in cortical region.

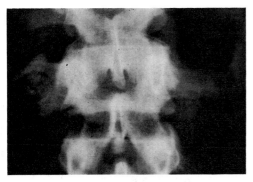

Figure 7-6. Osteoid osteoma of third lumbar transverse process. This lesion contained some of the more loosely arranged trabeculae, as seen in benign osteoblastoma. (Courtesy of Doctor J. E. Holmblad of Schenectady, New York.)

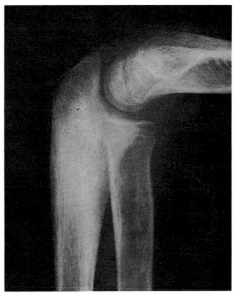

Figure 7-7. Partly because nidus was not visualized, this osteoid osteoma of ulna, with its diffuse subperiosteal new bone in layers, was mistaken for Ewing's sarcoma before operation.

mimic those of Ewing's tumor. One in this series had been treated by radiation else-where because of such mistaken diagnosis by roentgenogram.

In some cases, the typical clinical symptoms precede the onset of recognizable roentgenographic changes. It should also be emphasized that some osteoid osteomas, especially those in cancellous bone, show little or no perifocal sclerosis. This absence of sclerosis makes the roentgenographic appearance of ordinary osteoid osteoma merge with that of benign osteoblastoma, to be discussed in chapter 8.

Absence of significant sclerosis is usual for those osteoid osteomas near the end of a bone, especially if they abut an articular cartilage, and for those in a superficial subperiosteal location. Tumors near a joint may show osteoporosis only; those near the elbow may be especially difficult to localize.

Previous operation or the presence of a multifocal nidus may obscure details of the lesion. Angiography can help delineate the nidus.

Gross Pathology

Whether the osteoid osteoma is found in relatively nonsclerotic cancellous bone or buried in a large region of cortical sclerosis, the actual nidus, upon exposure, usually stands out as a discrete round or oval mass of tissue. It is ordinarily redder than the surrounding bone and can be lifted from its bed. The nidus itself varies in consistency from soft and granular to densely sclerotic, but sclerosis does not correlate with duration of symptoms. Sclerosis, when present, is usually most pronounced in the central portion of the nidus. Osteoid osteoma has, as previously noted, a peculiarly limited growth potential, which is an unusual feature of true neoplasms. Even when symptoms have been present several years, the nidus rarely exceeds 1 cm in greatest dimension. If the tumor proper is 2 cm or more in diameter, the general characteristics tend to overlap those of benign osteoblastoma.

When the sclerotic zone including the nidus is chiseled indiscriminately from an affected bone, it is difficult or impossible for the pathologist to find the all-important central mass of tumor tissue, without which the diagnosis cannot be established. It is important, therefore, that the surgeon remove the nidus intact for satisfactory pathologic appraisal. If the tumor is identified as such and is demonstrated to be completely removed, both the diagnosis and prognosis are established.

Radiographic guidance may help in locating the nidus in the excised specimen. The relatively rare multifocal nidus that may be present, especially after previous unsuccessful surgery, may be particularly difficult to localize.

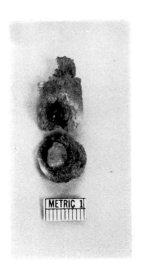
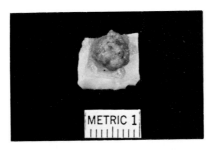
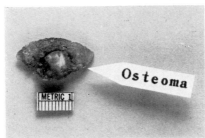
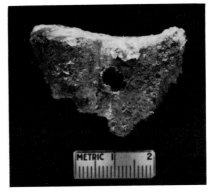

Figure 7-8. *Left.* Osteoid osteoma removed en bloc from neck of femur of twenty-one-year-old man who had had hip pain for one year. Photomicrographs of this lesion are shown in Figures 7-12 and 7-15.

Figure 7-9. *Top middle.* Nidus and whiter shell of bone. Lesion excised from near distal end of femur of fifteen-year-old boy.

Figure 7-10. *Bottom middle.* Typical osteoid osteoma from unusual site, the mandible. This occurred in twenty-six-year-old woman whose chief complaint was jaw pain.

Figure 7-11. *Right.* Red and granular osteoid osteoma, with very thin sclerotic rim, excised from os calcis of seven-year-old girl.

Histopathology

Microscopic examination reveals a distinct demarcation between the nidus and the surrounding bone. The surrounding bone may be densely sclerotic but otherwise shows no typical features.

The nidus itself consists of an interlacing network of osteoid trabeculae in which there is a variable amount of mineralization. The trabeculae are usually thin and arranged in a meaningless tangle that shows numerous anastomoses. The central part of the nidus ordinarily is the site of the most mineralization and may be converted into atypical bone. Within the trabecular framework, instead of bone marrow elements, there is a more or less vascular, fibrous connective tissue that contains variable numbers of benign giant cells. The osteoblasts that mantle the osteoid trabeculae in the zones of proliferation are too well differentiated to make one consider osteosarcoma except in rare instances; in these cases, the total pattern of osteoid osteoma including the small size of the nidus indicates the benign nature of the cells. The size of the trabeculae of these lesions varies from extremely small to rather broad bone beams. Cement lines may be prominent in the larger trabeculae. Cartilage is not present in this tumor.

Benign osteoblastoma typically contains broader and longer osteoid trabeculae. Further, it is, on the average, more vascular than is the ordinary osteoid osteoma.

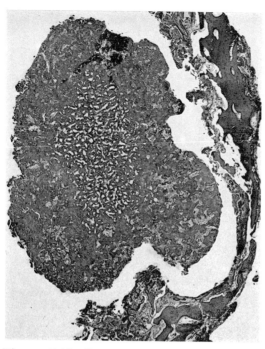

Figure 7-12. Section of entire osteoid osteoma shown in Figure 7-8. Tumor was covered by only thin rim of attenuated cortex. Lesion was in femoral neck of twenty-one-year-old man. (×12)

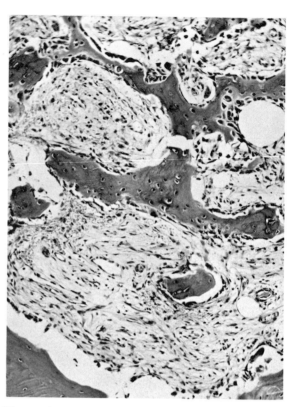

Figure 7-13. Osteoid osteoma with loosely arranged trabeculae. Adjacent bone is seen at bottom. (×160)

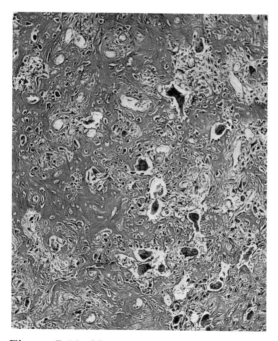

Figure 7-14. Numerous benign giant cells in typical ramifying trabeculae of slightly calcified osteoid osteoma. (×110)

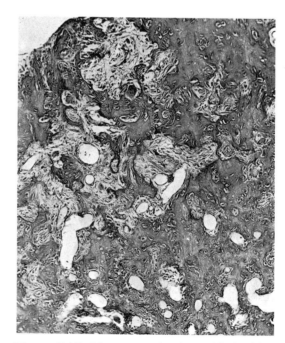

Figure 7-15. More completely ossified nidus with vascularity still prominent. (×90) This is from gross lesion seen in Figure 7-8 (left).

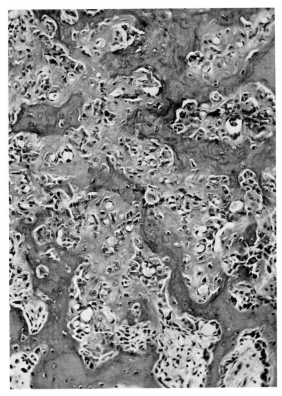

Figure 7-16. Osteoid osteoma of femoral neck. Some osteoblasts have prominent nuclei. Pagetoid seams are present in more mineralized trabeculae. Matrix of varied degrees of calcification is present. (×160)

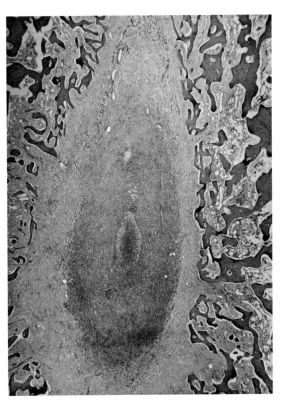

Figure 7-17. Rarefied area containing mainly plasma cells and lymphocytes. Surrounding bone is sclerotic. This is a "Brodie's" abscess, radiographically mimicking osteoid osteoma. (×16) (Case contributed by Doctor Edwin Pontius of Indianapolis, Indiana.)

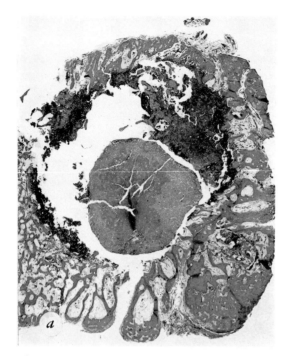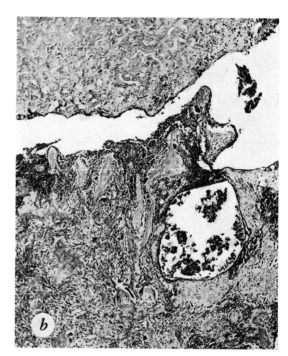

Figure 7-18. *a*. Cross-section of entire triangular bone illustrated in Figure 7-2. Surrounding the somewhat eccentric dense nidus is lesional tissue that is more vascular. (×7) *b*. Higher magnification of the same lesion to show dense, ordinary nidus of osteoid osteoma above and looser tissue like that of osteoblastoma below. Also present are large blood channels reminiscent of aneurysmal bone cyst. (×50)

Unfortunately, there is no clear line of distinction between these two tumors, and occasional borderline lesions might well be classed in either group. Careful review of the pertinent literature discloses that this is true, and the tumor illustrated in Figure 7-18 is a good example.

The bone adjacent to the nidus may contain scattered lymphocytes and plasma cells. Nearby synovium sometimes is thickened and shows a prominent infiltration, sometimes like that of rheumatoid synovitis, of similar chronic inflammatory elements.

Treatment

The treatment is complete surgical removal of the nidus. This is best accomplished by en bloc excision of it and some surrounding bone.

Roentgenographic guidance may be necessary at the time of operation. It is not necessary to remove all of the thickened bone around the osteoid osteoma proper, since this zone will resolve spontaneously if the entire nidus is gone.

Prognosis

Complete removal of the focus of tumor tissue results in cure. Incomplete removal of this focus may lead to recurrence of symptoms and the necessity for reoperation. Whether a true osteoid osteoma will resolve without surgical intervention is unknown. The cases in which such a course seems to have occurred have not had pathologic verification of the original diagnosis.

Sometimes the pathologist cannot identify a nidus of osteoid osteoma after thorough study of an excised specimen or of "shavings" from a region that clinically and by roentgenographic study was characteristic of osteoid osteoma. Interestingly, such patients are usually cured by the surgical procedure, which means that the nidus was somehow lost or that osteoid osteoma has a successful mimic. Recurrent symptoms strongly suggest the nidus was not found.

Multifocality of the nidus may explain persistence of symptoms in those with histologic verification of osteoid osteoma at the first operation.

Bibliography

1935 Jaffe, H. L.: "Osteoid Osteoma": A Benign Osteoblastic Tumor Composed of Osteoid and Atypical Bone. *Arch Surg, 31:*709-728.

1940 Jaffe, H. L., and Lichtenstein, L.: Osteoid-osteoma: Further Experience With This Benign Tumor of Bone: With Special Reference to Cases Showing the Lesion in Relation to Shaft Cortices and Commonly Misclassified as Instances of Sclerosing Non-suppurative Osteomyelitis or Cortical-bone Abscess. *J Bone Joint Surg, n.s., 22:*645-682.

1955 Rushton, J. G., Mulder, D. W., and Lipscomb, P. R.: Neurologic Symptoms With Osteoid Osteoma. *Neurology, 5:*794-797.

1956 Flaherty, R. A., Pugh, D. G., and Dockerty, M. B.: Osteoid Osteoma. *Am J Roentgenol, 76:*1041-1051.

1959 Freiberger, R. H., and Lortman, B. S.: Osteoid Osteoma. A Report of 80 Cases. *Am J Roentgenol, 82:*194-205.

1960 Lindbom, A., Lindvall, N., Soderberg, G., and Spjut, H.: Angiography in Osteoid Osteoma. *Acta Radiol, 54:*327-333 (November).

1961 Johnston, A. D.: Clinical Problems in Osteoid Osteoma. Evidence of Osteoclastic Aversion to Osteoid. *Bull Hosp Joint Dis, 23:*80-94.

1964 Fowles, S. J.: Osteoid Osteoma. *Br J Radiol, 37:*245-252.

1970 Giustra, P. E., and Freiberger, R. H.: Severe Growth Disturbance With Osteoid Osteoma: A Report of Two Cases Involving the Femoral Neck. *Radiology, 96:*285-288 (August).

1970 Lawrie, T. R., Aterman, K., and Sinclair, A. M.: Painless Osteoid Osteoma: A Report of Two Cases. *J Bone Joint Surg, 52A:*1357-1363 (October).

1970 Schulman, L., and Dorfman, H. D.: Nerve Fibers in Osteoid Osteoma. *J Bone Joint Surg, 52A:*1351-1356 (October).

1972 Mazabraud, A.: Remarques à propos de l'Ostéome-Ostéoïde et de l'Ostéoblastome. *Ann Anat Pathol (Paris), 17:*177-185 (April-June).

1973 Snarr, J. W., Abell, M. R., and Martel, W.: Lymphofollicular Synovitis With Osteoid Osteoma. *Radiology, 106:*557-560 (March).

1974 Corbett, J. M., Wilde, A. H., McCormack, L. J., and Evarts, C. M.: Intra-articular Osteoid Osteoma: A Diagnostic Problem. *Clin Orthop, 98:*225-230 (January-February).

1974 Greenspan, A., Elguezabel, A., and Bryk, D.: Multifocal Osteoid Osteoma: A Case Report and Review of the Literature. *Am J Roentgenol, 121:*103-106 (May).

1975 Sim, F. H., Dahlin, D. C., and Beabout, J. W.: Osteoid-Osteoma: Diagnostic Problems. *J Bone Joint Surg, 57:*154-159 (March).

1975 Keim, H. A., and Reina, E. G.: Osteoid-Osteoma as a Cause of Scoliosis. *J Bone Joint Surg, 57A:*159-163 (March).

1975 O'Hara, J. P. III, Tegtmeyer, C., Sweet, D. E., and McCue, F. C.: Angiography in the Diagnosis of Osteoid-Osteoma of the Hand. *J Bone Joint Surg, 57A:*163-166 (March).

1975 Norman, A., and Dorfman, H. D.: Osteoid-Osteoma Inducing Pronounced Overgrowth and Deformity of Bone. *Clin Orthop, 110:*233-238 (July-August).

Chapter 8

Benign Osteoblastoma (Giant Osteoid Osteoma)

THE LITERATURE concerning this rare, benign tumor is especially confusing. Its osteoblastic nature results in zones often quite like those of an osteoid osteoma, producing a histologic kinship that can scarcely be ignored. Benign osteoblastoma differs, however, in not sharing the markedly limited growth potential of the average osteoid osteoma. Further, it frequently lacks the characteristic pain and the halo of sclerotic bone of the latter tumor. Even so, one occasionally encounters a lesion whose composite features make it fall midway between the two lesions under discussion. McLeod and coworkers resolved this problem by arbitrarily regarding equivocal lesions as osteoblastoma when the lesion was more than 1.5 cm in diameter.

In the literature on neoplasms of the vertebral column, benign osteoblastoma is found under various diagnoses, including giant cell tumor, osteoid osteoma, osteogenic (or ossifying) fibroma, and sarcoma. An important reason for recognizing this entity is that it has commonly been mistaken for the much more aggressive, genuine giant cell tumor or even for sarcoma.

One may logically question whether benign osteoblastoma is correctly classed with true neoplasms since some of them regress or become arrested after incomplete surgical removal. Fields within some of these tumors resemble portions of aneurysmal bone cysts. This, coupled with a pronounced clinical similarity, suggests that both of these processes may be but different manifestations of a reaction to some as yet unknown agent.

The term "giant osteoid osteoma," introduced several years ago, was an attempt to recognize the pathologic similarity of this lesion to osteoid osteoma, at the same time indicating a difference, especially with respect to the size of the average tumor. Benign osteoblastoma nevertheless has become the most widely accepted designation for this tumor.

The problem is compounded by several features. Rarely, a lesion that is seemingly correctly called "osteoblastoma" develops into an osteosarcoma. Multifocality occurs in some tumors with variable amounts of reactive bone separating the zones of lesion; a large tumorous mass may result. These apparently separate zones of the lesion may actually represent wormlike permeation by a single tumor. Bizarre but apparently degenerating nuclei are seen in a very few benign osteoblastomas, and these may be mistaken for osteosarcoma.

The lesion called "cementoblastoma" at or around the root of a tooth is very similar to and has been included with osteoblastomas in this series.

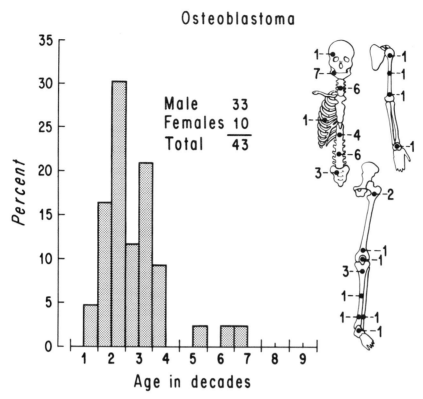

Figure 8-1. Skeletal, age, and sex distribution of benign osteoblastomas.

Incidence

This tumor accounted for less than 1 percent of the primary tumors of bone in the present series, but it is being diagnosed somewhat more frequently in recent years.

Sex

The marked predilection for males observed in the series has been noted in several other studies.

Age

The younger age-group is predominantly affected, and all but seven lesions in this series were in patients in the first three decades of life.

Localization

Benign osteoblastoma, in contrast to most other neoplasms of bone, manifests a distinct predilection for the vertebral column. Nineteen in this series affected the spinal column and sacrum. The remainder were in the long bones, except for one tumor of the patella, one in the talus, one in a carpal navicular, seven in the mandible (several of these might be called "cementoblastoma"), and one in the temporal bone. Other sites that have been reported involved include rib, scapula, innominate bone, maxilla, and the region of the base of the skull.

Symptoms

Pain, usually at the site of the tumor, is the cardinal symptom. In many instances, the pain is due to pressure on adjacent structures, notably the spinal cord or the emerging nerves, and it appears to lack the intrinsic severity of that caused by ordinary osteoid osteoma. Involvement of the spinal cord or nerves may result in weakness or even paraplegia. The pain may be referred to a site distant from the tumor. The lesion develops slowly; the average duration of pain in our original series was 25.8 months before the patient sought medical advice. If the affected bone is not covered by a thick layer of soft tissue, local swelling may be evident. Those patients with a lesion in the lower extremity may experience a limp. Patients with spinal tumors frequently had scoliosis, muscle spasm, and various neurologic symptoms.

Physical Findings

Physical examination is of little value in the definitive diagnosis of this lesion, but it may reveal a tender mass at the site of the tumor. Atrophy of the adjacent muscles is sometimes seen. Variable neurologic deficits may be noted, depending upon the degree of involvement of the spinal cord or emerging nerves.

Roentgenologic Features

The roentgenologic features are not as characteristic in this tumor as they are in ordinary osteoid osteoma. In some cases, one observes only bone destruction that is fairly well circumscribed which does not always suggest that the process is benign. In some instances, especially in the long bones, the lesional site is surrounded by a dense sclerotic zone similar to that seen in ordinary osteoid osteoma. The main difference from ordinary osteoid osteoma is that the region of the central nidus is almost always many times larger in these cases. Many benign osteoblastomas arise in bones that are predominantly cancellous, and this may account for the common absence of perifocal sclerosis. Occasionally, the tumor is surrounded by a thin layer of bone beneath an expanded periosteum, giving an appearance similar to that of aneurysmal bone cyst; some of Lichtenstein's benign osteoblastomas showed this feature. In older or previously treated lesions, ossification of tumor tissue may result in enough radiopacity to cause the roentgenologist to consider that the tumor is an osteoma. It may resemble chronic osteomyelitis.

McLeod and coworkers found that 76 percent of lesions in long bones were diaphyseal lesions. Nearly 40 percent contained mineral densities within the lesion. Nearly all of the appendicular tumors were associated with periosteal new bone formation. Their tumors varied in size and were up to 10 cm in greatest dimension.

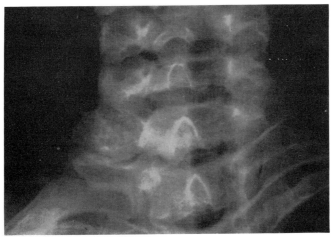

Figure 8-2. Example of tumor of this type. It has produced some expansion of the right transverse process of the seventh cervical vertebra. Excised specimen was 2 cm in diameter.

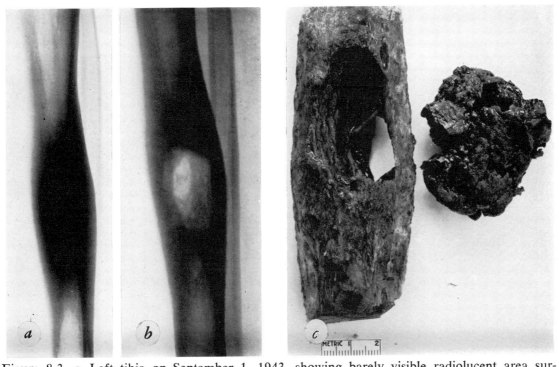

Figure 8-3. *a.* Left tibia on September 1, 1943, showing barely visible radiolucent area surrounded by dense sclerotic bone. *b.* Same lesion on January 17, 1946, after three drilling operations elsewhere, each of which brought temporary relief. *c.* Excised tumor and anterior half of tibia. Tumor showed classic features of benign osteoblastoma. (Reproduced with permission from: Dockerty, M. B., Ghormley, R. K., and Jackson, A. E.: *Ann Surg, 133:*77-89, 1951.)

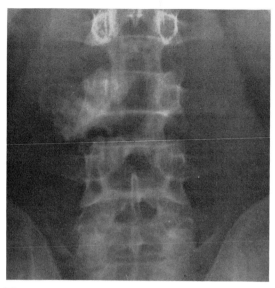

Figure 8-4. Completely lytic benign osteoblastoma 2.5 cm in diameter was removed eight years previously from site of this now sclerotic and asymptomatic tumor.

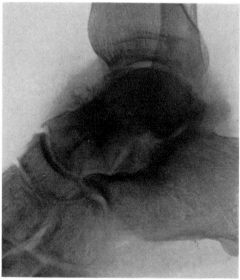

Figure 8-5. The 32 g tumor shown in Figure 8-9 was removed from this talus. (Reproduced with permission from: Dahlin, D. C., and Johnson, E. W., Jr.: *J Bone Joint Surg, 36A*:559-572, 1954.)

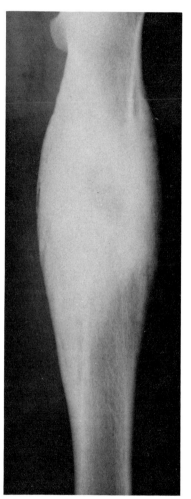

Figure 8-6. Osteoblastoma in nineteen-year-old man who had had pain for four-and-one-half years. Site had been "scraped out" five months prior to this roentgenogram. Central nidus was 2 cm in diameter.

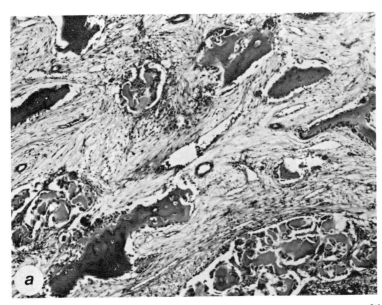

Figure 8-7. Multifocal osteoblastoma in seventeen-year-old man. *a.* Small islands of benign tumor are separated by broader trabeculae of bone and chronic inflammatory fibrous tissue. (×100) *b.* Same lesion shown in *a.* Bulk of this juxta-cortical mass is non-neoplastic. (Reproduced with permission from: McLeod, R. A., Dahlin, D. C., and Beabout, J. W.: *Am J Roentgenol, 126:*321-335, 1976.)

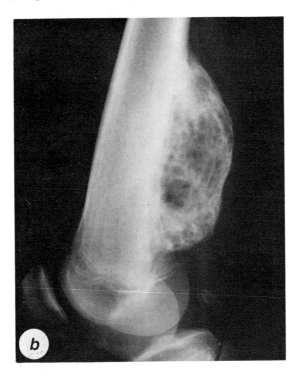

Gross Pathology

The gross pathologic features of this tumor are relatively characteristic. Entire gross specimens are rarely observed because the average lesion is removed by curettement. These tumors are, however, reasonably well circumscribed. The tumor tissue is hemorrhagic, granular, and friable, owing to its vascularity and its osteoid component, which shows variable calcification. In some of the older lesions, the consistency resembles that of cancellous bone, and decalcification is necessary before microscopic sections can be made. If the tumor bulges from and distorts the contour of the affected bone, its margins are sharply defined. Follow-up studies of some individual cases strongly suggest that young lesions are distinctly lytic, but that they may undergo progressive ossification.

As previously indicated, the bone adjacent to benign osteoblastoma often is not sclerosed. Around the tumor in some cases, there is a thin sclerotic rim, and around the tumor proper in others, especially those in the long bones of the extremities, there may be a zone of increased density that is as prominent as that associated with ordinary osteoid osteoma.

Reported tumors have varied up to 10 cm in greatest diameter. Sometimes the vascularity of osteoblastoma is such that hemostasis may be a problem for the surgeon.

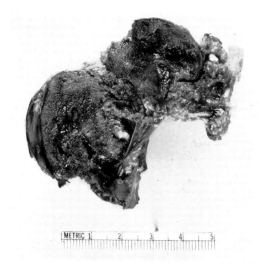

Figure 8-8. Cut surface of benign osteoblastoma removed from sacrum of twenty-two-year-old man who had had local pain for three years. Lesion was 4 by 3.5 by 3 cm. This predominantly lytic lesion involved left lower part of sacrum.

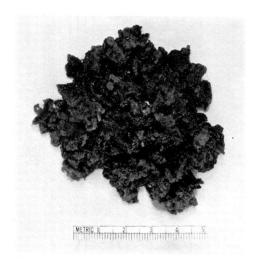

Figure 8-9. Curetted fragments of tumor for which the roentgenogram is illustrated in Figure 8-5. (Reproduced with permission from: Dahlin, D. C., and Johnson, E. W., Jr.: *J Bone Joint Surg, 36A*:559-572, 1954.)

Histopathology

Osteoblasts with regularly shaped nuclei containing little chromatin and often having fairly abundant cytoplasm produce interlacing trabeculae or discrete small islands of osteoid or bone.

The microscopic features of benign osteoblastoma are extremely variable and account for the confusion in the literature regarding this tumor. In what are apparently early lesions, one observes actively proliferating connective tissue that may show only slight osteoid formation and numerous giant cells. In older lesions, considerable ossification may be present. This variety accounts for the inclusion of cases of this type among the giant cell tumors, osteogenic fibromas, osteoid osteomas, and osteomas. In less mature lesions, mitotic figures are found in the actively proliferating cells, some of which may be obviously osteoblastic; hence the occasional confusion of this benign process with osteosarcoma. Most of the benign osteoblastomas contain numerous blood vessels, mainly of dilated capillary type, a feature that poses the question of vascular origin for this tumor.

Some of the lesions under discussion exhibit features of aneurysmal bone cyst. I have observed tumors in which some of the histologic sections were identical with those from an aneurysmal bone cyst, whereas other sections were typical of benign osteoblastoma. This reinforces the interesting speculation as to whether both of these two rather poorly understood processes are related, a possibility that is enhanced by the similar patient age and skeletal distribution of these two tumors and their similar response to therapy.

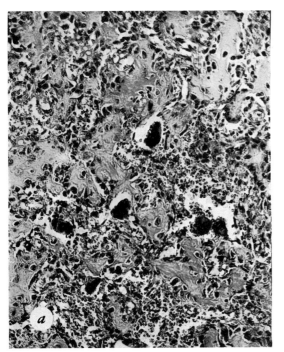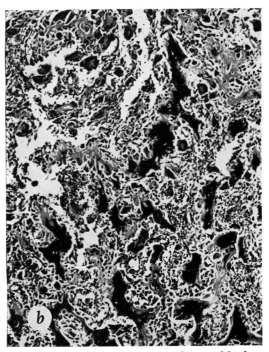

Figure 8-10. *a.* Benign osteoblastoma illustrated in Figure 8-9. Trabeculae of osteoid show no calcification in this area. Vascularity and benign giant cells are prominent. (×170) *b.* Black areas indicate calcification of trabeculae. Giant cells are present. (×100) (Reproduced with permission from: Dahlin, D. C., and Johnson, E. W., Jr.: *J Bone Joint Surg, 36A:*559-572, 1954.)

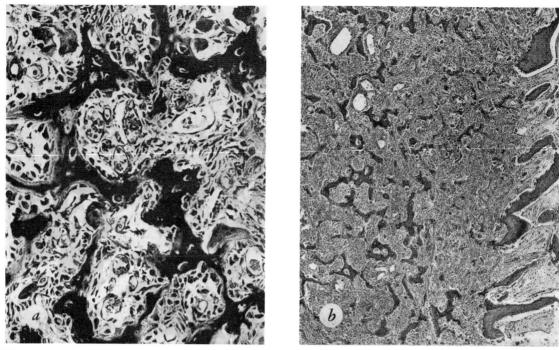

Figure 8-11. *a.* Benign osteoblastoma with partially ossified trabeculae and prominent vascularity. (×200) *b.* Vertebral tumor in this group, showing distinct demarcation from expanded and attenuated cortex on the right. (×35) (Reproduced with permission from: Dahlin, D. C., and Johnson, E. W., Jr.: *J Bone Joint Surg, 36A:559-572, 1954.*)

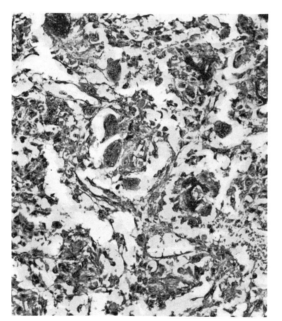

Figure 8-12. Extremely cellular benign osteoblastoma, presumably an early lesion. This type is likely to be mistaken for sarcoma. There is little osteoid production. (×175)

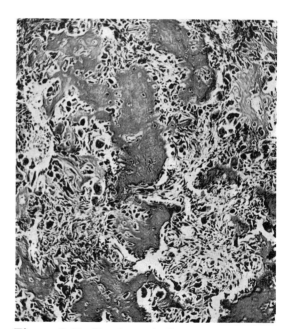

Figure 8-13. Pertinent lesion involving vertebra and showing, in this area, rather dense sclerosis. Giant cells are still abundant. (×110)

Multifocal osteoblastoma does not differ from the unifocal form except that non-neoplastic trabeculae separate the islands of tumor. The pseudomalignant tumors that microscopically contain bizarre but apparently degenerating cells are exceedingly rare and typically appear roentgenographically to be benign.

The lesion called "cementoblastoma" appears to be identical to some osteoblastomas not in the jaws. It tends to show nearly parallel peripheral trabeculae extending outward and discretely separated from adjacent tissue.

The malignant osteoblasts of some osteosarcomas are differentiated from the osteoblasts of osteoblastoma only with difficulty. The current concept of malignant osteoblastoma introduces a debatable and certainly controversial as well as difficult group of tumors.

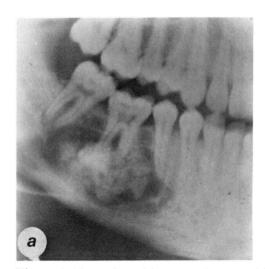
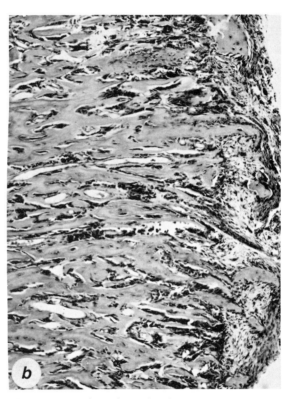

Figure 8-14. *a.* Osteoblastoma (cementoblastoma) at root of molar of thirteen-year-old girl. *b.* Such lesions often produce pain. Periphery of so-called cementoblastoma with extending rather fine trabeculae of new bone. Lesion is circumscribed by non-neoplastic fibrous tissue. (×100) Similiarity of lesions like this at and around roots of teeth to osteoblastomas in other parts of skeleton indicate their kinship to general groups of osteoblastomas. (Reproduced with permission from: McLeod, R. A., Dahlin, D. C., and Beabout, J. W.: *Am J Roentgenol, 126:*321-335, 1976.)

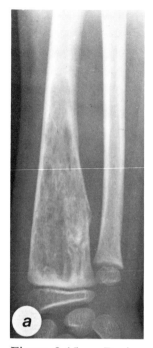
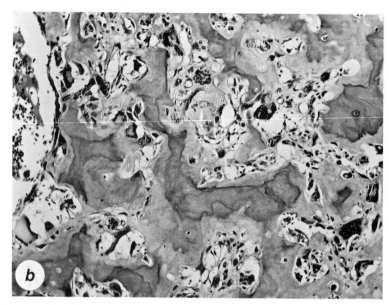

Figure 8-15. *a.* Benign osteoblastoma in nine-year-old boy with mistaken histologic diagnosis of osteosarcoma. Operation was necessary partly because of pathologic fracture. After conservative treatment, persistence of cystlike defects was seen roentgenographically, but patient was well more than five years after onset of symptoms. (Case contributed by Doctor F. Ricciarelli of Dubuque, Iowa.) *b.* This unusual osteoblastoma contained numerous large irregular hyperchromatic nuclei, as did radial lesion shown in *b.* These bizarre nuclei are probably degenerative like those in many benign neurilemmomas. Paucity of mitotic figures and benign appearance by roentgenogram aid in avoiding the pitfall of overdiagnosis of such tumors. (×160) (Reproduced by permission from: McLeod, R. A., Dahlin, D. C., and Beabout, J. W.: *Am J Roentgenol, 126:*321-335, 1976.)

Treatment

The benign nature of benign osteoblastoma dictates that conservative surgical treatment be used. This will usually entail removal of the entire lesion, or as much of it as possible, by curettement, with bone grafting of the defect if indicated. It is doubtful whether radiation therapy is helpful. In some of the cases in the present series, incomplete surgical removal of the lesional part has resulted in cure. The clinical course in the present cases suggests that until surgical intervention has been undertaken, the tumefaction usually increases; however, in a fourteen-year-old girl with an osteoblastoma involving the right half of the sacrum, no treatment was employed after biopsy, and she was asymptomatic fifteen years later. The tumor was not surgically accessible, and it was considered unwise to irradiate her pelvic region. Aegerter and Kirkpatrick described a very similar case.

Prognosis

Perhaps the main reason for recognizing this rare pathologic entity is that it is not malignant, and, as indicated, the response to treatment is nearly always good. Occasional tumors of this type that are incompletely removed will require more than one surgical procedure. The major problem likely to be encountered is that of involvement of the spinal column by a lesion; when this occurs, one must direct therapy to preservation of the integrity of the spinal cord and the emerging nerve roots.

Malignant change develops in a very few lesions thought to be correctly diagnosed as benign osteoblastomas. In rare cases with "borderline" malignancy, nearby soft tissue recurrence has developed.

The potential hazard of radiation therapy is indicated by one case in this series. A fatal fibrosarcoma developed in the same region ten years after roentgen therapy for osteoblastoma of the fifth cervical vertebra.

The diagnosis of benign osteoblastoma, despite the problems and exceptions presented, is a useful designation, and it indicates that the lesion can nearly always be cured by a relatively conservative surgical procedure.

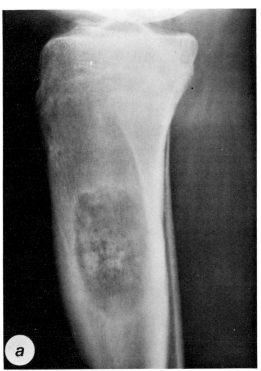 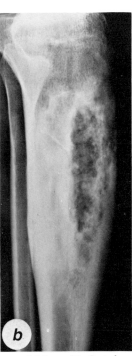

Figure 8-16. *a.* Benign osteoblastoma in sixteen-year-old boy in October 1968, when biopsy yielded material in Figure 8-17*a*. *b*. Recurrent lesion in same case. This roentgenogram taken February 17, 1972, was judged to show increased size of tumor and cortical perforation. Despite amputation for this lesion, pulmonary metastasis of osteosarcoma had developed by December 1973. (Reproduced with permission from: McLeod, R. A., Dahlin, D. C., and Beabout, J. W.: *Am J Roentgenol, 126:*321-335, 1976.)

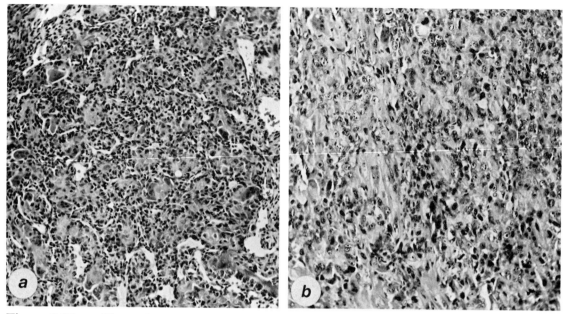

Figure 8-17. *a.* Tissue from October 1968 curettage of lesion shown in Figure 8-16*a.* It is characteristic of benign osteoblastoma. (×160) *b.* Tissue in March 1972 showing nuclear pleomorphism, anisocytosis, and osteoid production by malignant cells. (×160) (Reproduced with permission from: McLeod, R. A., Dahlin, D. C., and Beabout, J. W.: *Am J Roentgenol, 126:*321-335, 1976.)

Bibliography

1924 Lewis, D.: Primary Giant Cell Tumors of the Vertebrae: Analysis of a Group of Cases, With Report of Case in Which Patient Is Well Two Years and Nine Months After Operation. *JAMA, 83:*1224-1229.

1954 Dahlin, D. C., and Johnson, E. W., Jr.: Giant Osteoid Osteoma. *J Bone Joint Surg, 36A:*559-572.

1956 Jaffe, H. L.: Benign Osteoblastoma. *Bull Hosp Joint Dis, 17:*141-151.

1963 Salzer, M., and Salzer-Kuntschik, M.: Das Benigne Osteoblastom. *Langenbecks Arch Klin Chir, 302:*755-778.

1963 Marcove, R. C., and Alpert, M.: A Pathologic Study of Benign Osteoblastoma. *Clin Orthop, 30:*175-181.

1964 Lichtenstein, L., and Sawyer, W. R.: Benign Osteoblastoma. Further Observations and Report of Twenty Additional Cases. *J Bone Joint Surg, 46A:*755-765.

1967 Mayer, L.: Malignant Degeneration of So-Called Benign Osteoblastoma. *Bull Hosp Joint Dis, 28:*4-13 (April).

1968 Byers, P. D.: Solitary Benign Osteoblastomic Lesions of Bone: Osteoid Osteoma and Benign Osteoblastoma. *Cancer, 22:*43-57 (July).

1970 Schajowicz, F., and Lemos, C.: Osteoid Osteoma and Osteoblastoma: Closely Related Entities of Osteoblastic Derivation. *Acta Orthop Scand, 41:*272-291.

1974 Abrams, A. M., Kirby, J. W., and Melrose, R. J.: Cementoblastoma: A Clinical-Pathologic Study of Seven New Cases. *Oral Surg, 38:*394-403 (September).

1974 Yip, W.-K., and Lee, H. T. L.: Benign Osteoblastoma of the Maxilla. *Oral Surg, 38:*259-263 (August).

1975 Stutch, R.: Osteoblastoma—A Benign Entity? *Orthop Rev, 4:*27-33 (October).

1976 Mirra, J. M., Kendrick, R. A., and Kendrick, R. E.: Pseudomalignant Osteoblastoma Versus Arrested Osteosarcoma: A Case Report. *Cancer, 37:*2005-2014 (April).

1976 McLeod, R. A., Dahlin, D. C., and Beabout, J. W.: The Spectrum of Osteoblastoma. *Am J Roentgenol, 126:*321-335 (February).

1976 Schajowicz, F., and Lemos, D.: Malignant Osteoblastoma. *J Bone Joint Surg, 58B:*202-211 (May).

Chapter 9

Giant Cell Tumor (Osteoclastoma)

GIANT CELL TUMOR of bone is a distinctive neoplasm of poorly differentiated cells. The multinucleated giant cells apparently result from fusion of the proliferating mononuclear cells, and although they are a constant and prominent part of these tumors, they are likely of less significance than are the mononuclear cells. In fact, these osteoclastlike giant cells, with or without minor modifications, occur in a host of pathologic conditions of bone. The ubiquitous giant cell accounts for the confusion one finds in the older and in some of the recent literature on giant cell tumors. Authors have included conditions such as nonosteogenic fibroma, benign chondroblastoma, chondromyxoid fibroma, unicameral bone cysts with a cellular lining, giant cell reparative granuloma (epulis), aneurysmal bone cyst, hyperparathyroidism, giant-cell-containing osteosarcoma, and other entities in the general category of giant cell tumor. Inclusion of these "variants" with their widely divergent biologic behavior has greatly delayed understanding of the clinical features and response to treatment of true giant cell tumor. The exact cell of origin of this neoplasm is unknown.

In addition to the recognized conditions that have been confused with giant cell tumor, one occasionally encounters a benign, often fibrogenic, rarefying process that does not fit well into any of the known categories. These rare lesions which contain giant cells and variable amounts of proliferative new bone are likely to be found in the vertebrae or small bones of the hands and feet. They probably represent a peculiar reaction in bone and, fortunately, have a good prognosis.

Malignant giant cell tumor is the subject of Chapter 22. This malignant tumor cannot be diagnosed with assurance unless evidence of ordinary benign giant cell tumor exists within the lesion or has been demonstrated previously at the same site. If the stromal cells of a tumor that is rich in benign giant cells are malignant throughout, with features of either osteo- or fibrosarcoma, the tumor probably bears no relationship to giant cell tumor. The benign giant cells are but an incidental and confusing component. The clinical correlative studies by Troup and coworkers in 1960 have fortified this concept.

To further confuse the issue, giant cell tumor can produce metastasis even though cytologically benign. This occurrence is very rare, and only two such cases were found in the present series of 264 patients with giant cell tumors.

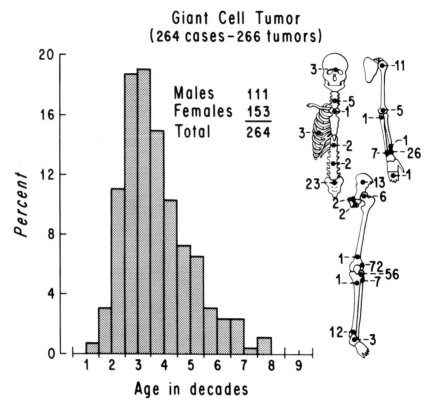

Figure 9-1. Skeletal, age, and sex distribution of giant cell tumors.

Incidence

The 264 cases in this series represented 4.2 percent of the total and 18.2 percent of the benign tumors.

Sex

In many of the recorded series, females have predominated. The ratio in the present series was 153 females to 111 males. This 57.9 percent incidence of females in the total group contrasts with the 74 percent incidence of females in the thirty-nine patients who were less than twenty years old. There is a preponderance of males in most series of other bone tumors.

Age

When the "variants" of giant cell tumor were excluded, 85 percent of the neoplasms occurred in patients beyond the age of nineteen years, with the peak incidence in the third decade of life. Most of those in the second decade were nearly twenty years of age. Eight were in the age-group of ten years through fourteen years. Two patients were only eight years old. The presence of many young persons in any series of giant cell tumors brings up the likelihood that "variants" are included.

Localization

Most giant cell tumors are found in the epiphyses of the long bones. More than half of the lesions in the present series occurred about the knee. The sphenoid and ribs accounted for three each, and the vertebrae above the sacrum for nine. This series reemphasizes that "variants" are more common than giant cell tumors in vertebrae above the sacrum. Seventeen lesions occurred in the pelvic bones and twenty-three in the sacrum. Three arose in tarsal bones, one in a phalanx, and one in the manubrium. It was not possible to segregate any unequivocal giant cell tumors from the numerous giant cell reparative lesions of jawbones.

Fourteen giant cell tumors of the sphenoid and eleven in the temporal bone were recorded to 1974. Especially in the latter area, variants such as giant cell reparative granuloma and even benign chondroblastoma must be considered.

Two patients in this series had two tumors each. Multiple tumors containing benign giant cells strongly suggest that the patient has another disease, such as a metabolic problem, rather than giant cell tumor.

A few giant cell tumors did not extend completely to the articular cartilage, although most of them did. In three instances, the tumors were completely metaphyseal.

Symptoms

Pain of variable severity is almost always the predominating symptom. More than three fourths of the patients in the present series had noted swelling in the affected region. Less common symptoms included weakness, limitation of motion of a joint, and signs of pathologic fracture.

Physical Findings

A hard, sometimes crepitant and sometimes painful mass is found in more than 80 percent of patients. There may be atrophy of muscles due to disuse, effusion into the adjacent joint, or local heat and redness.

Roentgenologic Features

According to Gee and Pugh, 1958, these features may be summarized as those of an expanding zone of radiolucency situated eccentrically in the end of a long bone of an adult. Such an appearance is neither specific for giant cell tumor nor produced by all such tumors. The roentgenographic appearance may have been altered by pathologic fracture or by previous therapy. The margin between tumor and normal bone is characterized by gradual alteration of density, and there is no reactive sclerosis at this junction in untreated tumors. Gee and Pugh were unable, after studying the available original roentgenograms of sixty-two of the patients in the present series, to correlate the roentgenographic features with the subsequent behavior of the tumors. A tumor not in the end of a tubular bone lacks specific roentgenographic signs.

Metaphyseal lesions are almost certainly not giant cell tumors, but three of the tumors in this series spared the epiphysis, and a very few similar cases have been reported.

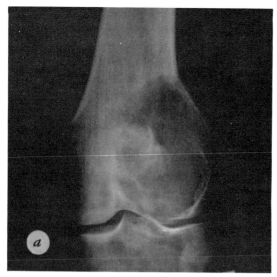 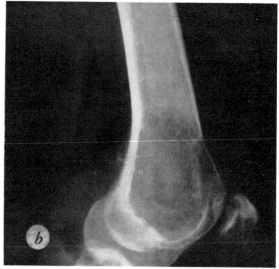

Figure 9-2, *a*. Giant cell tumor of lower end of femur of twenty-one-year-old woman who had noted local pain for nine months. *b*. Lateral view of same tumor.

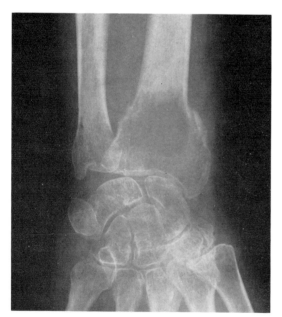 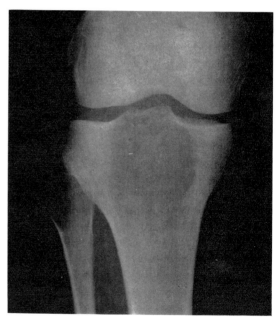

Figure 9-3. Giant cell tumor affecting sixty-one-year-old woman who had had local pain for 2.5 months.

Figure 9-4. Poorly defined giant cell tumor in thirty-two-year-old woman who had noted local pain for two months.

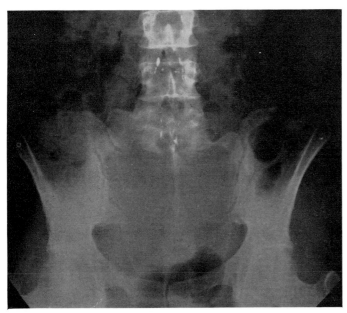

Figure 9-5. Extensive sacral destruction by giant cell tumor in thirty-six-year-old woman who had had low-back pain for nine months.

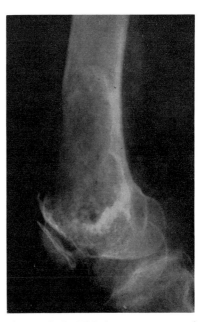

Figure 9-6. Third recurrence of benign giant cell tumor.

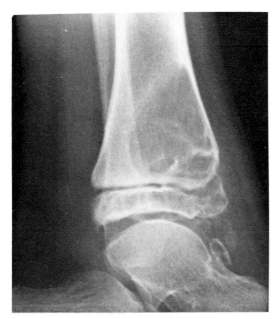

Figure 9-7. Giant cell tumor in epiphysis and in adjacent metaphysis in eight-year-old girl. Masses of tumor with ossified shells are in ankle joint.

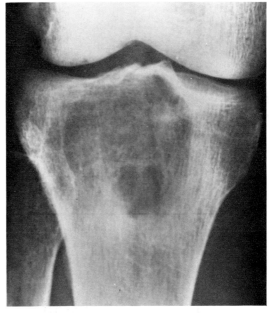

Figure 9-8. Metastatic adenoacanthoma resembling giant cell tumor in sixty-three-year-old woman. (Case contributed by Doctor M. Indech of Kitchener, Ontario, Canada.)

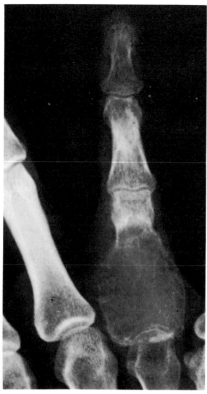

Figure 9-9. Giant cell tumor in unusual location, the first phalanx of fourth finger. (Case contributed by Doctor Richard Lester of Durham, North Carolina.)

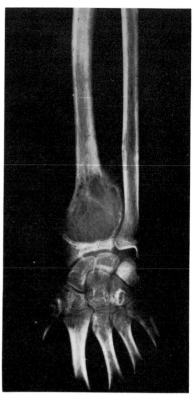

Figure 9-10. One of two metaphyseal giant cell tumors in present series. This occurred in eighteen-year-old man who had noted swelling for three months.

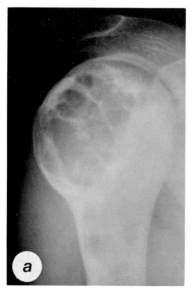

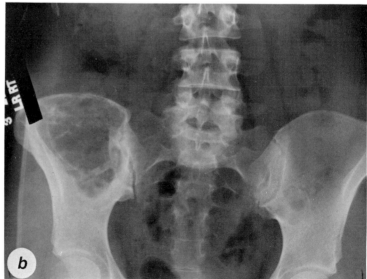

Figure 9-11. *a.* Giant cell tumor in twenty-one-year-old woman. This upper humeral tumor had been treated by curettage and grafting from ilium twenty-one months previously. *b.* At time of humeral recurrent tumor, she had this large second giant cell tumor of ilium. Lesion seemed to be located just posterior to area from which graft had been obtained. (Reproduced with permission from: Dahlin, D. C., Cupps, R. E., and Johnson, E. W., Jr.: *Cancer, 25:*1061-1070, 1970.)

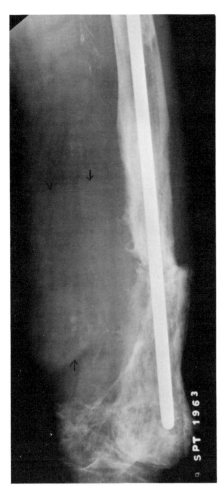

Figure 9-12. Giant cell tumor complicating Paget's disease of femur in eighty-four-year-old man. Note that, as might be expected, neoplasm does not involve the very end of bone. (Case contributed by Doctor R. E. Schulz of Ashland, Ohio.)

Benign giant cell tumors that implant into soft tissues or even when metastatic often produce a slightly ossified periphery.

Giant cell tumor may occur in a lesion of Paget's disease, a rare complication that seems to have a predilection for bones of the skull and face. Only one neoplasm in the present series, an iliac tumor, developed in osteitis deformans.

Other lesions, most notably fibrosarcoma, may produce roentgenologic features like those of giant cell tumor.

Gross Pathology

The tumor tissue is characteristically soft, friable, and gray to red. Firmer portions may be seen as the result of previous fracture, treatment, or degeneration, all of which may cause fibrosis and osteoid production. Small cystic or necrotic portions, sometimes filled with blood, may be present, but these ordinarily constitute an insignificant feature of untreated lesions not modified by previous fracture. This cystification may be sufficiently prominent in recurrent neoplasms to cause them to be confused with aneurysmal bone cysts. The aggressive nature of giant cell tumors accounts for their usually immense size when they have been neglected. Intact gross specimens show variable degrees of expansion of the bone with corresponding attenuation or destruction of the cortex. The remainder of the osseous structure in the region of the tumor is completely replaced. The tumor practically always extends to the articular cartilage, and its boundaries are only moderately well demarcated from adjacent bone and cartilage. Even with very large lesions, the periosteum is rarely breached.

Multicentric giant cell tumors are extremely rare; one patient in this series developed a giant cell tumor of the upper tibia sixteen months after excision of one from her sphenoid. In another patient, a recurrent tumor of the upper end of a humerus developed twenty-one months after curettage and grafting; coincident with the humeral tumor, she had a 9 by 8 by 5 cm giant cell tumor of her right ilium, and the mass seemed to be located posterior to the area from which the graft had been taken.

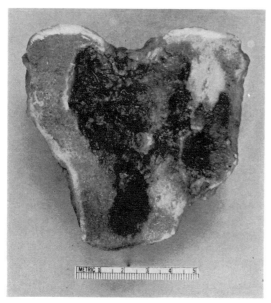

Figure 9-13. Excised giant cell tumor of lower part of femur. Tumor has been modified by two previous operations that included bone grafting, which accounts for white zones.

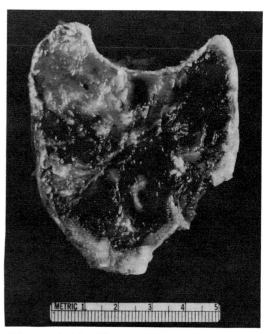

Figure 9-14. Giant cell tumor of distal end of radius. It had produced pain for 1.5 years and had not been treated. Dark zones were brown owing to hemosiderin pigment.

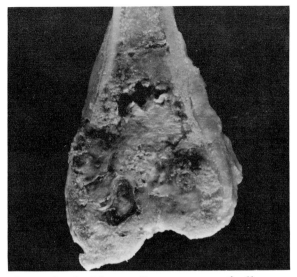

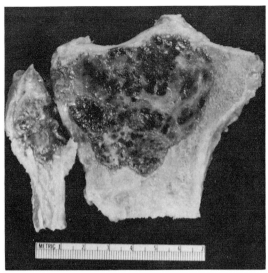

Figure 9-15. Giant cell tumor practically re-placed by grade 3 fibrosarcoma. This occurred fifteen years after curettage, cautery, and graft-ing of benign giant cell tumor, which was then recurrent seven years after similar treatment for primary lesion. Sarcoma produced death with metastasis in ten months despite amputa-tion.

Figure 9-16. Giant cell tumor in sixty-year-old man. This recurrent lesion, fifteen months after curettage and cautery, involved adjacent fibula. It was treated by amputa-tion because of degree of destruction of both bones.

Histopathology

The basic, proliferating cell has one round to oval or even spindle-shaped nu-cleus. In the fields that are diagnostic of true giant cell tumor, these nuclei are sur-rounded by an ill-defined cytoplasmic zone, and no discernible intercellular sub-stance is being produced. Mitotic figures can be found in practically every lesion, and in some, they are numerous. These nuclei lack the hyperchromatism and varia-tion in size and shape characteristic of sarcoma. However, one does occasionally encounter an osteosarcoma with unusually small malignant cells and an abundance of benign giant cells. Such tumors may pose a difficult problem in differentiation from giant cell tumor histologically, but they are nearly always metaphyseal in lo-cation and in a younger age-group. Histochemical and ultrastructural methods for differentiating giant cell tumor from its variants have not been of value, so the pathologist must make the differentiation on the basis of the sometimes subtle cytologic and histologic features correlated with the roentgenographic findings.

Evidence that the giant cells derive from fusion of the mononuclear cells includes the marked similarity of their nuclei. In certain areas, especially after fracture or unsuccessful treatment, some of the proliferating cells show metaplasia to a type capable of producing collagen or even osteoid tissue. Such osteoid and even bone is commonly seen in the periphery of soft-tissue implants or in metastatic deposits of benign giant cell tumor. Cartilaginous differentiation is unusual, and its presence is indicative of benign chondroblastoma, especially if it is disposed in discrete islands. Chondroid foci even indicate the possibility that one is dealing with an osteo-sarcoma. Zones containing numerous foam cells or phagocytized iron pigment apparently result from old hemorrhage or necrosis. Necrotic foci may be present and sometimes extensive. Tiny fragments of tissue containing a few giant cells are inadequate for verification of true giant cell tumor; thus, aspiration biopsy has limited usefulness in the diagnosis of this neoplasm.

A rich scattering of benign giant cells is usually prominent throughout viable zones, but giant cell tumors sometimes contain rather large fields with somewhat spindling mononuclear cells and devoid of multinucleated forms. Blood-filled spaces are sometimes prominent in giant cell tumor, especially after prior treatment or fracture; sometimes even after comparison with the roentgenogram, it may be difficult to differentiate such lesions from aneurysmal bone cyst.

It is not rare to find intravascular tumor at the periphery of giant cell tumor, but this does not seem to correlate with increased risk. When the roentgenographic changes are those of cell tumor, one can allow prominent mitotic activity and even worrisome cytopathology for this benign neoplasm.

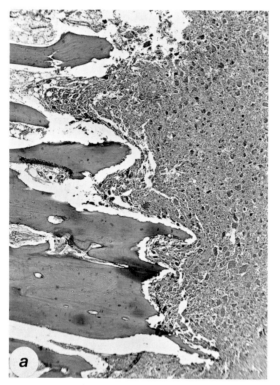 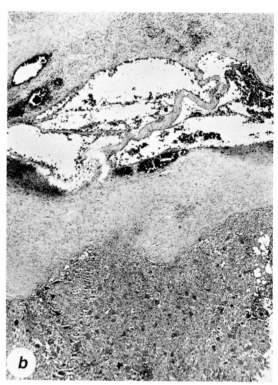

Figure 9-17. *a.* Giant cell tumor of radius showing typical irregular junction with adjacent bone. (×35) *b.* Regions with aneurysmal bone-cyst-like spaces in otherwise typical giant cell tumor. (×35) (Reproduced with permission from: Dahlin, D. C., Cupps, R. E., and Johnson, E. W., Jr.: *Cancer, 25:*1061-1070, 1970.)

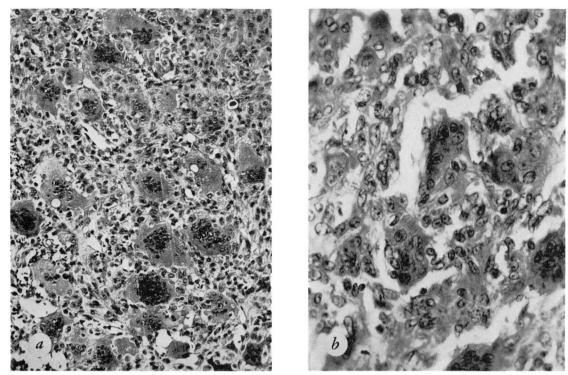

Figure 9-18. *a.* Typical benign giant cell tumor with no definite intercellular substance and with prominent multinucleated cells. (×160) *b.* Note marked similarity of nuclei of mononuclear and multinucleated cells. One can scarcely define boundaries of giant cells. (×420) (Reproduced with permission from: Williams, R. R., Dahlin, D. C., and Ghormley, R. K.: *Cancer, 7:*764-773, 1954.)

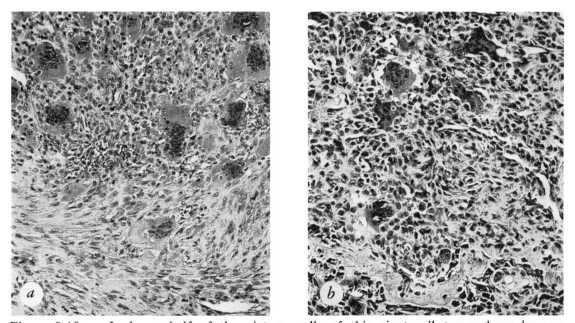

Figure 9-19. *a.* In lower half of the picture, cells of this giant cell tumor have become distinctly fibroblastic. Such fibrogenic zones that contain scattered multinucleated cells are seen in many conditions of bone. (×160) *b.* Osteoid trabecula in giant cell tumor. Such foci may be present even before therapy or fracture alters tumor. (×185) (Reproduced with permission from: Williams, R. R., Dahlin, D. C., and Ghormley, R. K.: *Cancer, 7:*764-773, 1954.)

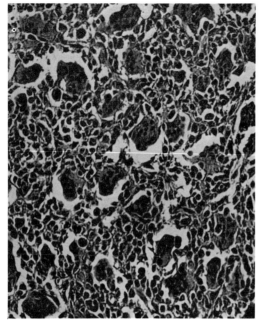

Figure 9-20. Sacral giant cell tumor. (×200) Tissue from case illustrated in Figure 9-5.

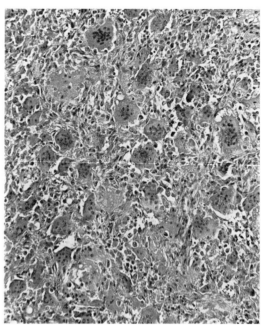

Figure 9-21. Classic giant cell tumor occurring in sphenoid of twenty-five-year-old woman. (×100)

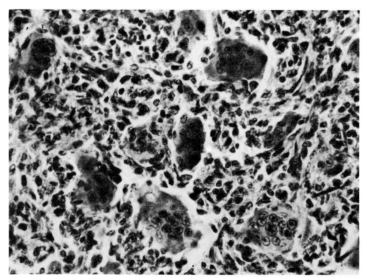

Figure 9-22. Giant cell tumor of dorsal vertebral body. Thorough sampling revealed no histologic evidence of variant such as aneurysmal bone cyst or osteoblastoma, both of which are considerably more common than true giant cell tumor in vertebrae above sacrum. (×365)

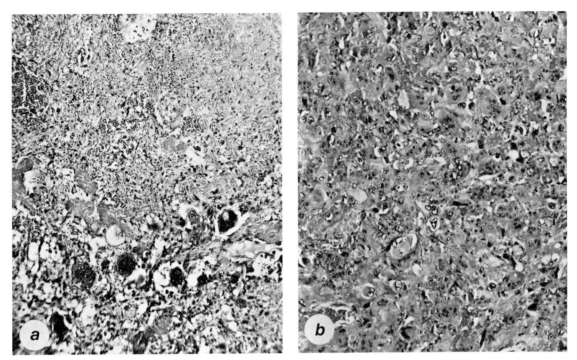

Figure 9-23. *a.* Giant cell tumor with large, nondiagnostic necrotic zone. (×100) *b.* Bizarre mononuclear cells in giant cell tumor of ilium. Patient was well five years after resection of lesion. (×160)

Malignant change in giant cell tumor is discussed under prognosis and in Chapter 22.

Grading of giant cell tumors has not been of value in our cases in helping predict those lesions likely to recur or even those likely to become sarcomatous eventually.

Treatment

Removal of the tumor by curettage is the most widely accepted type of therapy. Many advocate chemical or thermal cautery of the walls of the cavity, and the defect is ordinarily filled with bone chips. Total excision of the tumor and its surrounding shell of bone and periosteum is sometimes the treatment of choice, especially when a small bone such as the fibula or radius is involved. Some believe that total resection is indicated, even at the knee, although it may result in loss of function of the joint. Bone grafting or some replacement device may be required. In some of the massive lesions with extensive destruction of juxta-articular bone, primary amputation is necessary. After multiple recurrences, amputation or radical excision should be considered because of the hazard of malignant transformation.

Irradiation as primary or adjunctive therapy has its advocates but is becoming less acceptable because of its potential danger of inducing malignant transformation and the recognition that true giant cell tumors are relatively radioresistant. Irradiation should be reserved for those giant cell tumors not amenable to surgical excision.

When malignant change has occurred, the treatment is that indicated for radio-resistant sarcoma.

Prognosis

Long-term follow-up is essential in assessing the results of therapy for giant cell tumor, since malignant change has been known to develop nearly forty years after primary treatment. Several studies have shown that the recurrence rate is 50 percent or more, and sarcoma complicates the course in approximately 10 percent. These figures relate to tumors treated primarily by curettage and radiation.

Curettage was followed by recurrence in nearly 50 percent of the cases in the present series. Size of tumor, bone involved, preoperative duration of symptoms, cauterization of tumor cavity, bone grafting, cellular appearance, and adjunctive irradiation therapy have had no recognizable influence on the recurrence rate. Complete resection, now so often made possible with the newer replacement devices, should markedly improve the prognosis.

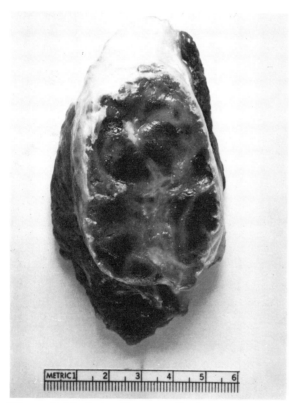 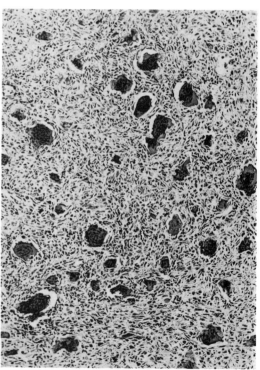

Figure 9-24. *Left.* Circumscribed recurrence of benign giant cell tumor excised from muscles adjacent to distal end of femur of twenty-two-year-old woman. There was no definite evidence of recurrence of primary lesion of distal portion of femur, which had been treated by curettage and grafting more than four years before, by irradiation during the ensuing year, and by curettage and grafting again a year prior to excision of this lesion. Such recurrence in soft tissues was unusual in this series. Interestingly, a thin shell of bone had developed from tumor cells at periphery of mass, a phenomenon that occurs sometimes in the rare metastasis of benign giant cell tumor. *Right.* Microscopic appearance of this recurrence in soft tissue appeared identical to that of original benign giant cell tumor of femur. (×110) (Reproduced with permission from: Johnson, E. W., Jr.: *Am J Surg, 109:*163-166, 1965.)

Amputation or total excision has been uniformly curative, but amputation is indicated as primary treatment only for huge, neglected giant cell tumors.

Secondary malignant change is usually in the form of pure fibrosarcoma or osteosarcoma. It was found in 20 of the 264 cases in the present series. Fifteen of the twenty malignant tumors in this series occurred an average of 9.4 years after the

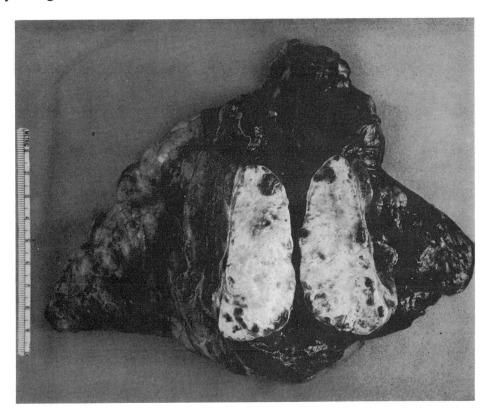

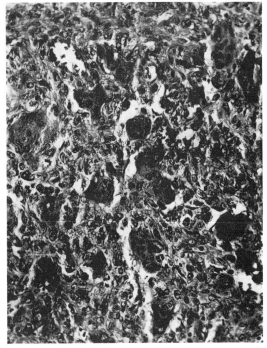

Figure 9-25. *Above.* Solitary metastatic benign giant cell tumor nodule excised with right lower pulmonary lobe and portion of attached diaphragm. This lesion appeared nearly six years after curettage, grafting, and irradiation of a giant cell tumor of distal end of radius. No residual tumor was present in radius. Patient has remained well for nearly eight years since pulmonary resection. *Right.* Pulmonary nodule that appeared identical to original benign giant cell tumor of radius. (×200) (Reproduced with permission from: Pan, P., Dahlin, D. C., Lipscomb, P. R., and Bernatz, P. E.: *Proc Staff Meet Mayo Clin, 39:*344-349, 1964.)

verification of benign giant cell tumor and therapy, which included irradiation in all but two instances. The mortality for patients with these sarcomas has been approximately 80 percent. Five patients had sarcomas present in portions of typical giant cell tumors at the time of their first operation.

Original sections from those benign giant cell tumors that recurred or from which secondary sarcomas developed were histologically indistinguishable from those cured by one surgical procedure. Grading of these tumors as to degree of malignancy has been of no prognostic value.

Metastasis from benign giant cell tumor, with the metastatic deposit appearing to be benign, has been documented adequately in somewhat more than a dozen cases, and only two instances were encountered in the present series.

Soft-tissue implantation of benign giant cell tumor near the osseous site of one is not unusual. This capability for implantation emphasizes the neoplastic quality of these lesions and underscores the precaution surgeons must employ in attempting to prevent this complication. Such soft-tissue masses often have a partially ossified peripheral shell. In a few instances, giant cell tumors have apparently been implanted from their original site to the location from which bone was procured for grafting.

A recently completed study of thirty-one giant cell tumors involving vertebrae above the sacrum indicated a prognosis better than one would expect judging from the experience with such tumors in more conventional sites. Although the mononuclear cells tended to be somewhat smaller and more spindling than in other giant cell tumors, these lesions did not have the characteristics of "variants" such as aneurysmal bone cysts or benign osteoblastomas.

Bibliography

1940   Jaff, H. L., Lichtenstein, L., and Portis, R. B.: Giant Cell Tumor of Bone: Its Pathologic Appearance, Grading, Supposed Variants and Treatment. *Arch Pathol, 30:*993-1031.

1949   Willis, R. A.: The Pathology of Osteoclastoma or Giant-Cell Tumour of Bone. *J Bone Joint Surg, 31B:*236-240.

1953   Shuffstall, R. M., and Gregory, J. E.: Osteoid Formation in Giant Cell Tumors of Bone. *Am J Pathol, 29:*1123-1131.

1953   Compere, E. L.: The Diagnosis and Treatment of Giant-cell Tumors of Bone. *J Bone Joint Surg, 35A:*822-830.

1953   Jaffe, H. L.: Giant-cell Tumor (Osteoclastoma) of Bone: Its Pathologic Delimitation and the Inherent Clinical Implications. *Ann R Coll Surg Engl, 13:*343-355.

1956   Dahlin, D. C., Ghormley, R. K., and Pugh, D. G.: Giant Cell Tumor of Bone: Differential Diagnosis. *Proc Staff Meet Mayo Clin, 31:*31-42.

1957   Bullock, W. K., and Luck, J. V.: Giant Cell Tumor-like Lesions of Bone. *Calif Med, 87:*32-36.

1958   Gee, V. R., and Pugh, D. G.: Giant-Cell Tumor of Bone. *Radiology, 70:*33-45.

1960   Troup, J. B., Dahlin, D. C., and Coventry, M. B.: The Significance of Giant Cells in Osteogenic Sarcoma: Do They Indicate a Relationship between Osteogenic Sarcoma and Giant Cell Tumor of Bone? *Proc Staff Meet Mayo Clin, 35:*179-186.

1961   Schajowicz, F.: Giant-Cell Tumors of Bone (Osteoclastoma). A Pathological and Histochemical Study. *J Bone Joint Surg, 43A:*1-29.

1961   Sherman, M., and Fabricius, R.: Giant-Cell Tumor in the Metaphysis in a Child. Report of an Unusual Case. *J Bone Joint Surg, 43A:*1225-1229.

1961 Goldner, J. L., and Forrest, J. S.: Giant Cell Tumor of Bone. *South Med J, 54:*121-133.

1962 Hutter, R. V. P., Worcester, J. N., Jr., Francis, K. C., Foote, F. W., Jr., and Stewart, F. W.: Benign and Malignant Giant Cell Tumors of Bone. A Clinicopathological Analysis of the Natural History of the Disease. *Cancer, 15:*653-690.

1963 Edeiken, Jack, and Hodes, P. J.: Giant Cell Tumors vs. Tumors with Giant Cells. *Radiol Clin North Am, 1:*75-100.

1964 Pan, P., Dahlin, D. C., Lipscomb, P. R., and Bernatz, P. E.: "Benign" Giant Cell Tumor of the Radius with Pulmonary Metastasis. *Proc Staff Meet Mayo Clin, 39:* 344-349.

1964 Jewell, J. H., and Bush, L. F.: "Benign" Giant-Cell Tumor of Bone with a Solitary Pulmonary Metastasis. A Case Report. *J Bone Joint Surg, 46A:*848-852.

1964 Tate, R. G.: Giant Cell Tumor of Bone. *Can J Surg, 7:*25-42.

1964 Bradshaw, J. D.: The Value of X-ray Therapy in the Management of Osteoclastoma. *Clin Radiol, 15:*70-74.

1964 Mnaymneh, W. A., Dudley, H. R., and Mnaymneh, L. G.: Excision of Giant-Cell Bone Tumor. *J Bone Joint Surg, 46A:*63-75.

1968 D'Aubigne, R. M., Thomine, J. M., Mazabraud, A., and Hannouche, D.: Évolution Spontanée et Post-Opératoire des Tumeurs à Cellules Géantes: Indications à Propos de 39 Cas dont 20 Suivis 5 Ans ou Plus. *Rev Chir Orthop, 54:*689-714 (December).

1970 Dahlin, D. C., Cupps, R. E., and Johnson, E. W., Jr.: Giant-Cell Tumor: A Study of 195 Cases. *Cancer, 25:*1061-1070 (May).

1970 Goldenberg, R. R., Campbell, C. J., and Bonfiglio, M.: Giant-Cell Tumor of Bone: An Analysis of Two Hundred and Eighteen Cases. *J Bone Joint Surg, 52A:*619-663 (June).

1972 D'Alonzo, R. T., Pitcock, J. A., and Milford, L. W.: Giant-Cell Reaction of Bone: Report of Two Cases. *J Bone Joint Surg, 54A:*1267-1271 (September).

1972 Jacobs, P.: The Diagnosis of Osteoclastoma (Giant-Cell Tumor): A Radiological and Pathological Correlation. *Br J Radiol, 45:*121-136 (February).

1972 Steiner, G. C., Ghosh, L., and Dorfman, H. D.: Ultrastructure of Giant Cell Tumors of Bone. *Hum Pathol, 3:*569-586 (December).

1973 Gresen, A. A., Dahlin, D. C., Peterson, L. F. A., and Payne, W. S.: "Benign" Giant Cell Tumor of Bone Metastasizing to Lung: Report of a Case. *Ann Thorac Surg, 16:*531-535 (November).

1974 Glasscock, M. E., and Hunt, W. E.: Giant-Cell Tumor of the Sphenoid and Temporal Bones. *Laryngoscope, 84:*1181-1187 (July).

1974 Miller, A. S., Cuttino, C. L., Elzay, R. P., Levy, W. M., and Harwick, R. D.: Giant Cell Tumor of the Jaws Associated With Paget Disease of Bone: Report of Two Cases and Review of the Literature. *Arch Otolaryngol, 100:*233-236 (September).

1975 Campanacci, M., Giunti, A., and Olmi, R.: Giant-Cell Tumors of Bone: A Study of 209 Cases With Long-Term Follow-Up in 130. *Ital J Orthop Traumatol, 1:*249-277 (August).

1975 Larsson, S.-E., Lorentzon, R., and Boquist, L.: Giant-Cell Tumor of Bone: A Demographic, Clinical, and Histopathological Study of All Cases Recorded in the Swedish Cancer Registry for the Years 1958 Through 1968. *J Bone Joint Surg, 57A:*167-173 (March).

1975 Tornberg, D. N., Dick, H. M., and Johnston, A. D.: Multicentric Giant-Cell Tumors in the Long Bones: A Case Report. *J Bone Joint Surg, 57A:*420-422 (April).

Chapter 10

Benign and Atypical Fibrous Histiocytoma

THIS TUMOR IS OF DEBATABLE nature and has been included with such lesions as monosteogenic fibroma and "xanthoma." The mononuclear cells tend to be fibrogenic and may contain lipid. This latter histiocytic capability is evident in the malignant counterpart to be described in Chapter 24. The fibrogenic zones may show a storiform or cartwheel pattern.

The general features of the process considered to be fibrous histiocytoma will be illustrated in the figures that follow.

Only 7 examples were found in this series of 6,221 bone tumors. One patient with a lesion of the middle part of the humerus required amputation two years after biopsy and was then lost to follow-up. One patient had pulmonary metastasis forty-nine months after excision of the primary tumor of the distal end of the femur. The other five patients have gotten along well after curettage, with grafting of the area when necessary.

The current concept is that this neoplasm results from a proliferation of cells that are capable of producing collagen or of assuming a histiocytic quality.

Incidence

Only 7 tumors of the 6,221 in this series were considered to be benign and atypical fibrous histiocytomas of bone.

Sex

Three women and four men were affected.

Age

All patients were adults, and their ages at diagnosis ranged from twenty-three to sixty years.

Localization

The distal part of a femur and of a tibia was involved in one case each. One tumor occurred in the middle part of a femur and another in the midportion of a humerus. One tumor affected the sacrum, one the ilium, and one was in both of these bones.

Symptoms

Local pain was the primary complaint of six of the seven patients. The duration of pain varied from four to twelve months. One patient with an iliac tumor had had the lesion for seven years. In one patient, the features of hypophosphatemic osteomalacia developed as the tumor of his femur became apparent. Symptoms of this disorder recurred when the tumor did and again when pulmonary metastasis occurred. It seems obvious that the cells of the neoplasm elaborated an obscure humoral substance.

Physical Findings

Most of these patients had no findings attributable to their tumors.

Roentgenologic Features

Generally, these tumors produced a well-defined zone of rarefaction. In two instances, the somewhat irregular edges were suggestive of a malignant tumor. Calcification was noted in one of the tumors.

Gross Pathology

The usual tissue was in irregular fragments. Sometimes it was slightly fibrous, and occasionally it was yellowish owing to its lipid content.

Histopathology

The similarity of this tumor to nonosteogenic fibroma has been mentioned. The fibrogenic quality may be manifested by interlacing bundles of cells. Benign giant cells are present in variable numbers, but they may be sparse. Some of the nuclei are indented or grooved, and this histiocytic quality may be associated with lipid, sometimes abundant, within the cells. Mitotic figures are rare. One tumor contained

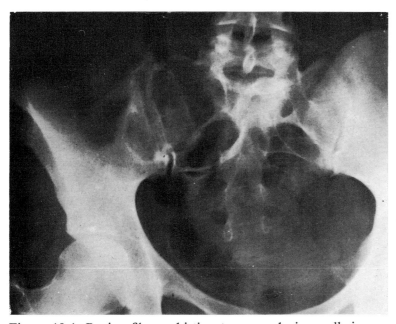

Figure 10-1. Benign fibrous histiocytoma producing well-circumscribed rarefaction in right side of sacrum and adjacent ilium of twenty-three-year-old woman who had noted sciatica for one year. She has remained well for thirty-six years after curettage of lesion, which weighed 100 g. Pathologic features are shown in Figures 10-5 and 10-8.

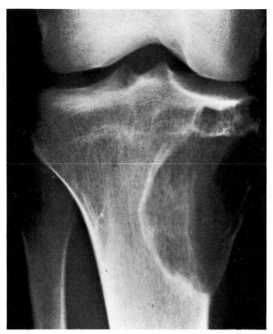

Figure 10-2. Fibrous histiocytoma in twenty-eight-year-old woman is well defined. Involvement of epiphysis and patient's age would both be unusual for nonosteogenic fibroma. Patient was well forty-two months after curettage and grafting. Histologic appearance of lesion is illustrated in Figure 10-6. (Case contributed by Doctor J. B. Wilks of Cincinnati, Ohio.)

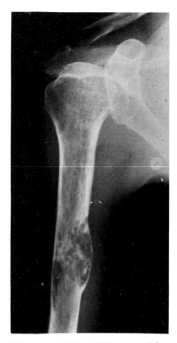

Figure 10-3. Fibrous histiocytoma in forty-nine-year-old man. This tumor had produced pain for eight months. Two years after biopsy, amputation was necessary, but details of this operation are unknown, and patient was lost to follow-up.

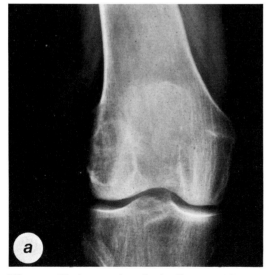

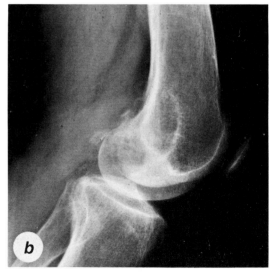

Figure 10-4. *a.* Atypical fibrous histiocytoma in forty-eight-year-old man. Implants in synovium of knee were removed thirty-four months after excision of histiocytoma. Amputation was performed for recurrence forty-one months after excision of lesion. Patient has had three operations for pulmonary metastasis from four to six years after excision but was alive and well eight years after first treatment. This is the patient who has had recurrent hypophosphatemic osteomalacia. *b.* Lateral view of same tumor.

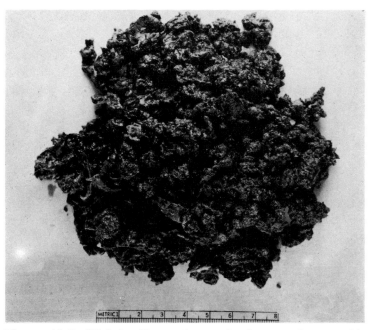

Figure 10-5. Slightly fibrous hemorrhagic-appearing xanthic material curetted from defect shown in Figure 10-1. This specimen is dark because it had been fixed prior to photography, but volume is apparent.

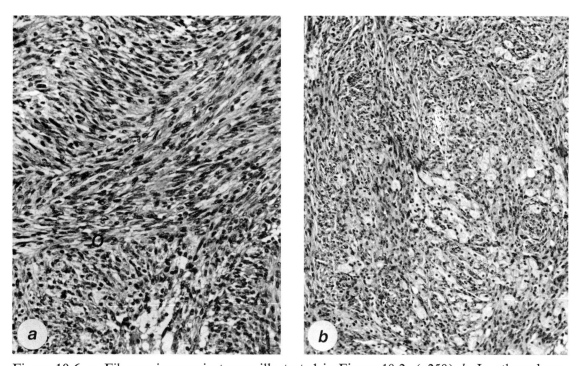

Figure 10-6. *a*. Fibrogenic zone in tumor illustrated in Figure 10-2. (×250) *b*. In other places, cells of this tumor assumed phagocytic quality and contained lipid. (×160)

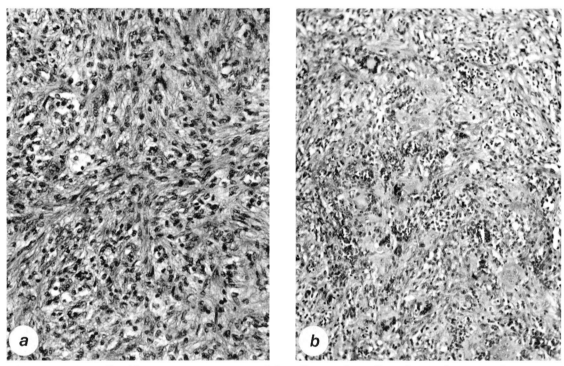

Figure 10-7. *a.* Storiform pattern suggested by fibrogenic cells of sacral tumor in twenty-seven-year-old woman who had had pain for seven months. She was well twenty-seven months after subtotal removal of mottled, yellowish lesion, which aggregated 6 cm in diameter. (×250) *b.* Scattered benign giant cells and some lipid-containing cells were present in tumor. (×160)

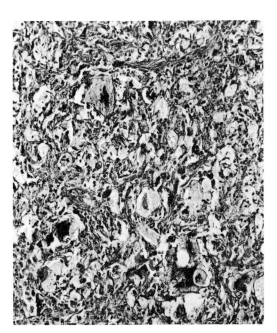

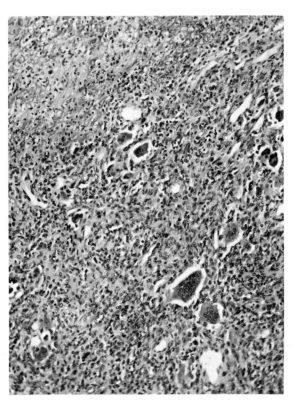

Figure 10-8. Markedly xanthic zone in tumor shown in Figures 10-1 and 10-5. (×125)

Figure 10-9. Hypophosphatemic-osteomalacia-producing tumor shown in Figure 10-4. Chondroid aura accounted for its original designation of atypical benign chondroblastoma. (×160)

poorly formed chondroid islands, some of which were lightly calcified; it had been considered to be an atypical benign chondroblastoma, and it is the lesion that produced recurrence, implants into the adjacent knee joint, and finally pulmonary metastasis.

Treatment and Prognosis

The few cases allow no firm conclusions. If the tumor is removed completely and no features of malignancy are recognized, a good result can be expected. The one patient with recurrence and later metastasis indicates that care must be exercised in the interpretation of such lesions.

Bibliography

1970 Pear, B. L.: The Histiocyte in Radiology: With Case Reports of Retroperitoneal Xanthogranuloma and Malignant Fibrous Xanthoma. *Am J Roentgenol, 110:*159-165 (September).

1972 Evans, D. J., and Azzopardi, J. G.: Distinctive Tumors of Bone and Soft Tissue Causing Acquired Vitamin-D-Resistant Osteomalacia. *Lancet, 1:*353-354 (February).

1972 Feldman, F., and Norma, D.: Intra- and Extraosseous Malignant Histiocytoma (Malignant Fibrous Xanthoma). *Radiology, 104:*497-508 (September).

1976 Renton, P., and Shaw, D. G.: Hypophosphatemic Osteomalacia Secondary to Vascular Tumors of Bone and Soft Tissue. *Skeletal Radiol, 1:*21-24 (September).

Chapter 11

Fibroma (Nonosteogenic Fibroma of Bone, Metaphyseal Fibrous Defect), Myxoma, Cortical Desmoid, Fibromatosis, and "Xanthoma"

THE FIRST THREE OF THE above terms all apply to the same basic histopathologic process in bone. The spontaneous resolution of most of these lesions and their relationship to the growing portions of bones support the concept that they represent faulty ossification rather than neoplasm. Roentgenographic evidence of cortical defects may be found in approximately one third of growing children, most commonly in the femur. A small fraction of these lesions pose a sufficient diagnostic problem or produce severe enough symptoms to require operation. Strangely, a few of these fibroblastic masses, histologically indistinguishable from the innocuous ones, continue to grow and may produce pathologic fracture of even a major tubular bone. Patients may have multiple fibrous defects in one or more extremities.

Despite the innocuous clinical behavior of this lesion, its component of benign multinucleated cells still frequently results in its being erroneously considered to be a genuine giant cell tumor of bone.

Three myxomas of bone have been sent in for consultation, but none was recognized in our series.

The so-called periosteal desmoid appears to be a hypocellular variant of this group of fibrous defects; perhaps it results from trauma or from a peculiarity of bone growth in the region. These abnormalities are most often near the end of the femoral shaft medially.

Congenital generalized fibromatosis, a rare condition, may produce rarefactions in bone, but these desmoplastic proliferations are quite different from the fibromas under discussion.

It is pertinent to point out that one occasionally sees fibrous defects of bone that lack the cellularity and roentgenologic features of typical fibroma. The exact nature of some of these is obscure. Some may result from old trauma, hemorrhage, or infection and some may represent the end stage or scar of an ordinary fibroma or of fibrous dysplasia. Several such lesions were encountered in the files of the Mayo Clinic, but they have been excluded from the data in Figure 11-1 and from the discussion which follows.

Xanthoma or xanthofibroma is a term that has been employed for some of the fibromas that have a prominent lipoid component. Aside from such fibromas, one occasionally encounters a small or large osseous lesion that is predominantly xanthic. Some aspects of this problem are indicated in this chapter and have been elaborated in Chapter 10.

Desmoplastic fibroma is a locally aggressive benign neoplasm that will be discussed in the chapter on fibrosarcoma of bone.

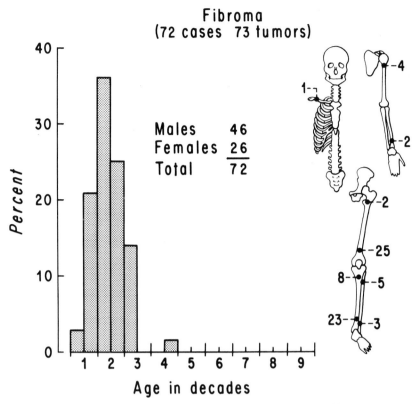

Figure 11-1. Skeletal, age, and sex distribution of fibromas.

Incidence

Although fibromas constituted only 5 percent of the benign bone tumors in this series, their true incidence is much greater because the vast majority of them never come to operation. The data in Figure 11-1, like the other data in this book, derive from surgical cases only.

Sex

Males predominated in the present series, which is in keeping with the findings of others. In my earlier series, which included some of the nondescript fibrous scars in bone, there was a female predominance.

Age

Fibroma in its classic form is almost exclusively a disease of childhood and adolescence. The oldest patient in this series was thirty-seven years old; the remainder were twenty-five years of age or less, and 85 percent were in the first two decades of life.

Localization

Every fibroma in this series was in the metaphyseal portion of a long bone of a limb except for one in the clavicle. Only four lesions were in an upper extremity. Some of the metaphyseal lesions, when found, were a considerable distance from the growth plate.

Symptoms

This lesion is commonly silent clinically and is discovered incidentally when a region is subject to roentgenographic study for unrelated reasons. Local pain, usually of short duration, is sometimes produced. Occasionally, especially in slender tubular bones such as the fibula, pathologic fracture ushers in the clinical symptoms.

Physical Findings

Physical examination is of little diagnostic value in fibroma of bone. In rare instances, slight swelling may be observed if the affected bone is near the surface of the body. One tibial lesion in this series produced compound fracture.

Roentgenologic Features

Most fibromas present a characteristic roentgenographic appearance that is virtually pathognomonic. When a large tubular bone is affected, the lesion is practically always eccentrically located and often produces some bulging of the cortical outline, which is usually very thin over the defect.

The tumor begins in the metaphysis, near or at the epiphyseal line, and appears to migrate toward the center of the bone as the epiphyseal region grows away from it. The inner boundary of the lesion often is demarcated by a thin or prominent scalloped line of sclerosis. Trabeculae frequently appear to traverse the defect and give it a multilocular appearance; these trabeculae are, however, nearly always incomplete, and the appearance is actually produced by the shadows of corrugations on the inner surface of the cavity housing the tumor. Sometimes a fibroma has a poorly delimited periphery with no surrounding sclerosis. In thin bones, the entire width of the bone may be involved. Central lesions may simulate fibrous dysplasia or simple bone cysts.

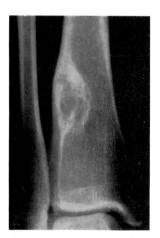 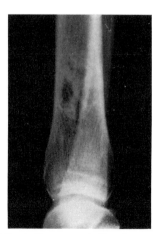 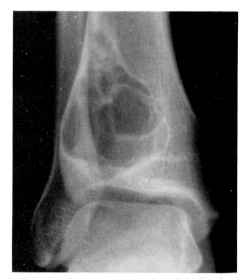

Figure 11-2. *Left and middle.* Fibroma of distal part of tibia in fourteen-year-old girl. Lesion was incidental finding at time of sprained ankle. Anteroposterior and lateral views. *Right.* Larger fibroma with characteristic loculated appearance and well-defined edges. This lesion occurred in eighteen-year-old man.

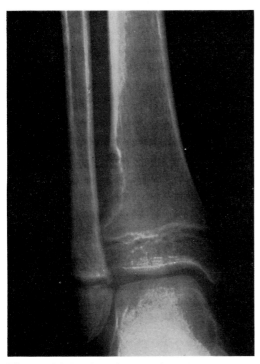

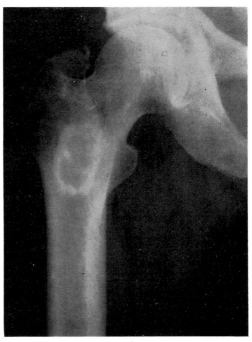

Figure 11-3. Another typical fibroma, although small. This one was found incidentally on roentgenographic study of ankle of eight-year-old girl.

Figure 11-4. This lesion was found incidentally in fifty-seven-year-old man and consisted of dense fibrous tissue with sclerosed border. Genesis of this process is obscure, and lesion was not included with fibromas.

Fracture through the lesion may occur if it is in a small bone or if it is very large.

Gross Pathology

As indicated by the roentgenogram, the cortex is ordinarily attenuated but intact over a fibroma unless fracture has occurred. The lesions vary in greatest diameter, some being 5 cm or more. The long axis tends to parallel that of the affected bone. The tumor itself is usually distinctly demarcated from the surrounding bone, and sometimes consists of multiple discrete lobules of soft tissue surrounded by walls of bone and showing confluence. The pathologist ordinarily receives curetted fragments of more or less fibrous, fleshy tissue. It may be completely or partially yellow, depending on its lipid content. It may contain enough hemosiderin to make it distinctly brown.

Histopathology

Microscopic examination reveals a dominant, cellular, fibroblastic connective-tissue background with the cells arranged in whorled bundles. The fibrogenic characteristic aids in differentiation from genuine giant cell tumors which, in sections from diagnostic portions, are not fibrogenic. Benign multinucleated cells, containing fewer nuclei on the average than do those of giant cell tumor, are irregularly

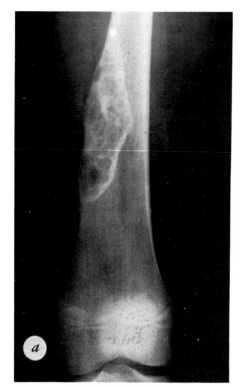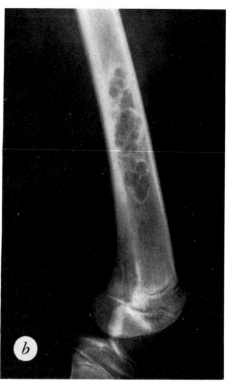

Figure 11-5. *a.* Unusually large fibroma in eleven-year-old girl. Its roentgeno-logic features, including appearance of trabeculation, bulging of cortical out-line, and distinct inner boundary, are typical. *b.* Lateral view of same lesion makes it appear to be a basically central one. (Roentgenograms of this case were provided through the courtesy of Doctors P. K. Odland, G. L. Thomas, and M. B. Llewellyn of Janesville, Wisconsin.)

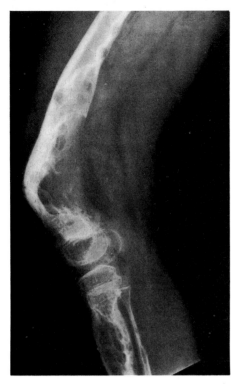

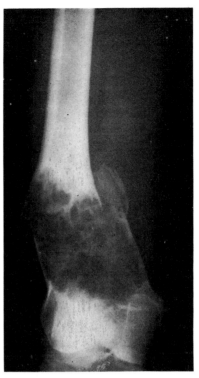

Figure 11-6. Multiple nonosteogenic fibromas that had produced multiple fractures of femur. Resultant deformity later necessitated amputation. Note that there is involvement of the tibia and fibula also.

Figure 11-7. Huge nonosteogenic fibroma with associated pathologic fracture of distal metaphyseal region of femur of fourteen-year-old girl. Curettage and grafting resulted in healing and some shortening of femur. (Case contributed by Doctor A. R. Haugen of San Bernardino, California.)

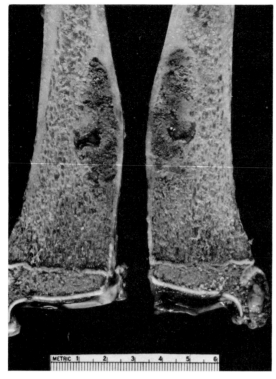

Figure 11-8. Fibroma in fifteen-year-old boy was incidental finding, amputation had been necessitated by trauma. Lesion had produced slight "expansion" of tibia, but its boundaries are discrete.

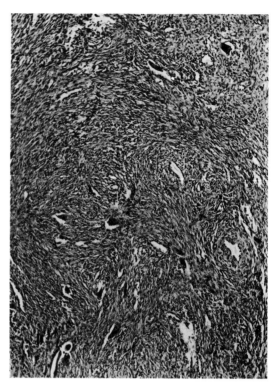

Figure 11-9. Classic appearance of non-osteogenic fibroma. Note cell-rich fibroblastic tissue disposed in somewhat whorled bundles. Giant cells are sparser than in average giant cell tumor. (×50)

distributed throughout the lesion. Nests of lipophages, which appear to be converted fibroblasts, are sometimes seen. They rarely dominate or even form a prominent part of the histologic pattern, although one encounters an occasional lesion in bone that has the roentgenographic appearance of fibroma but shows extreme lipidization. Giant cells are uncommon in the foci of foam cells. Hemosiderin pigmentation of variable degree is so commonly seen in the cytoplasm of the spindle-shaped cells that it aids in the recognition of nonosteogenic fibroma.

Occasional fibromas are active enough that mitotic figures may be found with comparative ease. The benign quality of the nuclei should allay the fear that one is dealing with a malignant tumor in such cases.

A fibroma associated with pathologic fracture may have undergone so much necrosis and hemorrhage that identification is difficult.

Small foci of osseous metaplasia may be found in some fibromas, even in some of those not complicated by fracture. This is contrary to much of what is reported in the literature, but this finding has led to the suggestion that fibroma and fibrous dysplasia are related processes.

Fibromas of bone may be large, as illustrated in this chapter, but histologically, such lesions are indistinguishable from the smaller tumors that are often referred

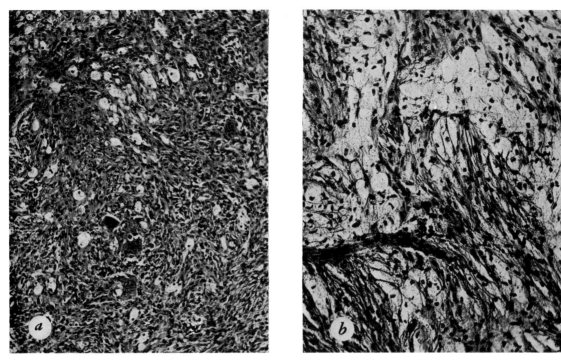

Figure 11-10. *a*. Essential features of fibroma, including fibroblastic connective tissue and benign giant cells. In addition, there are foam cells scattered throughout. (×110) *b*. Prominent nests of foam cells in fibroblastic stroma. (×200)

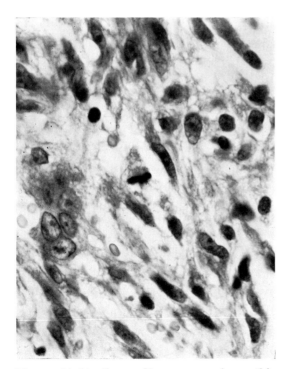

Figure 11-11. Some fibromas, such as this one, exhibit worrisome cellular activity, as evidenced by occasional mitotic figures. (×800)

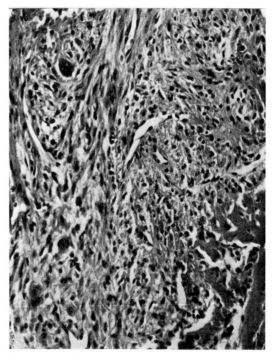

Figure 11-12. Rarely, fibromas produce foci of osteoid, as at lower right, even without previous fracture. (×210)

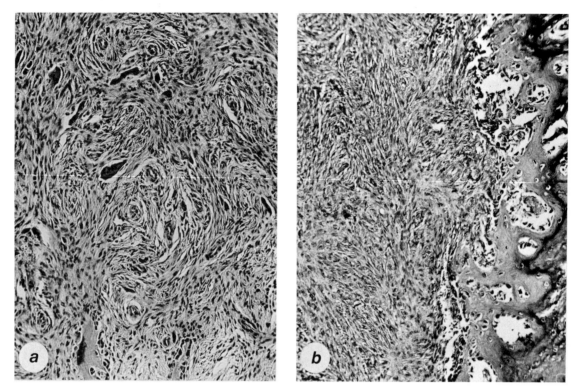

Figure 11-13. *a*. Nonosteogenic fibroma producing cystlike rarefaction in clavicle of seven-year-old boy. Lesion had no recognizable features of other lesions such as aneurysmal bone cyst. (×200) *b*. Edge of fibroma of femur showing good demarcation from adjacent bone. (×150)

to as metaphyseal fibrous defects. Although the so-called cortical desmoids may represent the most minimal form of metaphyseal fibrous defect, they show little, if any, of the cellular, whorled fibroblastic tissue or the benign giant cells of the classic lesion being described.

Benign giant cell tumor is often mistaken for nonosteogenic fibroma by the histopathologist. This mistake can nearly always be avoided if one pays attention to the fibrogenesis in the latter lesion. Furthermore, the age of the affected patient is usually different, and the roentgenograms are likewise different.

Treatment

If one is confident of the roentgenologic diagnosis and the structural integrity of the bone is not in question, no treatment need be employed and the progress of the lesion can be followed by repeat roentgenograms. If the diagnosis is uncertain, one can accomplish diagnosis and therapy with one surgical procedure. Nonosteogenic fibroma is readily eradicated by conservative surgical means, curettage ordinarily being employed. Bone grafting of the defect may be desirable if the lesion is large. Radiation therapy is contraindicated for two reasons, namely the inherent sarcoma-producing potential of this form of therapy and the frequent proximity of the fibroma to a growing epiphyseal line.

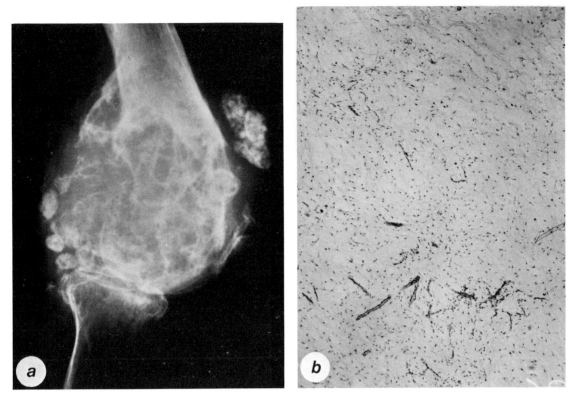

Figure 11-14. *a.* Myxoma of bone. The cystlike expanding rarefaction had produced pain for four years. Lesion contained no evidence that it was a degenerating chondroma or any tumor other than myxoma. Note that ossifying tumor is growing outside the bone, but some of the extraosseous mineralization is secondary to degenerative joint disease. *b.* Typical field showing only proliferating hypocellular myxomatous tissue. (×64) (Case contributed by Doctor D. S. Jacobs of Kansas City, Missouri.)

A competent radiologist can ordinarily recognize that the so-called periosteal desmoid is a "nontumor" and is not a malignant process requiring surgical assessment.

Prognosis

As indicated, conservative surgical treatment, when necessary, is curative. Many lesions have been shown to undergo spontaneous regression. It has been observed that fracture through one of these lesions heals but the defect in the bone usually persists.

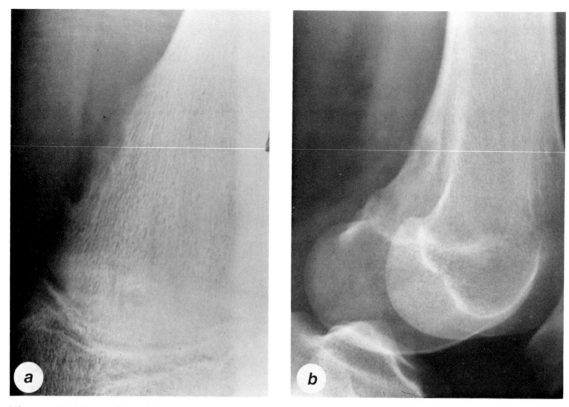

Figure 11-15. *a.* So-called cortical desmoid of medial side of distal femur. This area in twelve-year-old boy was associated with vague pain for two months. Resection was performed because of suggestion that lesion was malignant. *b.* Similar lesion, essentially an incidental finding, in fourteen-year-old girl.

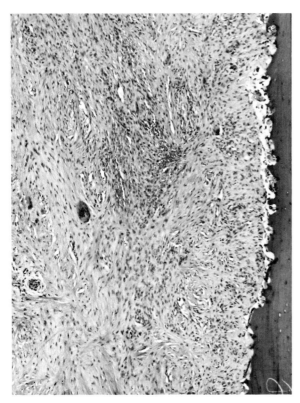

Figure 11-16. Another of these non-neoplastic zones, sometimes called "nontumors." Rather hypocellular fibrous tissue, sometimes containing a few benign giant cells, is next to somewhat irregular cortical bone. This, too, involved distal part of femoral shaft. (×100)

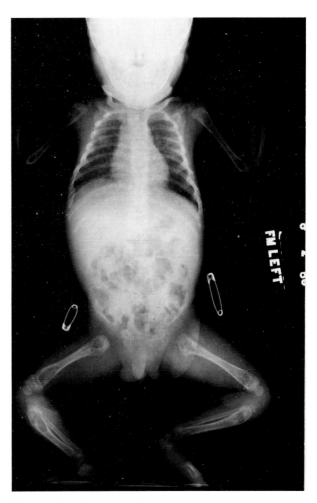

Figure 11-17. Congenital fibromatosis with metaphyseal defects in many bones of three-month-old boy. Patient had evidence of cutaneous and visceral disease and died shortly after this roentgenogram was made. Patients may recover, especially if they have predominantly skeletal lesions.

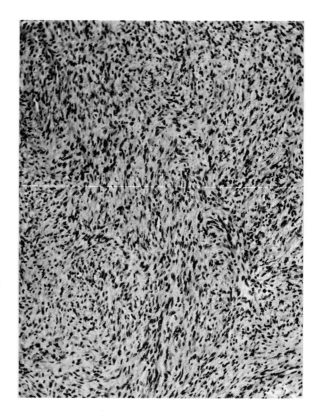

Figure 11-18. Material from tibial defect in another example of fibromatosis. Four-month-old boy had numerous skeletal metaphyseal defects much like those seen in roentgenogram in Figure 11-17. Interlacing bundles of spindle-shaped cells without anaplasia are characteristic. At sixteen months, patient had developed compression fractures of several vertebrae. At five years of age, he was healthy, except for slightly short neck and kyphosis. Lesions in bones had nearly completely resolved. (×160) (Case contributed by Doctors W. Weiseth of Eugene, Oregon, and Doctor V. D. Sneeden of Portland, Oregon.)

"Xanthoma" of Bone

In the total series of bone tumors were twenty-two that were composed predominantly of xanthic material in the form of masses of cholesterol and clusters of lipophages. These lesions often contained considerable hemosiderin. Fairly definite clinical and roentgenologic evidence indicated that a few of these were fibromas (fibrous defects) of bone, and portions of the histologic pattern supported this concept. Four lesions were in the correct location and patient age-group for giant cell tumor and were so categorized; zones within them supported this diagnosis microscopically. These four lesions suggest that giant cell tumor may sometimes become degenerative and quiescent. A few of these "xanthomas" were undoubtedly markedly degenerative and probably ancient lesions of fibrous dysplasia. Some were likely simple bone cysts altered by time and organization of hematomas within them. This group of "xanthomas" provided evidence to suggest that aneurysmal bone cyst may become senescent, lose its typical features, and contain nondescript, lipid-laden fibrous tissue. Lesions of hyperparathyroidism may show marked fatty degeneration. Several of these tumors had no features by which their fundamental nature could be surmised. Sometimes prior surgical or radiation therapy masked the basic pathologic changes. Five of the seven tumors now called "benign or atypical fibrous

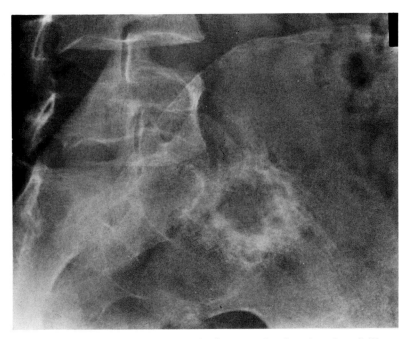

Figure 11-19. "Xanthoma" producing rarefaction in ala of ilium. This was an incidental, asymptomatic finding in sixty-year-old man. Xanthic fibrotic central rarefied zone was surrounded by bone showing nonspecific sclerosis.

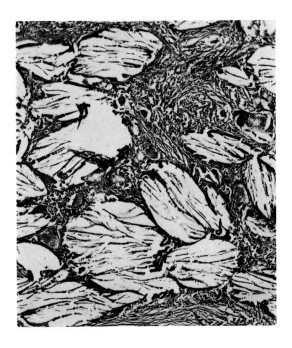

Figure 11-20. Another "xanthoma" of bone was curetted out in pieces, aggregating 7 cm in diameter, from ilium of thirty-one-year-old man. Cholesterol clefts and benign giant cells were prominent throughout. Patient was well fifteen years later. (×65)

histiocytoma" and described in some detail in Chapter 10 had been included originally in the "xanthoma" group.

With recognition of the likelihood that "xanthoma" of bone is always a secondary phenomenon in some preexisting process, it is necessary to acknowledge that one may encounter such tumors. They are not related to the lipid-storage disorders such as Gaucher's disease nor are they part of the histocytosis X complex which includes eosinophilic granuloma, Schüller-Christian disease, and Letterer-Siwe syndrome.

These "xanthomas" are benign, and conservative surgical treatment has been effective for almost all of them. A very few resemble the so-called fibrous xanthomas or histiocytomas; even the malignant variant of this ill-defined neoplasm is suggested by an occasional tumor.

Bibliography

1942	Jaffe, H. L., and Lichtenstein, L.: Non-osteogenic Fibroma of Bone. *Am J Pathol, 18:* 205-221.

1945	Hatcher, C. H.: The Pathogenesis of Localized Fibrous Lesions in the Metaphyses of Long Bones. *Ann Surg,122:*1016-1030.

1949	Ponseti, I. V., and Friedman, B.: Evolution of Metaphyseal Fibrous Defects. *J Bone Joint Surg, 31A:*582-585.

1951	Kimmelstiel, P., and Rapp, I.: Cortical Defect Due to Periosteal Desmoids. *Bull Hosp Joint Dist, 12:*286-297.

1955	Caffey, J.: On Fibrous Defects in Cortical Walls of Growing Tubular Bones. *Adv Pediatr, 7:*13-51.

1955	Devlin, J. A., Bowman, H. E., and Mitchell, C. L.: Non-osteogenic Fibroma of Bone: A Review of the Literature With the Addition of Six Cases. *J Bone Joint Surg, 37A:*472-486.

1956	Cunningham, J. B., and Ackerman, L. V.: Metaphyseal Fibrous Defects. *J Bone Joint Surg, 38A:*797-808.

1956	Maudsley, R. H., and Stansfeld, A. G.: Non-osteogenic Fibroma of Bone. (Fibrous Metaphyseal Defect). *J Bone Joint Surg, 38B:*714-733.

1961	Kauffman, S. L., and Stout, A. P.: Histiocytic Tumors(Fibrous Xanthoma and Histiocytoma) in Children. *Cancer, 14:*469-482.

1961	Condon, V. R., and Allen, R. P.: Congenital Generalized Fibromatosis. Case Report, with Roentgen Manifestations. *Radiology, 76:*444-448.

1963	Teng, P., Warden, M. J., and Cohn, W. L.: Congenital Generalized Fibromatosis (Renal and Skeletal) With Complete Spontaneous Regression. *J Pediatr, 62:*748-753 (May).

1964	Gordon, I. R. S.: Fibrous Lesions of Bone in Childhood. *Br J Radiol, 37:*253-259 (April).

1964	Morton, K. S.: Bone Production in Non-osteogenic Fibroma: An Attempt to Clarify Nomenclature in Fibrous Lesions of Bone. *J Bone Joint Surg, 46B:*233-243 (May).

1967	Perou, M. L., Kolis, J. A., Zaeske, E. V., and Borja, S. R.: Myxoma of the Toe: Case Report. *Cancer, 20:*1030-1034 (June).

1973	Baer, J. W., and Radkowski, M. A.: Congenital Multiple Fibromatosis: A Case Report With Review of the World Literature. *Am J Roentgenol, 118:*200-205 (May).

1974	Barnes, G. R., Jr., and Gwinn, J. L.: Distal Irregularities of the Femur Simulating Malignancy. *Am J Roentgenol, 122:*180-185 (September).

1974	Drennan, D. B., Maylahn, D. J., and Fahey, J. J.: Fractures Through Large Non-ossifying Fibromas. *Clin Orthop, 103:*82-88 (September).

1974	Steiner, G. C.: Fibrous Cortical Defect and Nonossifying Fibroma of Bone: A Study of the Ultrastructure. *Arch Pathol, 97:*205-210 (April).

Chapter 12

Benign Vascular Tumors

Hemangiomas of bone have a minor role in a consideration of lesions requiring surgical procedures for diagnosis or therapy. The alterations commonly interpreted as hemangiomas of the vertebrae by the roentgenologist are practically always asymptomatic and are probably zones of telangiectasis rather than true hemangiomas. Most bona fide hemangiomas in bone are solitary lesions. Hemangiomas may affect two or more bones of a single extremity, sometimes involving the overlying soft tissues as well, and sometimes producing serious malformation and dysfunction. Diffuse skeletal hemangiomatosis (Wallis and coworkers, 1964) is a rare disorder with the lesions most commonly seen in the spine, ribs, pelvis, skull, and shoulders. When such hemangiomatosis affects soft tissues as well as bones, the prognosis is poor; otherwise, the osseous process tends to become stabilized with variable degrees of lytic and sclerotic change.

"Disappearing" or "phantom" bone disease, also called massive osteolysis and Gorham's disease, is now linked with the angiomas of bone. This relatively rare condition, which usually occurs in children or young adults, is characterized by the dissolution, in whole or in part, of one or several adjacent bones. The affected bones show a cavernous angiomatous permeation as the prominent pathologic feature. The process is self-limited, but the extent of progression is unpredictable.

Hemangioendothelioma or hemangiosarcoma of bone encompasses a somewhat nebulous group of tumors that vary from debatably malignant capillary and cavernous proliferations to highly lethal endothelial sarcomas sometimes of multicentric origin.

Hemangiopericytoma, another rather poorly understood neoplasm with poorly defined histologic delineation, occurs as a very rare primary lesion of bone. Chapter 27 elaborates the problem of malignant vascular tumors in bone.

Lymphatic vascular proliferations are also described as producing solitary or multiple zones of rarefaction of the skeleton. A problem is that when blood escapes from the spaces of a hemangioma, the spaces resemble those of lymphangioma; conversely, if blood is introduced into lymphatic spaces, the features resemble those of hemangioma. Perhaps both types of vascular malformation coexist in some cases.

Glomus tumor may erode bone or even arise within it.

The foregoing statements suggest the wide range of the clinical and pathologic spectrum of vascular proliferations in bone. A well-defined and lucid classification of these disorders is not available. Accordingly, portions of the brief discussion to follow will be in general terms.

The bibliography indicates the wide spectrum of vascular disorders affecting bone.

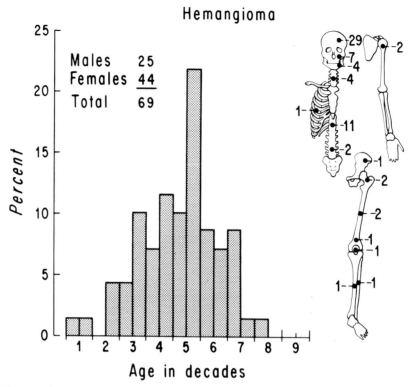

Figure 12-1. Skeletal, age, and sex distribution of solitary hemangiomas.

Incidence

The sixty-nine solitary hemangiomas in the present series comprised only 1.1 percent of the total series. The total series included seven examples of massive osteolysis (disappearing bone disease), twenty-five hemangioendotheliomas (*see* Chapter 27), and five hemangiopericytomas, which will be described in Chapter 27 also.

Sex

Nearly twice as many females as males had hemangioma.

Age

According to most reports, hemangiomas are usually found in adults. In this series, nearly one third of the patients were in the fifth decade of life.

Localization

Two thirds of the hemangiomas were in the cranium or vertebrae. Eleven affected the jaws. Three patients had multiple bones involved; one of these had involvement of a fibula and nearby tarsals and metatarsals, one had three separate defects in the skull, and one had involvement of three separate vertebrae. Two of the seven patients with massive osteolysis had the pelvic region affected, one a leg and part of the pelvis, one a leg, two the thoracic region, and one the forearm.

Symptoms

Many of the hemangiomas of the calvarium in this series were asymptomatic and were discovered during roentgenographic study for other reasons. Hemangiomas that produce expansion of bone and new bone formation may result in notable swelling. Local pain is sometimes a feature. There may be fractures, including compression fractures of vertebrae. Severe hemorrhage may be encountered during surgical procedures. Patients with massive osteolysis have pain and disability commensurate with the degree of osseous involvement. Malignant vascular tumors have the nonspecific pain and swelling common to all malignant processes in bone.

Physical Findings

Physical examination usually contributes no specific information. Occasionally, soft-tissue or cutaneous hemangiomas provide evidence suggesting the nature of the osseous disease. It should be remembered, however, that such nonosseous hemangiomas are also part of the Maffucci syndrome, which includes skeletal chondromatosis.

Roentgenologic Features

Hemangiomas in vertebrae characteristically cause rarefaction with exaggerated vertical striations or a coarse honeycombed appearance. In the skull, hemangiomas produce a well-circumscribed zone of rarefaction, which may have a honeycombed appearance and is often associated with outward expansion of the bony profile. This expanded zone may show striations of bone radiating outward from the center of the lesion. In other bones, hemangiomas produce rarefactions that may have features like those described above. When hemangioma of soft tissues coexist, it may contain phleboliths. The defects in diffuse skeletal hemangiomatosis often contain sclerotic foci. Massive osteolysis does not respect boundaries, and adjacent bones often disappear. A diagnostic sign is a tapering down of the bone at the edge of the zone of complete resorption. Diffuse hemangiomas, especially when they involve more than one bone, may produce a pattern much like that of massive osteolysis.

Localized hemangiomas of soft tissues in a periosteal location are associated, in rare instances, with considerable sclerosis and deformity of nearby but uninvolved bone.

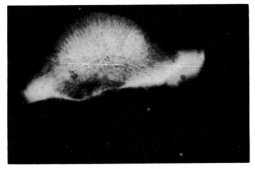 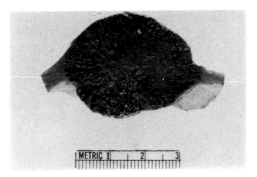

Figure 12-2. *Left.* Roentgenogram of hemangioma excised from calvarium. Expansion inwardly as well as outwardly has occurred, and striations are prominent. *Right.* Specimen of same hemangioma, showing honeycombing and radiating spicules of bone.

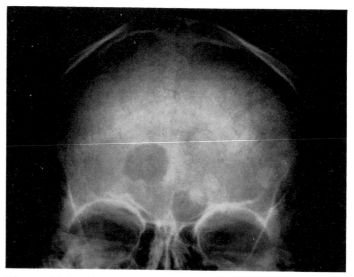

Figure 12-3. Characteristic, fairly sharply delimited defect produced by cavernous hemangioma of skull. Although sunburst appearance has been attributed to hemangiomas that have expanded bone, such an ominous appearance has been unusual in the experience of the Mayo Clinic.

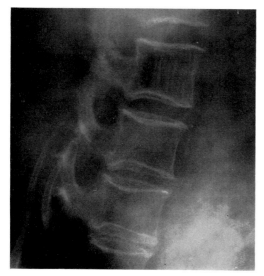

Figure 12-4. Rarefaction of vertebral body with exaggerated vertical striation, changes commonly attributed to hemangioma in this location. (Reproduced with permission from: Pugh, D. G.: *Roentgenologic Diagnosis of Diseases of Bones.* Baltimore, Williams & Wilkins, 1954, pp. 559AS-559AV.)

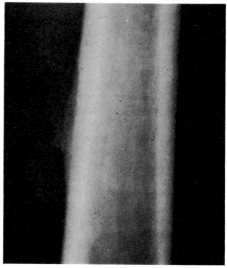

Figure 12-5. Painful subperiosteal cavernous hemangioma near midshaft of femur. In this unusual location, lesion has eroded cortex slightly and caused some reactive new bone.

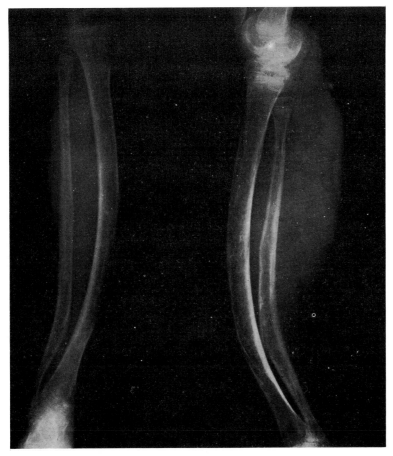

Figure 12-6. Massive diffuse hemangioma of deep soft tissues of leg associated with multicentric cavernous hemangioma of tibia, fibula, and bones of foot in eight-year-old girl. Amputation was necessary because of increasing disability and failure to control tumor by other means.

Gross Pathology

On exposure, a hemangioma is likely to be blue, and a honeycombed feature may be obvious. A firm, fleshy appearance without obvious vessels suggests that one is dealing with a cellular and possibly malignant tumor. Bony trabeculae may be produced and even give the "sunburst" effect.

Histopathology

Interpretation of vascular lesions of bone is complicated by the difficulty in knowing when a conglomeration of vascular channels is a hemangioma instead of a hamartomatous malformation. Assessing the literature is made all but impossible because of the large number of unconvincing photomicrographs. If the blood has escaped, hemangioma can simulate lymphangioma to further complicate the problem. In fact, hemangioma and lymphangioma may coexist as I have observed in examples of massive osteolysis. Most hemangiomas of bone are basically cavernous, although sometimes a capillary component is present and may even be dominant.

Some angiosarcomas of bone with their component of spindle-shaped vasoformative cells are readily recognizable as such, but the borderline between benign and malignant capillary proliferations is not always easily drawn.

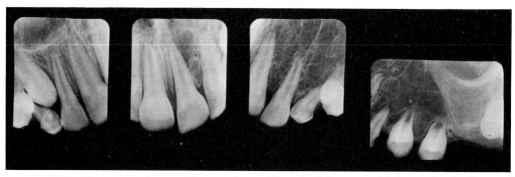

Figure 12-7. Cavernous hemangioma of maxilla of eight-year-old boy who had noted swelling for eight months. Tumor bled freely during thorough curettage of angiomatous spongy bone. Patient was well sixteen years after this treatment. (From: Lund, B. A., and Dahlin, D. C.: *J. Oral Surg. 22,* 3:234-242, 1964. Copyright by the American Dental Association. Reprinted by permission.)

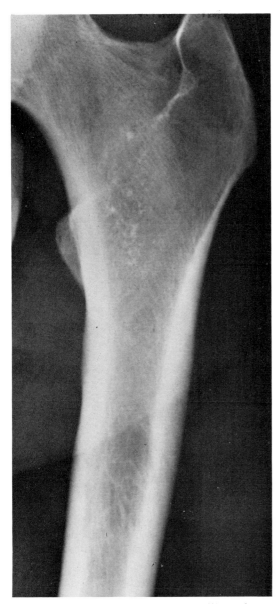

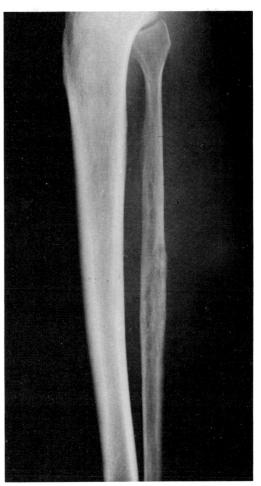

Figure 12-8. Cavernous and capillary hemangioma in forty-one-year-old woman, producing central rarefaction. Thorough curettage was followed by pathologic fracture that healed, and patient was well one year later.

Figure 12-9. Cavernous hemangioma of middle portion of fibula of fifty-two-year-old woman. Lesion was resected because it produced pain, and it was considered to be probably reticulum cell sarcoma. Patient was well eleven years later.

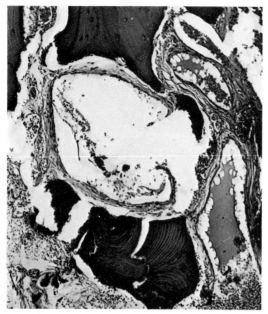

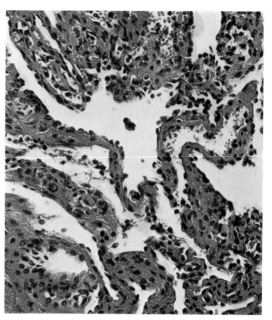

Figure 12-10. Cavernous hemangioma of skull. Thin-walled large blood vessels are interspersed among osseous trabeculae. (×95) This is same case as that represented in Figure 12-3.

Figure 12-11. Mixed capillary and cavernous hemangioma that had expanded ascending ramus of mandible. This lesion was originally classed erroneously as hemangiopericytoma. (×200)

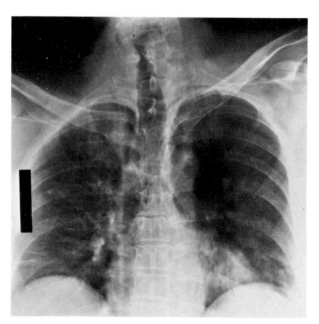

Figure 12-12. Hemangioma of vertebral bodies, especially T3 through T6 in fifty-nine-year-old man who had had biopsy-demonstrated tumor in this location ten years previously. Symptoms were mainly pain and numbness and were slowly progressing.

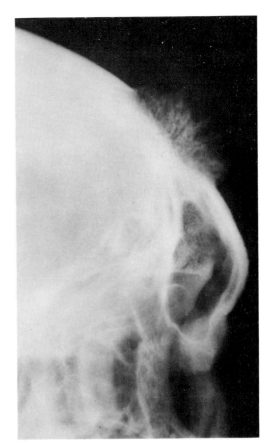

Figure 12-13. Capillary and cavernous hemangioma that had produced tumefaction for five years in seventy-year-old man. Patient died of unrelated disease seven years after excision of hemangioma.

Figure 12-14. "Phantom" or "disappearing" bone disease also called "massive osteolysis." Twenty-seven-year-old woman had pathologic fracture of rib. Eight years after onset, having lost all or part of most of her right ribs and ninth, tenth, and eleventh thoracic vertebrae, she died from the effects of this destruction of her thoracic cage.

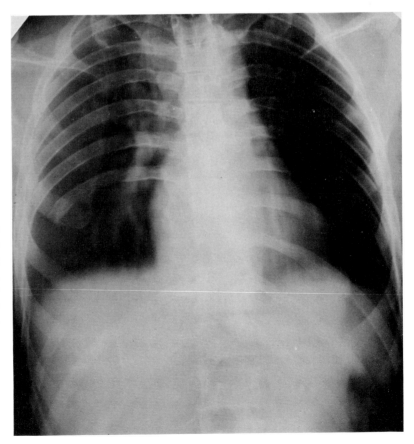

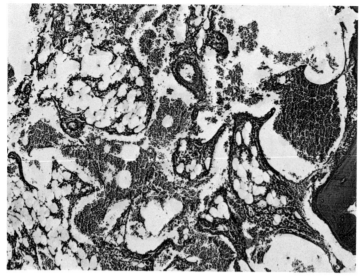

Figure 12-15. "Phantom" bone disease. This cavernous hemangioma pattern was found in one of the ribs procured for biopsy in case illustrated in Figure 12-14. This histologic appearance is characteristic of that found routinely in massive osteolysis or "phantom" bone disease. (×65)

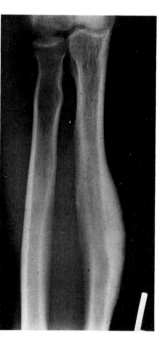

Figure 12-17. Local swelling had been noted by twenty-three-year-old man for eleven years. Sclerosis of ulna was non-neoplastic, and response to benign cavernous hemangioma 1 by 1.5 by 1.5 cm in adjacent periosteal tissues. Marked alteration of adjacent bone has been seen with various soft-tissue neoplasms including hemangioma.

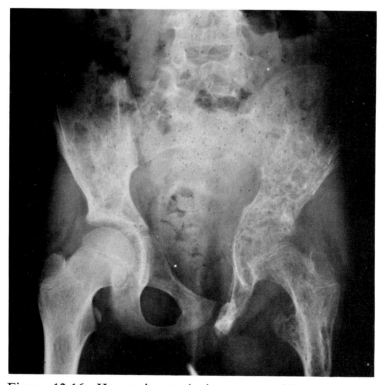

Figure 12-16. Hemangiomatosis in ten-year-old boy. Patient had skeletal and soft-tissue hemangiomas that had necessitated amputation below left knee. His problem illustrates relationship of hemangiomas to massive osteolysis (Gorham's disease).

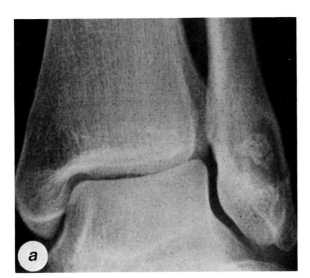

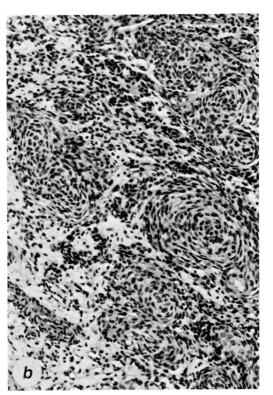

Figure 12-18. *a.* Glomus tumor in distal shaft of fibula of twenty-one-year-old woman. Patient had no complaints twenty-two months after its excision. *b.* Tumor is composed of whorls of slightly spindling benign cells often disposed around capillaries. Central density seen by x-ray is not explained. (×250) (Case contributed by Doctor P. Mao of Phoenix, Arizona.)

Treatment

Hemangiomas usually respond well to conservative surgical procedures. Radiation may be required for lesions that are in inaccessible sites. The unpredictable course of massive osteolysis has made the results of treatment difficult to assess, but reconstructive surgical procedures and radiation have been employed. The reader is referred to pertinent references in this chapter for additional information.

Bibliography

1942 Thomas, A.: Vascular Tumors of Bone: A Pathological and Clinical Study of Twenty-seven Cases. *Surg Gynecol Obstet 74:*777-795.

1954 Pugh, D. G.: *Roentgenologic Diagnosis of Diseases of Bones.* Baltimore, Williams & Wilkins, pp. 559AS-559AV.

1955 Gorham, L. W., and Stout, A. P.: Massive Osteolysis (Acute Spontaneous Absorption of Bone, Phantom Bone, Disappearing Bone): Its Relation to Hemangiomatosis. *J Bone Joint Surg, 37A:*985-1004.

1955 Cohen, J., and Craig, J. M.: Multiple Lymphangiectases of Bone. *J Bone Joint Surg, 37A:*585-596.

1957 Kleinsasser, O., and Albrecht, H.: Die Hämangiome und Osteohämangiome der Schädelknochen. *Langenbecks Arch Chir, 285:*115-133.

1958 Jaffe, H. L.: *Tumors and Tumorous Conditions of the Bones and Joints.* Philadelphia, Lea & Febiger, pp. 224, 341.

1961 Hayes, J. T., and Brody, G. L.: Cystic Lymphangiectasis of Bone: A Case Report. *J Bone Joint Surg, 43A:*107-117 (January).

1961 Koblenzer, P. J., and Bukowski, M. J.: Angiomatosis (Hamartomatous Hem-lymph-angiomatosis): Report of a Case With Diffuse Involvement. *Pediatrics, 28:*65-76 (July).

1961 Krueger, E. G., Sobel, G. L., and Weinstein, C.: Vertebral Hemangioma With Compression of Spinal Cord. *J Neurosurg, 18:*331-338.

1961 Lidholm, S.-O., Lindbom, A., and Spjut, H. J.: Multiple Capillary Hemangiomas of the Bones of the Foot. *Acta Pathol Microbiol Scand, Fasc. 1, 51:*9-16.

1961 Sherman, R. S., and Wilner, D.: The Roentgen Diagnosis of Hemangioma of Bone. *Am J Roentgenol, 86:*1146-1159.

1962 Goidanich, I. F., and Campanacci, M.: Vascular Hamartomata and Infantile Angio-ectatic Osteohyperplasia of the Extremities. *J Bone Joint Surg, 44A:*815-842.

1962 Spjut, H. J., and Lindbom, A.: Skeletal Angiomatosis. Report of Two Cases. *Acta Pathol Microbiol Scand, Fasc. 1, 55:*49-58.

1962 Hartmann, W. H., and Stewart, F. W.: Hemangioendothelioma of Bone. Unusual Tumor Characterized by Indolent Course. *Cancer, 15:*846-854.

1964 Halliday, D. R., Dahlin, D. C., Pugh, D. G., and Young, H. H.: Massive Osteolysis and Angiomatosis. *Radiology, 82:*637-644.

1964 Lund, B. A., and Dahlin, D. C.: Hemangiomas of the Mandible and Maxilla. *J Oral Surg, 22:*234-242.

1964 Wallis, L. A., Asch, T., and Maisel, B. W.: Diffuse Skeletal Hemangiomatosis. Report of Two Cases and Review of Literature. *Am J Med, 37:*545-563.

1965 Bundens, W. D., Jr., and Brighton, C. T.: Malignant Hemangioendothelioma of Bone. Report of Two Cases and Review of the Literature. *J Bone Joint Surg, 47A:*762-772.

1969 Campanacci, M., Cenni, F., and Giunti, A.: Angectasie, Amartomi, e Neoplasmi Vascolari dello Scheletro ("Angiomi," Emangioendotelioma, Emangiosarcoma). *Chir Organi Mov, 58:*472-496.

1971 Dorfman, H. D., Steiner, G. C., and Jaffe, H. L.: Vascular Tumors of Bone. *Hum Pathol, 2:*349-376 (September).

1971 Unni, K. K., Ivins, J. C., Beabout, J. W., and Dahlin, D. C.: Hemangioma, Hemangiopericytoma, and Hemangioendothelioma (Angiosarcoma) of Bone. *Cancer, 27:*1403-1414 (June).

1973 Brower, A. C., Culver, J. E., Jr., and Keats, T. E.: Diffuse Cystic Angiomatosis of Bone: Report of Two Cases. *Am J Roentgenol, 118:*456-463 (June).

1974 Asch, M. J., Cohen, A. H., and Moore, T. C.: Hepatic and Splenic Lymphangiomatosis With Skeletal Involvement: Report of a Case and Review of the Literature. *Surgery, 76:*334-339 (August).

1976 Sugiura, I.: Intra-osseous Glomus Tumor: A Case Report. *J Bone Joint Surg, 58B:*245-247 (May).

Chapter 13

Lipoma and Liposarcoma

DESPITE THE ABUNDANCE of adipose connective tissue in bone marrow, lipomas of bone are extremely rare. Moorefield and coworkers collected twenty-six cases from the literature in 1976. Lipomas of soft tissues adjacent to bone, sometimes even apparently arising in or under the periosteum, may cause erosion of bone, but such is rare. Discrete, small collections of adipose connective tissue that might possibly be considered neoplastic are sometimes seen in vertebrae.

Liposarcoma of bone can occur. Schwartz and coworkers described the fourteenth probable or proved case in the literature in 1970. Goldman in 1964 described a case and accepted only three of those reported after Dawson's study as being adequately documented. No unequivocal liposarcoma of bone was found in the present series. In one case, there was extensive malignant destruction of a humerus by liposarcoma, but the patient had a large retroperitoneal mass that may have been the primary site. Liposarcomas of soft-tissue origin sometimes produce skeletal metastasis that may mimic primary sarcoma of bone.

Tumors containing the large, sometimes vacuolated, pleomorphic cells that make one think of liposarcoma have been included among the osteosarcomas or the fibrous histiocytomas in the Mayo Clinic series. This was done because foci of simi-

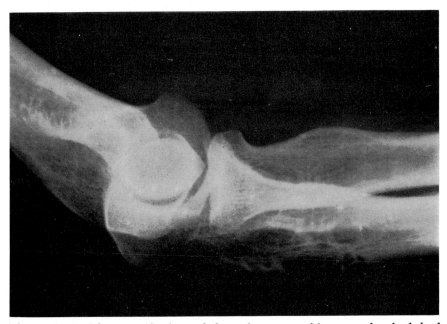

Figure 13-1. Lipoma of ulna of forty-four-year-old man who had had a lump in region of involvement for thirty years. He had no complaints referable to the lesion. Roentgenologist interpreted process as probably neoplastic and suggested possibility of its being malignant. (Reproduced with permission from: Caruolo, J. E., and Dahlin, D. C.: *Proc Staff Meet Mayo Clin*, 28:361-363, 1953.)

149

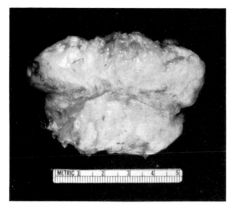

Figure 13-2. *Above.* Lipoma excised from region of involvement shown in Figure 13-1. Tumor was found beneath periosteum and had produced irregular, partially loculated erosion of cortex.

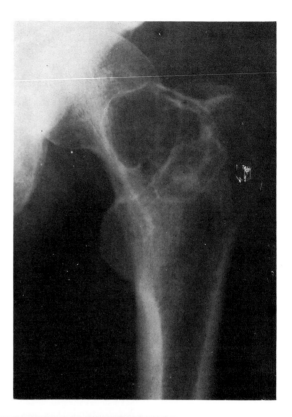

Figure 13-3. *Right.* Lipoma of neck and trochanteric region of femur. Note sclerotic discrete borders. This occurred in sixty-two-year-old man who had had hip pain for five months. Patient was well four years after curettage and bone grafting. (Case contributed by Doctor J. A. Holbert of Coos Bay, Oregon.)

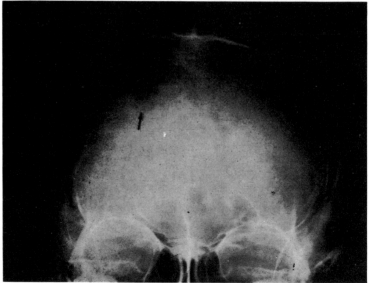

Figure 13-4. Lipoma involving left frontal bone of thirty-one-year-old man. This lesion, which was 1.5 by 1.5 by 0.4 cm when excised, was apparently an incidental finding on roentgenogram taken because of patient's complaint of headache of two years' duration.

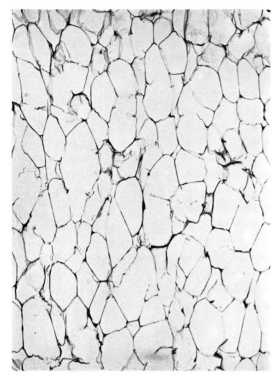

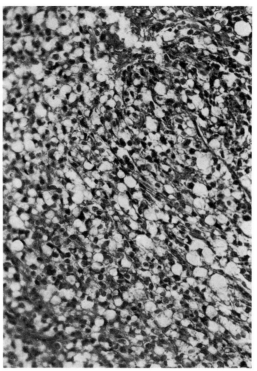

Figure 13-5. Typical histologic appearance of lipoma is representative of tissue seen in cases depicted in Figures 13-1, 13-2, 13-3, and 13-4. (×120)

Figure 13-6. Liposarcoma that had destroyed upper half of right humerus of thirty-eight-year old woman. She also had an abdominal mass that may have been the primary site. Vacuolated cells took a strongly positive stain for fat. (×200)

lar pleomorphic cells occur in many tumors that are obviously osteosarcomas and in others that fit the current criteria for malignant fibrous histiocytoma.

Only five lipomas were found in this total series of bone tumors, making the incidence less than 1 per 1,000 cases. Two of the lesions produced radiolucent zones, each 1.5 cm in maximal diameter, in a parietal and a frontal bone respectively. The third lesion may have represented merely a localized focus of osteoporosis. It had produced a poorly defined 4 by 3 cm region of rarefaction visible in the roentgenogram of the upper part of the shaft of a femur. The fourth, illustrated in Figures 13-1 and 13-2, was located beneath the periosteum of the ulna. The fifth lesion was in a rib. The ages of the five patients (three men and two women) ranged from thirty-one to seventy-one years. Four of the lipomas were incidental findings, but the ulnar example produced a mass.

Treatment

Treatment of the rare lipoma that one may encounter in bone should be conservative. The necessity for surgical intervention is ordinarily dictated by failure to make a correct preoperative diagnosis.

The available evidence indicates that prompt ablative surgical treatment is the one of choice for liposarcoma. There are too few reported cases to provide statistics on prognosis.

Bibliography

1953 Fairbank, H. A. T.: A Parosteal Lipoma. *J Bone Joint Surg, 35B:*589.

1953 Caruolo, J. E., and Dahlin, D. C.: Lipoma Involving Bone and Simulating Malignant Bone Tumor: Report of Case. *Proc Staff Meet Mayo Clin, 28:*361-363.

1955 Child, P. L.: Lipoma of the Os Calcis: Report of a Case. *Am J Clin Pathol, 25:*1050-1052.

1955 Dawson, E. K.: Liposarcoma of Bone. *J Pathol Bacteriol, 70:*513-520.

1956 Mastragostino, S.: Tumori Lipoblastici Primitivi dello Scheletro. *Chir Organi Mov, 44:*18-36.

1957 Mastromarino, R., and Assennato, G.: Lipoma intraosseo. *Ortop Traumatol, 25:*1077-1084.

1957 Newman, C. W.: Fibrolipoma of the Mandible. Report of Case. *J Oral Surg, 15:*251-252.

1957 Smith, W. E., and Fienberg, R.: Intraosseous Lipoma of Bone. *Cancer, 10:*1151-1152.

1957 Skinner, B. G., and Fraser, R. G.: Medullary Lipoma of Bone. *J Can Assoc Radiol, 8:*19-21.

1959 Kauffman, S. L., and Stout, A. P.: Lipoblastic Tumors of Children. *Cancer, 12:*912-925.

1961 Retz, L. D.: Primary Liposarcoma of Bone. Report of a Case and Review of the Literature. *J Bone Joint Surg, 43A:*123-129.

1962 Fleming, R. J., Alpert, M., and Garcia, A.: Parosteal Lipoma. *Am J Roentgenol, 87:*1075-1084.

1963 Catto, M., and Stevens, J.: Liposarcoma of Bone. *J Pathol Bacteriol, 86:*248-253.

1964 Moon, N., and Marmor, L.: Parosteal Lipoma of the Proximal Part of the Radius. A Clinical Entity With Frequent Radial-Nerve Injury. *J Bone Joint Surg, 46A:*608-614.

1964 Goldman, R. L.: Primary Liposarcoma of Bone. Report of a Case. *Am J Clin Pathol, 42:*503-508.

1965 Salzer, M., and Salzer-Kuntschik, M.: Zur Frage der Sogenannten Zentralen Knochenlipome. *Beitr Pathol Anat, 132:*365-375 (December).

1968 Ross, C. F., and Hadfield, G.: Primary Osteo-Liposarcoma of Bone (Malignant Mesenchyoma): Report of a Case. *J Bone Joint Surg, 50B:*639-643 (August).

1970 Schwartz, A., Shuster, M., and Becker, S. M.: Liposarcoma of Bone: Report of a Case and Review of the Literature. *J Bone Joint Surg, 52A:*171-177 (January).

1974 Freiberg, R. A., Air, G. W., Glueck, C. J., Ishikawa, T., and Abrams, N. R.: Intraosseous Lipomas With Type-IV Hyperlipoproteinemia: A Case Report. *J Bone Joint Surg, 56A:*1729-1732 (December).

1976 Moorefield, W. G., Jr., Urbaniak, J. R., and Gonzalvo, A. A. A.: Intramedullary Lipoma of the Distal Femur. *South Med J, 69:*1210-1211 (September).

Chapter 14

Neurilemmoma and Related Tumors

NEUROGENIC TUMORS of bone are rare. Thirty-six well-documented cases of neurilemmoma arising in bone were collected from the literature and their own material by Fawcett and coworkers in 1967. The foci with myxoid change and lipid-laden histiocytes interspersed with fibrogenic cells, often showing pallisading of nuclei, usually but not always distinguishes neurilemmoma from the neurofibroma characteristic of Recklinghausen's disease.

Neurofibromatosis was associated with various skeletal changes that occurred in approximately half of a large group of cases studied at the Mayo Clinic by Hunt and Pugh in 1961. These changes included erosive defects in bone caused by contiguous neurogenic tumors, disorders of bone growth associated with hypertrophy of overlying soft tissues, dysplasia of vertebral bodies with scoliosis, defects of the posterior orbital wall, congenital bowing, and pseudarthrosis. Intraosseous neurofibromas are distinctly rare. Some of the osseous defects described in patients with Recklinghausen's disease have been coincidental, unrelated processes.

Malignant tumors of neurogenic origin (malignant schwannomas) have rarely been described as arising in bone, and the evidence in reported cases is not alto-

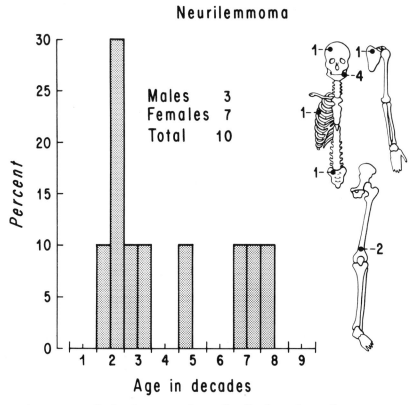

Figure 14-1. Skeletal, age, and sex distribution of neurilemmomas.

gether convincing. The inherent characteristics of a malignant growth make it difficult to verify the exact tissue of origin in a questionable case. Gross relationship to a nerve is important in establishing the neurogenic origin of a sarcoma. In any event, the problem is academic since the treatment for such a sarcoma would be the same as for fibrosarcoma of bone.

Incidence

Neurilemmoma is a rare primary bone tumor. These ten cases accounted for less than 1 percent of the primary benign tumors of bone in our series.

Sex

Seven of the ten patients were female.

Age

A wide age range was represented, but four of the patients were in the second decade of life.

Localization

Four of the tumors were in the mandible, and the remainder affected a wide variety of bones. The marked mandibular predilection mirrors the reported experience with this tumor, with nearly half of the reported neurilemmomas involving this bone.

Symptoms

Many neurilemmomas of bone are asymptomatic, a few produce significant pain, and some result in local tumefaction.

Physical Findings

There are no specific features unless the patient has neurofibromatosis.

Roentgenographic Features

Well-defined cystlike rarefactions, sometimes with a slightly sclerotic border, are produced by neurilemmomas. When in a major tubular bone, these rarefactions occur typically in the shaft and often near its end. Sometimes the defect appears to be bubbly because of irregular corrugations of the wall of the cavity housing the lesion. In neurofibromatosis, an elongated defect occurs in the course of an affected nerve.

Gross Pathology

Material removed from a neurilemmoma of bone, like that of its soft-tissue counterpart, is a relatively firm mass of fibroblastic tissue. It may be somewhat gelatinous or myxoid, and yellow or brownish discoloration is sometimes present. Re-

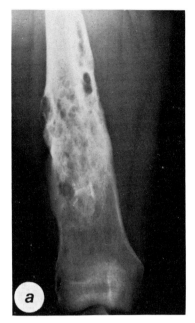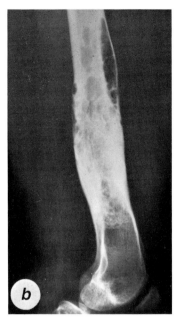

Figure 14-2. *a* and *b*. Neurilemmoma extensively involving shaft of femur of sixteen-year-old girl. Four and one-half years earlier, she had suffered a fracture through a cystlike defect in area; defect was slightly smaller than the lesion shown. This tumor was not treated and showed essentially no progression 1.5 years later.

lationship to a nerve or its canal, if such can be established, is an important diagnostic feature. The lesion may be partially cystic.

Histopathology

The component spindling cells are basically fibrogenic. Pallisading as in Figures 14-3 and 14-5 is characteristic but may be found only with some difficulty. The lesion may contain prominent areas of myxoid-appearing cells with a sprinkling of mononuclear, sometimes histiocytic, chronic inflammatory cells. As with neurilemmomas of soft-tissue localization, the nuclei may be irregular in size, dark-staining, and bizarre probably owing to degeneration. Although these nuclei may strongly suggest that the lesion is malignant, the virtual absence of mitotic figures and the benign roentgenographic appearance indicate the benign quality of the neoplasm.

Secondary bony changes due to erosion by a neurilemmoma of soft-tissue origin, especially along the spinal column or in the cranium, are sometimes seen.

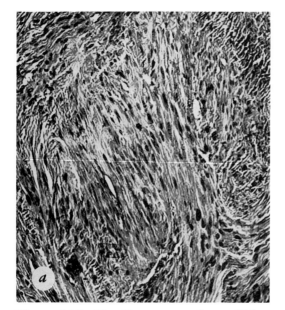
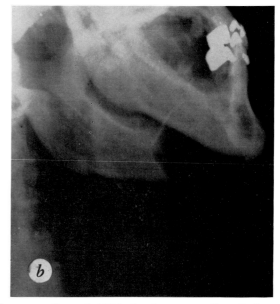

Figure 14-3. Neurilemmoma of mandible. *a.* Tissue section. (×180) *b.* An expanding lesion is evident. This neurilemmoma was found in sixty-four-year-old woman, and clinical history suggested that it had been present for twenty years.

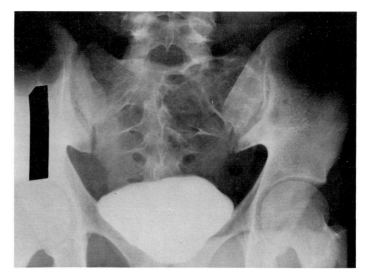

Figure 14-4. Neurilemmoma of sacrum occurred in sixteen-year-old boy who had had leg-length discrepancy for four years (short left leg) and slight back pain for three months. He was well 2.5 years after excision of the lesion.

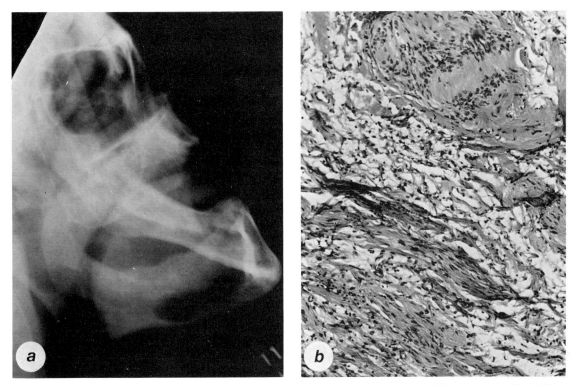

Figure 14-5. *a*. Neurilemmoma in mandibular canal in sixty-five-year-old man with Reckling-hausen's neurofibromatosis. Lesion surrounded nerve. *b*. Features of neurofibroma were present in part of tumor. (×100)

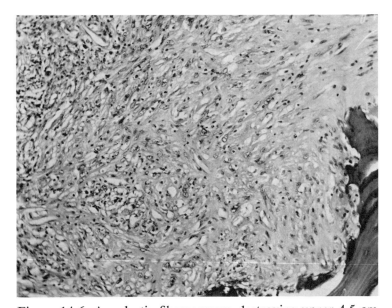

Figure 14-6. Anaplastic fibrosarcoma destroying upper 4.5 cm of left tibial metaphysis and epiphysis of sixty-six-year-old woman with neurofibromatosis. There were no histologic stigmata to prove whether sarcoma was neurofibrosarcoma or an incidental fibrosarcoma, not neurofibroma related. (×160)

Treatment

Conservative local removal is indicated. Stigmata of neurofibromatosis may dictate the amount of tissue that should be removed.

Prognosis

A good result is to be expected. The consequence of neurofibromatosis, if that disease is present, may influence the long-term results.

Bibliography

1934 Peers, J. H.: Primary Intramedullary Neurogenic Sarcoma of the Ulna. Report of a Case. *Am J Pathol, 10:*811-819.

1939 Gross, P., Bailey, F. R., and Jacox, M. W.: Primary Intramedullary Neurofibroma of the Humerus. *Arch Pathol, 28:*716-718.

1940 De Santo, D. A., and Burgess, E.: Primary and Secondary Neurilemmoma of Bone. *Surg Gynecol Obstet, 71:*454-461.

1943 Green, W. T., and Rudo, N.: Pseudarthrosis and Neurofibromatosis. *Arch Surg, 46:*639-651.

1950 McCarroll, H. R.: Clinical Manifestations of Congenital Neurofibromatosis. *J Bone Joint Surg, 32A:*601-617.

1952 Güthert, H.: Ein Malignes Neurinom des Knochens. *Zentralbl Allg Pathol, 88:*185-188.

1953 Jones, H. M.: Neurilemmoma of Bone. *Br J Surg, 41:*63-65.

1953 Adams, J. P., and Golden, J. L.: Fibrous Lesions of Bone. *South Med J, 46:*529-536.

1954 Bruce, K. W.: Solitary Neurofibroma (Neurilemmoma, Schwannoma) of the Oral Cavity. *Oral Surg, 7:*1150-1159.

1957 Wilber, M. C., and Woodcock, J. A.: Ganglioneuromata in Bone. *J Bone Joint Surg, 39A:*1385-1388.

1958 Jaffe, H. L.: *Tumors and Tumorous Conditions of the Bones and Joints.* Philadelphia, Lea & Febiger, pp. 240-255.

1960 Samter, T. G., Vellios, F., and Shafer, W. G.: Neurilemmoma of Bone. Report of 3 Cases with a Review of the Literature. *Radiology, 75:*215-222.

1961 Hunt, J. C., and Pugh, D. G.: Skeletal Lesions in Neurofibromatosis. *Radiology, 76:*1-20.

1962 Ackerman, L. V., and Spjut, H. J.: Tumors of Bone and Cartilage. In *Atlas of Tumor Pathology,* Section II, Fascicle 4. Washington, D.C., Armed Forces Institute of Pathology, National Research Council, pp. 247-249.

1967 Fawcett, K. J., and Dahlin, D. C.: Neurilemmoma of Bone. *Am J Clin Pathol, 47:*759-766 (June).

1974 Vicas, E., Bourdua, S., and Charest, F.: Le Neurilemmome du Sacrum: Présentation d'un Cas. *Union Med Can, 103:*1057-1060 (June).

1975 Polkey, C. E.: Intraosseous Neurilemmoma of the Cervical Spine Causing Paraparesis and Treated by Resection and Grafting. *J Neurol Neurosurg Psychiatry, 38:*776-781 (August).

1976 Gordon, E. J.: Solitary Intraosseous Neurilemmoma of the Tibia: Review of Intraosseous Neurilemmoma and Neurofibroma. *Clin Orthop, 117:*271-282 (June).

Chapter 15

Myeloma

THIS TUMOR of hematopoietic derivation is the most common neoplasm of bone in the present series. Furthermore, its relative incidence is increasing; nearly 53 percent of the 1,812 patients with malignant bone tumors seen and verified pathologically at the Mayo Clinic in the 11 years from 1964 through 1975 had myeloma. This neoplasm is composed of plasma cells showing variable degrees of differentiation. The neoplastic process is usually multicentric and often involves bone marrow so diffusely that it may be diagnosed in the great majority of cases by marrow aspiration.

Most patients with myeloma have predominant hematologic problems, and their therapy is managed by hematologists or by cancer chemotherapists and radiotherapists. The discussion in this chapter is oriented toward the problems as encountered in surgical material. The complex hematologic and protein disturbances will not be elaborated, but some of the pertinent literature is indicated in the bibliography.

Extraskeletal infiltrates of myeloma cells in a wide variety of tissues may occur in patients with multiple myeloma, but they are rarely a prominent feature. The tumors of solitary extramedullary myeloma (plasmacytoma), of which nearly 80 percent occur in the upper air passages and oral cavity, is curable in most cases by local therapy, which has included electrocoagulation, excision, irradiation, or combinations of these. Some patients with these extramedullary plasma cell tumors develop multiple myeloma.

Renal involvement with manifestations of renal insufficiency is an important complication of myeloma that may be the immediate cause of death. Not myelomatous infiltration, but blockage of the tubules by proteinaceous casts is the usual histologic finding. Much less important is the occasional development of renal amyloidosis, "metastatic" calcification of the kidneys in those with severe skeletal demineralization, or pyelonephritis.

"Solitary" Myeloma

Occasionally, one sees a single osseous focus of myeloma that is associated with normal sternal marrow and with few or none of the abnormal laboratory findings so characteristic of multiple myeloma. Patients with such lesions usually develop multiple myeloma, but sometimes only after a latent period of five to ten years or even longer. Some become long-term "cures." "Solitary" myeloma in bone must be distinguished from a focus of chronic osteomyelitis with abundant plasma cells. The distinction is aided by the proliferation of fibroblasts and capillaries as part of the response to inflammation and the sprinkling of polymorphonuclear leukocytes and histiocytes in the latter condition.

Myeloma

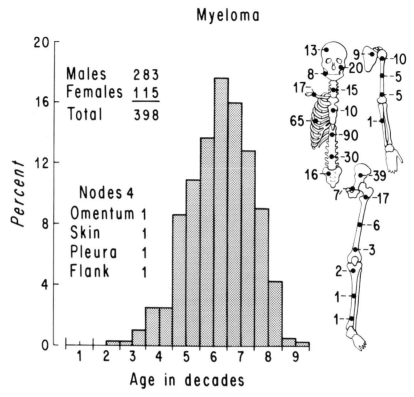

Males 283
Females 115
Total 398

Nodes 4
Omentum 1
Skin 1
Pleura 1
Flank 1

Percent

Age in decades

Figure 15-1. Skeletal, age, and sex distribution of 398 surgical cases (1,847 cases diagnosed by marrow aspiration not included).

Incidence

The total of 2,245 myelomas of bone comprised 47 percent of the malignant bone tumors in this series. The major reasons for operation in the surgical series included the presence of an indeterminate osseous lesion or compression of the spinal cord.

Sex

Of the 398 patients who underwent surgery, 71 percent were men.

Age

The well-known rarity of myeloma before the fifth decade of life was shown in this series. Essentially, the same percentage of lesions considered to be "solitary" were in patients less than fifty years old, as in the overall group. Of the twenty-eight patients with myeloma of jaw bones, the youngest were two patients in the third decade of life.

Localization

The bones that contain hematopoietic marrow in adults harbor most of the recognizable myeloma nodules. Although the data tabulated above are selected, since they are based on surgical cases only, the distribution shown is similar to that observed at autopsy except that the skull is usually involved by the time myeloma has caused the patient's death. The group of "solitary" myelomas had a skeletal distribution much like that depicted above, but 55 percent of eighty-seven cases were vertebral examples, indicating a predilection for this area. In a few of those listed as maxillary tumors, it was difficult to be certain that the neoplasm began in bone.

Symptoms

Pain of an increasing nature is the most common complaint of patients with myeloma, and it is most often centered in the lumbar or thoracic spinal regions. On the average, the pain is of less than six months' duration before the time the patient is admitted, but sometimes it has been present for several years. Weakness and loss of weight occur during the course of the disease in nearly every case of myeloma. Pathologic fracture, with abrupt onset of symptoms, is common, and most such fractures involve the vertebral column. Neurologic symptoms, usually from disease of the spinal cord or nerve roots secondary to pathologic fracture or extraosseus extension of the neoplastic tissue, are frequently observed. Complaints referable to renal involvement may be encountered. Less common symptoms include palpable tumor, hemorrhagic tendency, anemia, and fever. It is not uncommon for myeloma to produce features of an intrathoracic tumor by extension from a nearby osseous focus.

In rare instances, other neoplasms coexist with myeloma, and myeloma is occasionally familial.

Physical and Laboratory Findings

Physical findings may reflect secondary changes resulting from generalized malignant disease with replacement of bone marrow. Local pain or tenderness, with or without palpable tumor, and neurologic dysfunction may be elicited.

Smears of peripheral blood often show excessive rouleau formation and have been reported as containing myeloma cells in from 10 to 73 percent of cases. Rarely, plasma cell leukemia develops. Generally, there is moderate to severe anemia. Erythrocyte sedimentation rate is notoriously rapid. Hypercalcemia occurs in from 20 to 50 percent of patients. Eventually, Bence Jones proteinuria can be found in more than half of the patients. Evidences of renal insufficiency or amyloidosis, which may be generalized, sometimes develop. Levels of serum alkaline phosphatase are rarely elevated.

Electrophoretic studies of serum and urinary proteins provide critical diagnostic information because of elevation of various globulin fractions. Kyle, in a study of 869 cases, found skeletal roentgenographic abnormalities in 79 percent. Serum protein electrophoresis showed a spike in 76 percent, hypogammaglobulinemia in 9 percent, and minor or no abnormalities in 15 percent; a globulin spike was seen in 75 percent of urinary electrophoretic patterns. Serum immunoelectrophoresis revealed only a monoclonal heavy chain in 83 percent and a monoclonal light chain in 8 percent (Bence Jones proteinemia). Amyloidosis was found in 7 percent of the patients. There is an interrelationship among amyloidosis, Waldenströms macroglobulinemia, and myeloma. The complexities of these protein studies have been elaborated by Osserman and Takatsuki (1963).

Roentgenologic Features

These features result from replacement of osseous structures by the myelomatous masses. The first and most extensive changes usually occur in the ribs, vertebrae, skull, and pelvis. Classically there are "punched-out" areas of bone destruction that vary up to 5 cm in diameter and about which there is no surrounding zone of sclerosis. Expansion of the affected bone may produce a "ballooned-out" appearance, especially in the ribs. Variable osteoporosis is common, and pathologic fracture, especially of vertebrae, is often seen. From 12 to 25 percent of patients with myeloma have no discernible foci of bone destruction. Some of these, on close scrutiny, will be found to have diffuse demineralization of portions of the skeleton. Metastatic carcinoma, reticulum cell sarcoma, and hyperparathyroidism can produce bone lesions that simulate those of myeloma. "Solitary" myeloma lesions of bone are classically destructive, but they too may produce expansion of the bone's contour. Only three patients in this series had sclerosing lesions. Predominantly sclerosing lesions in myeloma are extremely rare. Pugh has stated that sclerosing areas in the roentgenogram of a patient with myeloma are usually due to some process other than myeloma. Osteosclerotic myeloma may be associated with peripheral neuropathy.

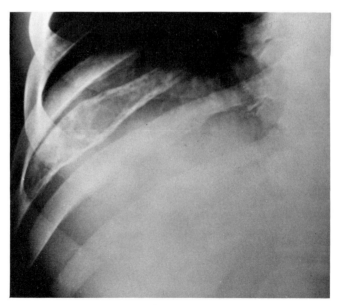

Figure 15-2. "Solitary" myeloma expanding the rib of forty-five-year-old man. Patient was well ten years after resection of this tumor.

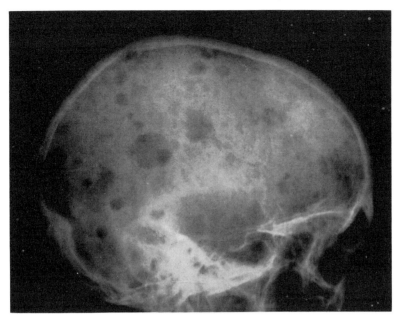

Figure 15-3. Myeloma in one of the most commonly affected sites. There are numerous discrete foci of osseous destruction.

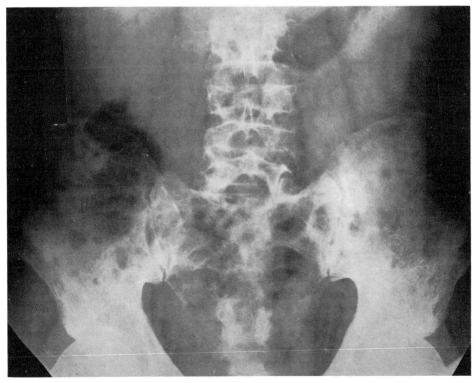

Figure 15-4. Another classic example of multiple myeloma. As in preceding illustration, discrete foci of rarefaction are not associated with sclerosis of bone. (Reproduced with permission from: Pugh, D. G.: *Roentgenologic Diagnosis of Diseases of Bones*. Baltimore, Williams & Wilkins, 1954, pp. 487-492.)

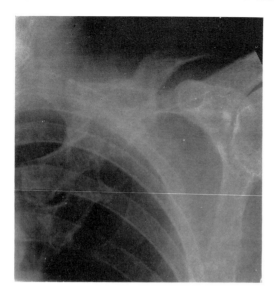

Figure 15-5. *Left.* Expansile lesion of clavicle. This proved to be myeloma of the "solitary" type. A fracture, apparently pathologic, occurred through this region in September 1950 and again in January 1953. Clavicle was excised in April 1953. Patient died of unrelated cause and without evidence of myeloma fourteen years later, at age seventy-two years. *Below.* Excised specimen from case illustrated at left.

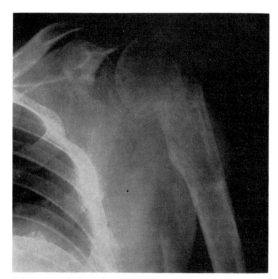

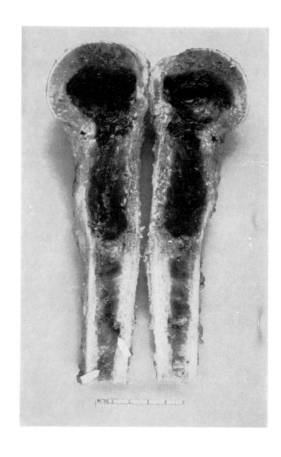

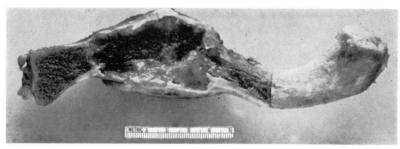

Figure 15-6. *Above.* Destruction of humerus produced by "solitary" myeloma. Forequarter amputation was performed on November 11, 1953. Sixteen months later, signs of dissemination were present. An erroneous diagnosis of reticulum cell sarcoma was made at time of amputation. *Right.* Gross specimen in same case. This lesion dramatically demonstrated occasional difficult problem of differentiating myeloma from reticulum cell sarcoma. *See also* Figure 15-10.

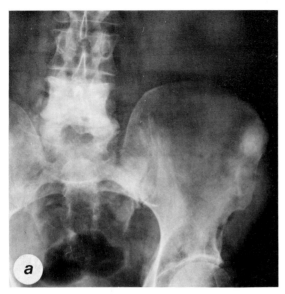
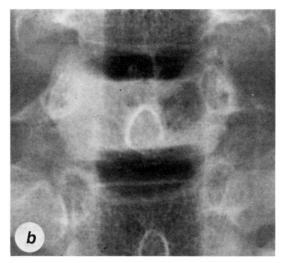

Figure 15-7. *a.* Sclerosing lesions of myeloma in sixty-two-year-old man who also had Cushing's disease. Myelomatous deposit studied at autopsy is shown in Figure 15-11. *b.* Sclerosing and lytic lesion of "solitary" myeloma in seventh cervical vertebra of thirty-two-year-old man.

Gross-Pathology

The myelomatous masses are classically soft, gray, and friable, resembling the tissue of a malignant lymphoma. As with other invasive tumors, more marrow often will be seen to be involved than is indicated by the roentgenologic changes. Expansion of the affected bone and, even more commonly, extraosseous extension of the tumor contribute to damage to adjacent structures. Extraosseous lesions are sometimes grossly discernible in other portions of the hematopoietic system, notably in the lymph nodes and spleen. Nodes containing myeloma were removed from eight patients, and an infiltrated testis was removed from one patient in this surgical series. As indicated, pathologic fracture may be present and often results in damage to the spinal cord. In very rare instances, enough amyloid is formed by the tumor to be grossly obvious. An unusual combination of sclerosis and lysis involved almost an entire femur in this series; amputation was performed for plasma cell myeloma that complicated chronic osteomyelitis of forty years' duration.

Histopathology

Typically, one sees sheets of closely packed cells with little intercellular substance. These cells have abundant cytoplasm which tends to be granular and basophilic. The cell outlines are distinct, and the nucleus is characteristically round or oval and eccentric. Two or even three nuclei are sometimes observed. When one studies a series of cases of myeloma, gradations are found to exist, these apparently reflecting the maturity or degree of differentiation of the cells. At one extreme are tumors with cells closely resembling the plasma cells seen in inflammatory conditions; these show prominent clumping of chromatin, sometimes producing the "wheel-spoke" appearance. With decreasing differentiation, nucleoli become large and clumping of chromatin is less marked. Cytoplasmic vacuoles increase in prom-

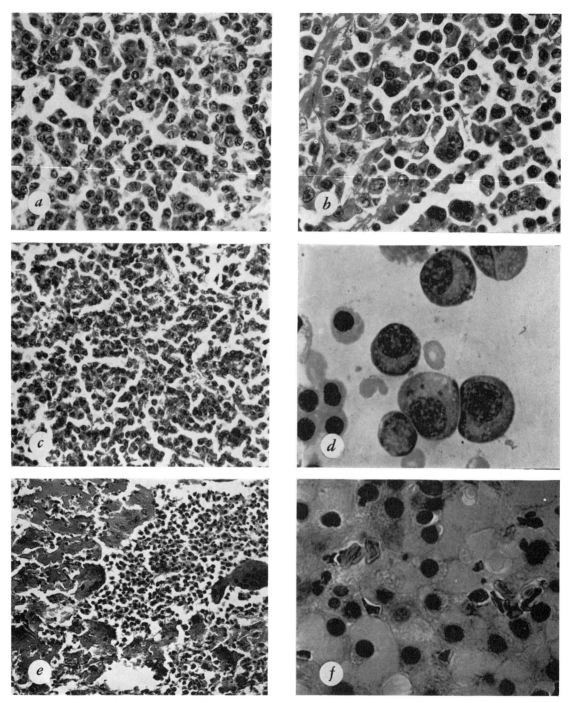

Figure 15-8. *a*. Relatively well differentiated myeloma with characteristic eccentric nuclei and abundant cytoplasm. (×380) *b*. Highly malignant myeloma at same magnification as in *a*. Note large nuclei and multinucleated giant cells. (×380) *c*. Same tumor as illustrated in *a*. (×265) *d*. Wright-stained smear of sternal marrow containing typical myeloma cells. (×850) *e*. Amyloid masses in myeloma nodule. Note benign giant cell reaction commonly seen around amyloid masses. (×175) *f*. Myeloma cells that contain amyloid or precursor. This is extremely rare finding. (×800) (Figure 15-8*e* reproduced with permission from: Dahlin, D. C., and Dockerty, M. B.: *Am J Pathol, 26:*581-593, 1950.)

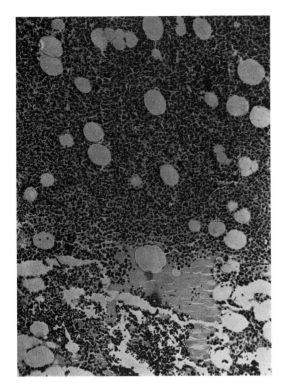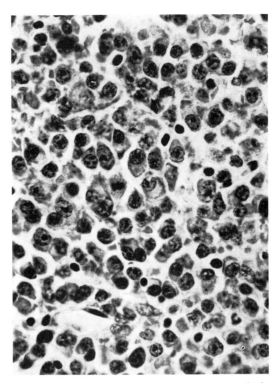

Figure 15-9. *Left.* Myeloma nodule in section of bone marrow has replaced hematopoietic elements and most of the fat. (×100) *Right.* Higher magnification showing characteristic well-defined cytoplasm of myeloma cells and nuclear anaplasia as manifested by large nucleoli. (×700)

inence and the cell boundary becomes indistinct. Finally, the nuclei may have grooves and lobules. At the other extreme is a tumor that may be indistinguishable from reticulum cell sarcoma. In fact, some myelomas have foci that are quite like reticulum cell sarcoma, and some even contain multinucleated cells of such size that the diagnosis of Hodgkin's sarcoma may be considered. The occasional shading together of these tumors should not be surprising, since all three very likely are basically of reticuloendothelial derivation.

Mitotic figures are rare in the average myeloma. The similarity of the cells comprising the solid sheets in this tumor contrasts with the multiplicity of cell types in the occasional chronic inflammatory focus that superficially resembles myeloma. The inflammatory pseudoneoplasm often contains a prominent capillary network that aids in differentiation.

Amyloidosis is related to the altered proteins as evidenced by its occurrence in approximately 10 percent of patients with myeloma. Its distribution with generalized deposition simulates that of primary systemic amyloidosis, a diagnosis that depends on the exclusion of myeloma as well as the more obvious causes of amyloidosis. Amyloid deposits are sometimes found within the myelomatous proliferations and may be so abundant as to mask the neoplasm. Amyloid with no demonstrable myeloma very rarely produces lytic defects in bone. In 1948, Bayrd described the cytologic details of myeloma cells as seen in marrow smears. Maldonado and coworkers described the ultrastructural features of the myeloma cell.

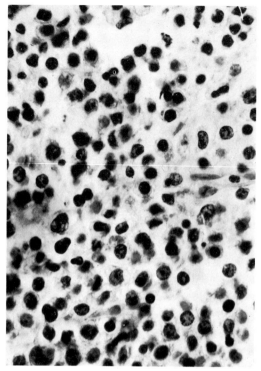

Figure 15-10. Anaplastic tumor with cytologic features suggesting either malignant lymphoma or myeloma. In rare instances, an absolute distinction cannot be made on a single specimen of tissue. (×525)

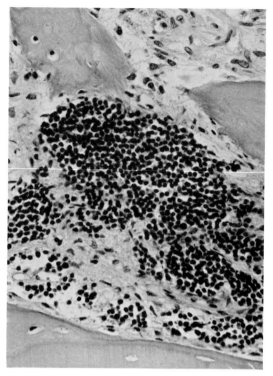

Figure 15-11. Island of myeloma cells in sclerotic bone at autopsy of patient illustrated in Figure 15-7a. (×400)

Treatment

The mode of treatment in myeloma varies, depending upon whether the disease is "solitary" or disseminated.

For localized myeloma, irradiation is the treatment of choice. Excision (total if possible) or at least diagnostic biopsy should precede irradiation. At the Mayo Clinic, aspiration biopsy has been used successfully in the diagnosis of a number of patients who had vertebral involvement. In the patients with severe neurologic symptoms, decompression of the spinal cord may be necessary prior to irradiation. Therapy must be directed at preservation of the spinal cord since many patients with a "solitary" lesion may live several years before dissemination occurs. Amputation may have to be considered for patients with a solitary lesion of myeloma in an extremity.

Chemotherapy has now proved to be of value in the management of patients with multiple myeloma. Various chemical agents have been able to effect subjective and objective improvement. It may be desirable to use irradiation in conjunction with chemotherapy if focal myelomatous proliferations produce a significant problem in a patient with multiple myeloma. General supportive measures are necessary.

Prognosis

Inanition, anemia, involvement of the spinal cord, and renal failure are the major factors contributing to the death of patients with disseminated myeloma, and many patients die within two years after diagnosis. In an earlier series of surgical cases in which the disease was not in a solitary focus at the time of diagnosis, somewhat more than 10 percent survived at least five years. Accurate prediction of survival time in a given case is not possible. Some have found that those with more undifferentiated myeloma cells in smear preparations have a poorer prognosis than the average.

Occasional patients die from the effects of a complicating systemic amyloidosis.

"Solitary" myeloma, as many authors have stressed, is the forerunner of disseminated myelomatosis. The current series reemphasizes that such dissemination may be long delayed and perhaps is not inevitable. Of thirty-four patients with "solitary" skeletal myelomas treated before 1960, eighteen were alive five years later. Seven of these died at intervals that ranged from five to twenty years after diagnosis, and eleven were alive at intervals that ranged from seven to twenty-four years. This series attests to the value of local therapy for this disease. Cohen and coworkers (1964) have elaborated some facets of the problem in a study of vertebral myelomas not as strictly localized as the "solitary" lesions in the current study. They found that the degree of cellular anaplasia did not affect the patient's chance of prolonged survival and that elevated serum globulin levels and Bence Jones proteinuria were not necessarily associated with short survival.

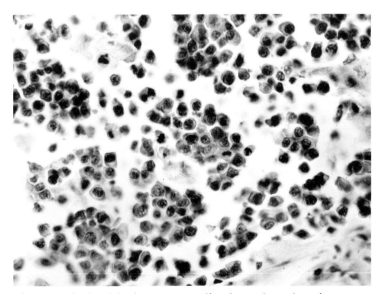

Figure 15-12. Myeloma complicating the chronic osteomyelitis illustrated in Figures 15-13 and 15-14. Only immature plasma cells comprised this malignant tumor. (×550)

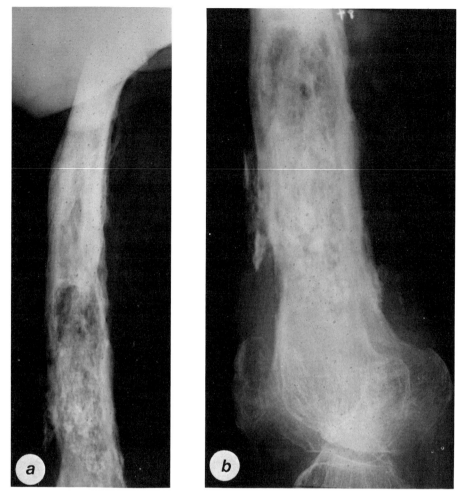

Figure 15-13. *a* and *b*. Osteomyelitis of forty years' duration and recently complicated by myeloma in fifty-three-year-old man. Wound, after disarticulation at hip, showed myeloma and patient died four months after amputation. Sarcoma is rare complication of chronic osteomyelitis compared with considerably more common squamous cell carcinoma.

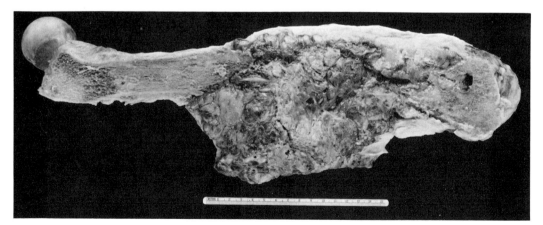

Figure 15-14. Myeloma lesion in case illustrated in Figure 15-13 was 23 by 15 by 15 cm and had destroyed more than half of chronically infected femur. In addition, one case of malignant lymphoma and one of fibroblastic osteosarcoma complicating chronic osteomyelitis were found in this entire series.

Bibliography

1948 Bayrd, E. D.: The Bone Marrow on Sternal Aspiration in Multiple Myeloma. *Blood, 3:*987-1018.

1950 Dahlin, D. C., and Dockerty, M. B.: Amyloid and Myeloma. *Am J Path, 26:*581-593.

1950 Churg, J., and Gordon, A. J.: Multiple Myeloma: Lesions of the Extra-osseous Hematopoietic System. *Am J Clin Pathol, 20:*934-945.

1953 Svien, H. J., Price, R. D., and Bayrd, E. D.: Neurosurgical Treatment of Compression of the Spinal Cord Caused by Myeloma. *JAMA, 153:*784-786.

1953 Bruce, K. W., and Royer, R. Q.: Multiple Myeloma Occurring in the Jaws. A Study of 17 Cases. *Oral Surg,* 6:729-744.

1954 Pugh, D. G.: *Roentgenologic Diagnosis of Diseases of Bones.* Baltimore, Williams & Wilkins, pp. 487-492.

1955 Carson, C. P., Ackerman, L. V., and Maltby, J. D.: Plasma Cell Myeloma: A Clinical, Pathologic and Roentgenologic Review of 90 Cases. *Am J Clin Pathol, 25:*849-888.

1959 Glenchur, H., Zinneman, H. H., and Hall, W. H.: A Review of Fifty One Cases of Multiple Myeloma: Emphasis on Pneumonia and other Infections as Complications. *AMA Arch Int Med, 103:*173-183.

1960 Engels, E. P., Smith, R. C., and Krantz, S.: Bone Sclerosis in Multiple Myeloma. *Radiology, 75:*242-247.

1960 Kyle, R. A., Bayrd, E. D., McKenzie, B. R., and Heck, F. J.: Diagnostic Criteria for Electrophoretic Patterns of Serum and Urinary Proteins in Multiple Myeloma. *JAMA, 174:*245-251.

1960 Feinleib, M., and MacMahon, B.: Duration of Survival in Multiple Myeloma. *J Natl Cancer Inst, 24:*1259-1269.

1961 Kyle, R. A., and Bayrd, E. D.: "Primary" Systemic Amyloidosis and Myeloma. Discussion of Relationship and Review of 81 Cases. *Arch Intern Med, 107:*344-353 (March).

1962 Silverman, L. M., and Shklar, G.: Multiple Myeloma: Report of a Case. *Oral Surg, 15:*301-309.

1962 Webb, H. E., Harrison, E. G., Masson, J. K., and ReMine, W. H.: Solitary Extramedullary Myeloma (Plasmacytoma) of the Upper Part of the Respiratory Tract and Oropharynx. *Cancer, 15:*1142-1155.

1963 Osserman, E. F., and Takatsuki, K.: Plasma Cell Myeloma: Gamma Globulin Synthesis and Structure. A Review of Biochemical and Clinical Data, With the Description of a Newly Recognized and Related Syndrome, "H-Gamma-2-Chain (Franklin's) Disease." *Medicine, 42:*357-384.

1964 Baitz, T., and Kyle, R. A.: Solitary Myeloma in Chronic Osteomyelitis: Report of Case. *Arch Intern Med, 113:*872-876 (June).

1964 Cohen, D. M., Svien, H. J., and Dahlin, D. C.: Long-Term Survival of Patients With Myeloma of the Vertebral Column. *JAMA, 187:*914-917.

1965 Herskovic, T., Andersen, H. A., and Bayrd, E. D.: Intrathoracic Plasmacytomas. Presentation of 21 Cases and Review of Literature. *Dis Chest, 47:*1-7.

1966 Griffiths, D. L.: Orthopaedic Aspects of Myelomatosis. *J Bone Joint Surg, 48B:*703-728 (November).

1966 Maldonado, J. E., Brown, A. L., Jr., Bayrd, E. D., and Pease, G. L.: Ultrastructure of the Myeloma Cell. *Cancer, 19:*1613-1627 (November).

1966 Osman, R., and Morrow, J. W.: Myeloma of the Testicle: A Case Report. *J Urol, 96:*352-355 (September).

1966 Suissa, L., LaRosa, J., and Linn, B.: Plasmacytoma of Lymph Nodes: A Case Report. *JAMA, 197:*294-296 (July).

1967 Grossman, R. E., and Hensley, G. T.: Bone Lesion in Primary Amyloidosis. *Am J Roentgenol, 101:*872-875 (December).

1967 Lowell, D. M.: Amyloid-Producing Plasmacytoma of the Pelvis: Case Report and Review of the Literature. *Arch Surg, 94:*899-903 (June).

1967 Moossy, J., and Wilson, C. B.: Solitary Intracrainal Plasmacytoma. *Arch Neurol, 16:*212-216 (February).

1968 Poole, A. G., and Marchetta, F. C.: Extramedullary Plasmacytoma of the Head and Neck. *Cancer, 22:*14-21 (July).

1969 Elias, E. G., Gailani, S., Jones, R., Jr., and Mittelman, A.: Extraosseous Multiple Myeloma: A Cause of Intestinal Obstruction. *Ann Surg, 170:*857-861 (November).

1970 Markel, S. E., and Theros, E. G.: RPC of the Month From the AFIP: Plasma-cell Granuloma of Pelvis and Femora. *Radiology, 95:*679-686 (June).

1971 Remigio, P. A., and Klaum, A.: Extramedullary Plasmacytoma of Stomach. *Cancer, 27:*562-568 (March).

1972 Kotner, L. M., and Wang, C. C.: Plasmacytoma of the Upper Air and Food Passages. *Cancer, 30:*414-418 (August).

1972 Pear, B. L.: Radiographic Studies of Amyloidosis. *CRC Crit Rev Radiol Sci, 3:*425-451 (August).

1972 Oberkircher, P. E., Miller, W. T., and Arger, P. H.: Nonosseous Presentation of Plasma-Cell Myeloma. *Radiology, 104:*515-520 (September).

1974 Meyer, J. E., and Schulz, M. D.: "Solitary" Myeloma of Bone: A Review of 12 Cases. *Cancer, 34:*438-440 (August).

1974 Getaz, P., Handler, L., Jacobs, P., and Tunley, I.: Osteosclerotic Myeloma With Peripheral Neuropathy. *S Afr Med J, 48:*1246-1250 (June).

1975 Berman, H. H.: Waldenstrom's Macroglobulinemia With Lytic Osseous Lesions and Plasma-Cell Morphology: Report of a Case. *Am J Clin Pathol, 63:*397-402 (March).

1975 Kyle, R. A.: Multiple Myeloma: Review of 869 Cases. *Mayo Clin Proc, 50:*29-40 (January).

1975 Perry, M. C., and Kyle, R. A.: The Clinical Significance of Bence Jones Proteinuria. *Mayo Clin Proc, 50:*234-238 (May).

1976 Kyle, R. A., and Elveback, L. R.: Management and Prognosis of Multiple Myeloma. *Mayo Clin Proc, 51:*751-760 (December).

Chapter 16

Malignant Lymphoma of Bone
(Reticulum Cell Sarcoma)

PRIOR TO THE CLASSIC article by Parker and Jackson in 1939, reticulum cell sarcomas of bone were generally "lumped" with Ewing's tumors. The remarkably better prognosis as well as clinical implications makes it important to recognize this special tumor. The discussion in this chapter is oriented to the problems of lymphoma of the skeleton as encountered by the surgical pathologist, the surgeon, and the therapist. Detailed considerations of lymphoma in general and of leukemia are purposely avoided.

Although the term "reticulum cell sarcoma" is commonly employed for the tumor under discussion, it is a misnomer since relatively few pertinent tumors are composed solely of this type of cell. A mixture of reticulum cells, lymphoblasts, and lymphocytes is so common in these neoplasms that it is a diagnostic aid. Furthermore, lymphocytic and Hodgkin's lymphomas can produce primary lesions in bone. For these reasons, the term "malignant lymphoma" better categorizes the entire group. These tumors are morphologically identical to their soft-tissue counterparts.

When malignant lymphoma is responsible for an osseous lesion, one of three clinical conditions may be found. First, careful study of the patient may reveal no evidence of distant disease, and the osseous lesion can be presumed to be primary. Of the 327 cases in this series, 150 could be placed in this category. This "primary" variety affords the best opportunity for successful therapy. Second, similar disease may be found in other osseous or in soft-tissue sites, and one must assume that the bony lesion in question may be a region of secondary involvement. This category contained one hundred thirty cases of this series. Third, a patient with known lymphomatous disease not in bone may have tissue removed from a metastatic osseous focus for one reason or another. Although such obviously secondary skeletal involvement is commonly seen at autopsy, especially in reticulum cell sarcoma and Hodgkin's disease, only forty-seven examples were encountered in this surgical series.

Focal infiltrates in leukemia may mimic the histologic appearance of malignant lymphoma. Osseous manifestations are likely to be prominent in acute leukemias, especially in childhood. In nearly 10 percent of patients with acute leukemia, the clinical course is dominated by symptoms referable to the bones and joints. The lower extremities are most commonly affected. Juxtaepiphyseal rarefactions, focal or extensive osteolytic zones, periosteal elevation with new bone deposition, and generalized rarefaction are among the roentgenographic findings.

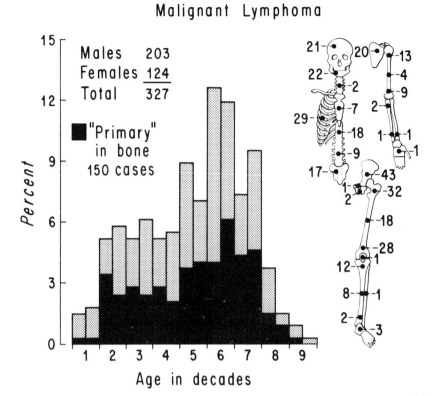

Malignant Lymphoma

Males 203
Females 124
Total 327

"Primary" in bone 150 cases

Figure 16-1. Skeletal, age, and sex distribution of malignant lymphomas of bone.

Incidence

Malignant lymphoma comprised 6.8 percent of the malignant group in this series. The 150 that were "primary" in bone comprised only 3.1 percent.

Sex

Males predominated in a ratio of approximately 3 : 2 in the "primary" and in the total group. This is in general agreement with the literature.

Age

This neoplasm can occur at any age but is rare in the very young. The age distribution for those presumably primary in bone parallels that of the overall group.

Localization

When a malignant lymphoma arises in certain specific sites such as the antrum or along the spinal column, it is often impossible to prove an osseous origin. Many patients with involvement of the antrum and one or more of its bony walls are excluded from the above data because an origin from bone could not be verified. Likewise, most surgical patients with lymphoma affecting the spinal cord or its emerging nerves are excluded because proof of osseous disease was not available. The distribution of the "primary" cases was similar to that of the entire group. A fibular tumor of the earlier series was excluded because its anaplasia made categorization of it uncertain.

Symptoms

Pain, swelling, and subsequent disability are the cardinal features of any malignant tumor of bone, including lymphoma. Pain of variable intensity is practically a constant feature, and occasionally it has been present for several years, although ordinarily its duration is measured in months. Neurologic symptoms commonly occur when these tumors affect the spinal column. Many have emphasized that patients with even extensive solitary malignant lymphomas have a surprising sense of well-being and absence of general complaints so commonly associated with malignant disease. Pathologic fracture may occur. One patient in this series developed malignant lymphoma in a focus of old chronic osteomyelitis of the tibia.

Physical Findings

A mass in the region of the tumor, which may be tender or warm, is the main finding, and this is often associated with disability of the affected part. Enlarged regional lymph nodes may be found. One should search for signs of disseminated malignant lymphoma, such as involvement of multiple bones, distant lymph nodes, and other soft-tissue structures. Because of the occasional similarity of tumefactions due to malignant lymphomas and those due to leukemia, it is important to study the peripheral blood of these patients.

Roentgenologic Features

Roentgenologically, the lesions frequently appear to be very extensive, often involving 25 to 50 percent of the affected bone and in some cases involving the entire shaft. Bone destruction is the predominant feature of primary reticulum cell sarcoma. The areas of destruction give the bone a mottled and patchy appearance in many cases, and sometimes its outline is entirely lost. The diseased bone blends imperceptibly with the adjacent normal bone. Approximately half of the patients in this series had evidence of some reactive proliferation of new bone that is not laid down by the tumor cells themselves. Nearly every malignant lymphoma destroys cortical bone, and approximately 25 percent are associated with some thickening of the cortex. There is often obvious soft-tissue extension of the tumors, and sometimes there is calcification in the soft-tissue mass. Approximately one fourth of the patients have evidence of pathologic fracture.

Irregular sclerosis of the affected site is sometimes a marked feature and adds to the confusion of reticulum cell sarcoma with chronic osteomyelitis that sometimes occurs. Disseminated malignant lymphomatous involvement of the skeleton may simulate osteoblastic metastatic carcinomatosis. Sclerosis may precede the diagnosis by several years and even resemble Paget's disease of bone.

Wilson and Pugh, who studied the Mayo Clinic series, concluded that the roentgenograms varied so much that their appearance could not be regarded as characteristic. Although the radiologist suspects frequently the diagnosis of reticulum cell sarcoma, other lesions including metastatic carcinoma, osteosarcoma, Ewing's tumor, eosinophilic granuloma, and chronic osteomyelitis cannot always be excluded with certainty.

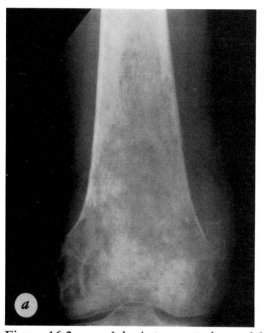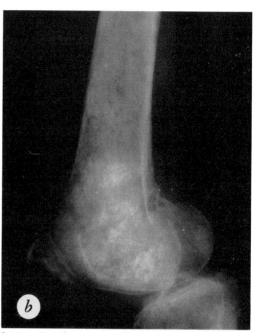

Figure 16-2. *a* and *b*. Anteroposterior and lateral views of primary malignant lymphoma destroying lower portion of femur of twenty-six-year-old woman. There is blotchy sclerosis in areas of destruction. Patient died eleven years later with evidence of disseminated disease. (Reproduced with permission from: Ivins, J. C., and Dahlin, D. C.: *J Bone Joint Surg, 35A*: 835-842, 1953.)

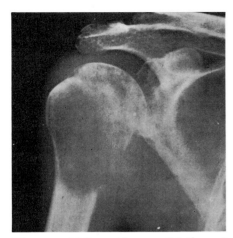

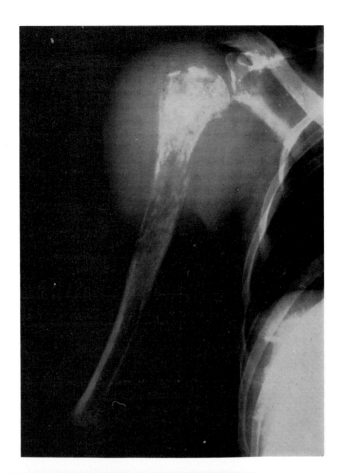

Figure 16-3. *Above.* Malignant lymphoma containing elements resembling multinucleated Reed-Sternberg cells. Although lesion was apparently "solitary," forty-year-old patient died with dissemination eight months later. *Right.* Nearly all cells of this sarcoma were immature reticulum cells (histiocytes). This radiosensitive tumor recurred and necessitated forequarter amputation eight months after radiation, and the twenty-eight-year-old man died two months after amputation.

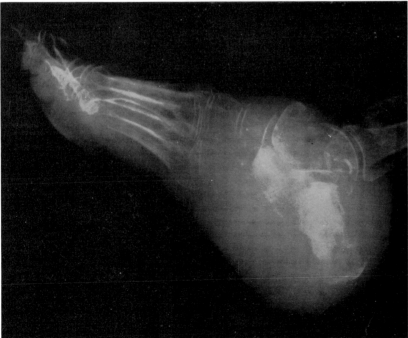

Figure 16-4. Reticulum cell sarcoma producing extensive destruction of tarsal bones of sixty-five-year-old woman. Inguinal nodes were enlarged, and biopsy material from one of these presented characteristic pattern of malignant lymphoma of reticulum cell type. Patient died with widespread disease in less than one year.

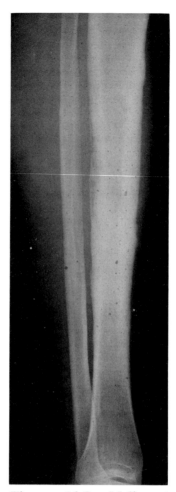

Figure 16-5. Malignant lymphoma in forty-three-year-old man. Features suggest Paget's disease. Above-knee amputation was followed by sixteen-year survival and then death from unrelated hepatitis.

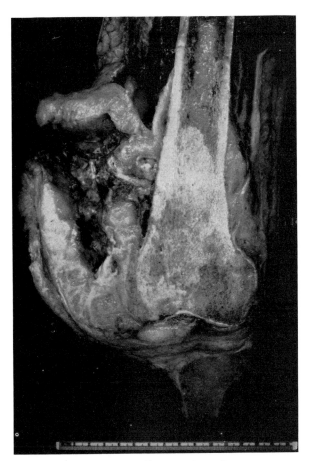 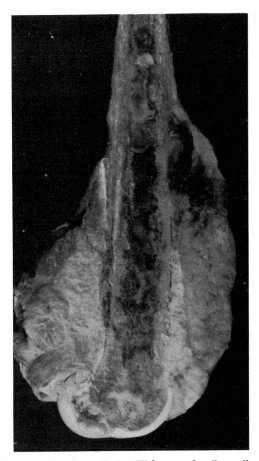

Figure 16-6. Two malignant lymphomas removed by amputation. *Left.* This nearly "pure" reticulum cell sarcoma had been considered an "inflammatory" lesion at time of previous biopsy. At time of amputation, it had grown through the skin. Despite postoperative radiation therapy to groin and pelvis, patient died in two years. *Right.* This malignant lymphoma of mixed-cell type, also involving lower portion of femur, was treated the same way, and patient survived twenty-seven years. (Reproduced with permission from: McCormack, L. J., Ivins, J. C., Dahlin, D. C., and Johnson, E. W., Jr.: *Cancer, 5:*1182-1192, 1952.)

Gross Pathology

The gross features of primary malignant lymphoma of bone are not pathognomonic, but some of them warrant mention. Although any portion, and frequently a large part, of a long bone may be involved, the main mass of the tumor and its extraosseous extension, if present, are most often in or near the metaphyseal region. A variable amount of soft-tissue extension is practically always present by the time diagnosis is made. The bone itself at the affected site is destroyed to a variable extent, and not infrequently one sees white areas of necrosis or zones of secondary sclerosis. Residual osseous trabeculae are frequently admixed with tumor, imparting a firm and gritty consistency. When a reticulum cell sarcoma extends into the soft tissues, it produces a soft mass that is friable and simulates the appearance of malignant lymphomas arising in soft tissues. The margins of a malignant lymphoma in the bone as well as in the adjacent soft tissues are ordinarily indistinct. Regional lymph nodes may be involved, and as indicated above, there may be any of the gross pathologic evidences of disseminated malignant lymphoma.

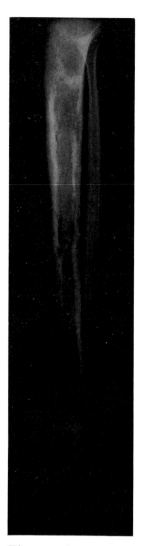 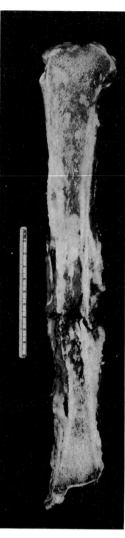 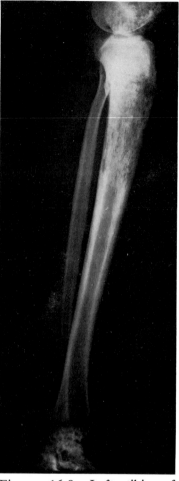

Figure 16-7. *Left.* Predominantly reticulum-cell type of malignant lymphoma of right tibia. *Right.* Specimen shows that, although nearly entire tibia is involved, there is little soft-tissue extension of tumor.

Figure 16-8. Left tibia of same patient as in Figure 16-7 showing similar involvement three years after amputation for first tumor. Patient died with disseminated disease fourteen months after second osseous lesion developed.

Histopathology

The basic proliferating cell in tumors of this type is the reticulum cell. Characteristically, it has a grooved or folded nucleus, one or more distinct nucleoli, and indistinct, irregular cytoplasmic boundaries. Cytoplasmic processes may extend outward from the cell bodies. Reticulum cells overshadow all others in some of these tumors, but the great majority contain variable numbers of lymphoblasts and lymphocytes, and sometimes these cells dominate the histologic pattern. On rare occasions, one encounters a pure lymphocytic malignant lymphoma that is apparently primary in bone. Occasional highly malignant reticulum cell sarcomas of bone contain multinulceated cells of the Reed-Sternberg type, and these tumors quite logically fall into the category of Hodgkin's sarcoma. Even the granulomatous form of

Hodgkin's disease can present as a primary tumor of bone. In 19 of the 327 patients, Reed-Sternberg cells were present, and several of the patients had tumors that were clinically primary in bone.

Since the cells of the average malignant lymphoma lie in a reticular framework, there is a tendency for an alveolar grouping, a feature that is often prominent even under low magnification. This helps differentiate reticulum cell sarcoma from Ewing's tumor, in which large masses of cells are associated with no fibrillar intercellular material. Special stains for reticulum accentuate the network in which the cells lie. In my experience, however, this stain has been of little value for diagnosis because those tumors that appear atypical when stained with ordinary dyes contain an equivocal amount of stainable reticulum. An absence of granules that stain positive with periodic acid-Schiff stain helps differentiate this sarcoma from Ewing's tumor, stainable granules usually being present in the latter lesion. I have been unable to discern a difference between a malignant lymphoma that begins in bone from such a tumor that begins elsewhere in the body.

The large numbers of lymphocytic cells present in some of these tumors may lead to the diagnosis of an inflammatory process, an error especially likely to occur if one has only a small amount of material for biopsy or if the tumor is infected, as it is likely to be in malignant lymphoma of the jaws.

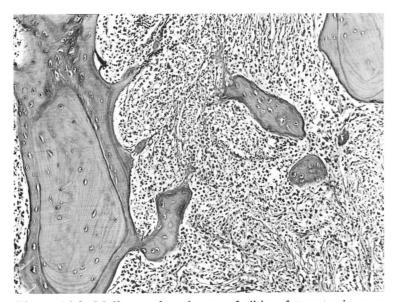

Figure 16-9. Malignant lymphoma of tibia of twenty-six-year-old woman. This is from lesion shown in Figures 16-7 and 16-8. Pleomorphic malignant cellular tumor has infiltrated between preexisting trabeculae of bone. Considerable appositional new bone has been produced around trabecula at left, and there are a few strands of new bone within tumor. Fibrillar intercellular framework is prominent in this tumor. (×100)

Certain anaplastic small cell tumors are in a gray zone between lymphoma and Ewing's sarcoma. A practical plan is to make the diagnosis of Ewing's sarcoma if the cells are so anaplastic that they cannot be categorized in the reticulum-cell-lymphocyte series with certainty. The histiocytes of histiocytosis X may be difficult to differentiate from reticulum cell sarcoma, especially if cytologic features are distorted by decalcification, but generally, the cells of histiocytosis X are obviously benign, lacking the pleomorphism and hyperchromatism of malignant cells.

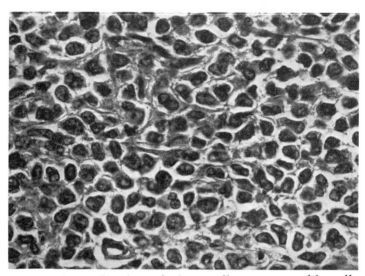

Figure 16-10. Classic reticulum cell sarcoma with cells showing grooved and indented nuclei, indistinct cytoplasmic borders, and reticular framework that is easily seen, even with this hematoxylin-eosin stain. (×650)

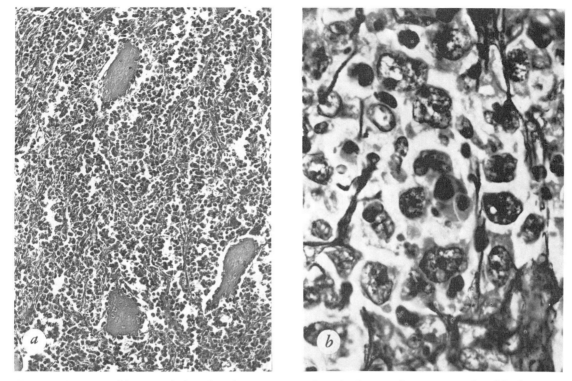

Figure 16-11. *a.* Characteristic alveolar pattern of reticulum cell sarcoma, in this instance invading and destroying trabeculae of normal bone. (×125) *b.* Higher magnification to show nuclear detail and strands of reticulin (reticulin stain). (×800) (Reproduced with permission from: Ivins, J. C., and Dahlin, D. C.: *J Bone Joint Surg, 35A:*835-842, 1953.)

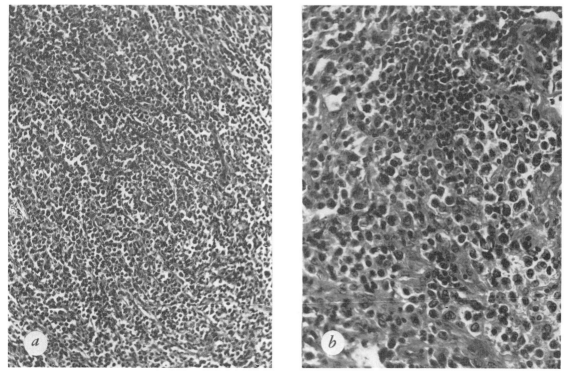

Figure 16-12. *a.* Typical alveolar pattern of reticulum cell sarcoma. Even at this magnification, reticular framework is visible. (×115) *b.* In this field are seen lymphoblasts and lymphocytes, cells commonly found in primary malignant lymphomas in bone. (×300)

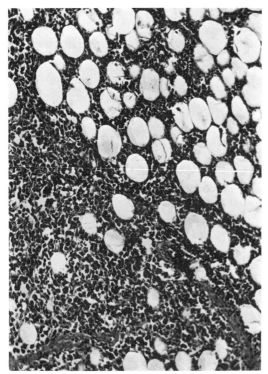

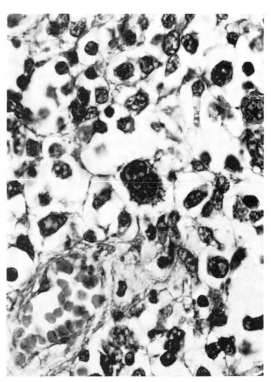

Figure 16-13. Reticulum cell sarcoma with invasion into adjacent fat, a feature that accounts for poorly defined border ordinarily seen on gross inspection of one of these lesions. (×150) (Reproduced with permission from: McCormack, L. J., Ivins, J. C., Dahlin, D. C., and Johnson, E. W., Jr.: *Cancer, 5:*1182-1192, 1952.)

Figure 16-14. Hodgkin's type of malignant lymphoma manifesting itself as a destructive tumor of sternum with invasion of structures behind and in front of manubrium. Note centrally located Reed-Sternberg cell. (×700)

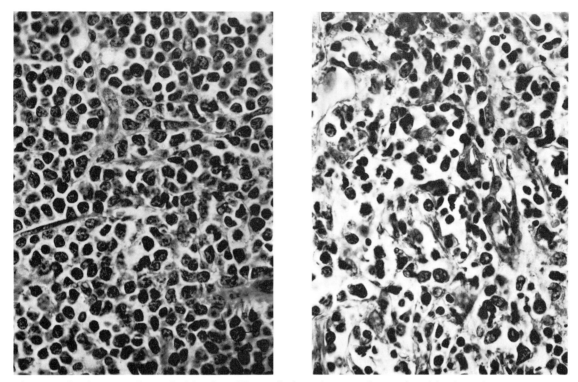

Figure 16-15. *Left*. Lymphoblastic differentiation is prominent in this lymphoma. (×600) *Right*. Lymphoma showing alveolar grouping and variation in size and shape of cells. (×425)

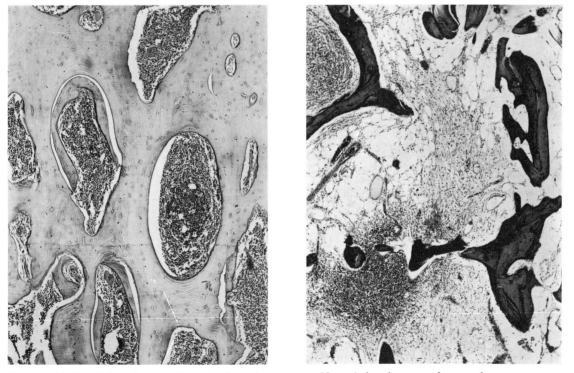

Figure 16-16. Sclerotic reaction to lymphoma manifested by layers of new bone on pre-existing trabeculae. *Left*. Tumor permeating skull. (×80) *Right*. Sclerosing reaction at and even beyond periphery of lymphoma of ilium. (×60)

Treatment

The accumulated experience with primary malignant lymphomas that are apparently solitary in bone does not yet allow one to be dogmatic regarding the treatment of choice. The consensus now favors irradiation for control of the primary lesion. Sometimes amputation becomes necessary because irradiation either results in local necrosis that is disabling or fails to halt the growth of the primary tumor. These facts have suggested to some that primary abaltive surgical procedures should be used, especially for tumors below the midfemur level. Regional lymph nodes require attention, and radiation therapy is likely most efficacious for these. Irradiation is indicated for those tumors not amenable to surgical removal. Chemotherapy provides subjective and objective relief for many patients with disseminated lymphoma; focal lesions in such patients may require radiation therapy. Bone-marrow study is important in evaluating the extent of disease, and it seems likely that lymphangiogram for the study of pelvic and retroperitoneal nodes is desirable in the assessment of these patients with a lesion in bone.

Prognosis

Most reports indicate that reticulum cell sarcoma has the best prognosis of any of the primary malignant tumors of bone. Five-year survival rates of 40 to 50 percent and even higher have been reported. In a series that we studied recently (Fig. 16-17), 44 percent of the patients with primary lymphoma have survived five years. Many of these, unfortunately, succumb later. No rule applies in an individual case because of the well-known vagaries of the malignant lymphomas. Patients with one lesion adequately treated may have, in a period of months or many years, a tumor in another bone, in a distant lymph node, or in other soft tissue, or they subsequently may even have a leukemic blood picture, as was seen in several instances in the present series.

The prognosis for the group with pure reticulum cell sarcoma was not unlike that for the much larger group with cytologically mixed lesions. The small groups with Hodgkin's and lymphocytic types appear to have a poorer outlook.

Figure 16-17 shows that primary tumors of the pelvic girdle region were associated with a significant probability of long-term survival.

Most of the small group of patients with mandibular tumors in the present series have become long-term survivors. The locally invasive and basically inoperable lymphomas of the maxillary region, not included in this series, can be cured in a gratifying percentage of cases by appropriate radiation therapy (Steg and co-workers, 1959).

Whether chemotherapy treatment ancillary to radiation is desirable for patients with primary malignant lymphoma of bone is not yet a settled issue.

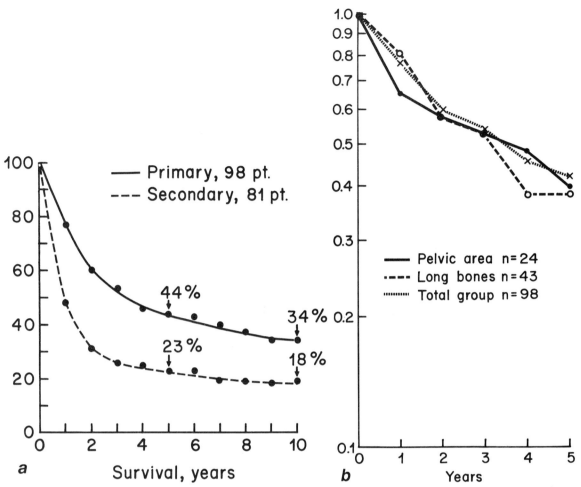

Figure 16-17. *a.* Probability of survival for patients with primary and with secondary lymphoma of bone. *b.* Semilogarithmic graph shows probability of survival for patients having primary lymphoma of innominate bone and sacrum (pelvic area) compared with patients having tumors of long bones and with patients in total group. (Reproduced with permission from: Boston, H. C., Jr., Dahlin, D. C., Ivins, J. C., and Cupps, R. E.: *Cancer, 34:*1131-1137, 1974.)

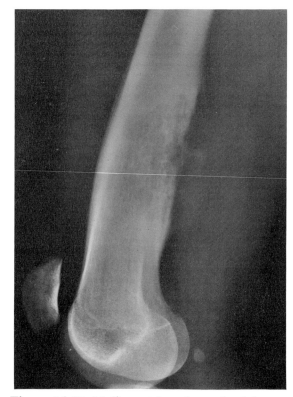

Figure 16-18. Malignant lymphoma in eighteen-year-old man. Patient was well sixty-four months after biopsy and radiation therapy.

Bibliography

1934 Craver, L. F., and Copeland, M. M.: Lymphosarcoma in Bone. *Arch Surg, 28:*809-824.

1939 Parker, Frederic, Jr., and Jackson, Henry, Jr.: Primary Reticulum Cell Sarcoma of Bone. *Surg Gynecol Obstet, 68:*45-53.

1947 Jackson, H., and Parker, F., Jr.: *Hodgkin's Disease and Allied Disorders.* New York, Oxford U. Pr., pp. 1-177.

1952 McCormack, L. J., Ivins, J. C., Dahlin, D. C., and Johnson, E. W., Jr.: Primary Reticulum-cell Sarcoma of Bone. *Cancer, 5:*1182-1192.

1952 Valls, J., Muscolo, D., and Schajowicz, F.: Reticulum-Cell Sarcoma of Bone. *J Bone Joint Surg, 34B:*588-598.

1954 Francis, K. C., Higinbotham, N. L., and Coley, B. L.: Primary Reticulum Cell Sarcoma of Bone: Report of 44 Cases. *Surg Gynecol Obstet, 99:*143-146.

1955 Bethge, J. F. J.: Die Ewingtumoren oder Omoblastome des Knochens. Differential-diagnostische und Kritische Erörterungen. *Ergeb Chir Orthop, 39:*327-425.

1955 Wilson, T. W., and Pugh, D. G.: Primary Reticulum-cell Sarcoma of Bone, With Emphasis on Roentgen Aspects. *Radiology, 65:*343-351.

1958 Ullrich, D. P., and Bucy, P. C.: Primary Reticulum Cell Sarcoma of the Skull. *Am J Roentgenol, 79:*653-657.

1959 Steg, R. F., Dahlin, D. C., and Gores, R. J.: Malignant Lymphoma of the Mandible and Maxillary Region. *Oral Surg, 12:*128-141.

1961 Thomas, L. B., Forkner, C. E., Jr., Frei, E., III, Besse, B. E., Jr., and Stabenau, J. R.: The Skeletal Lesions of Acute Leukemia. *Cancer, 14:*608-621.

1963 Silverstein, M. N., and Kelly, P. J.: Leukemia With Osteoarticular Symptoms and Signs. *Ann Intern Med, 59:*637-645.

1968 Wang, C. C., and Fleischli, D. J.: Primary Reticulum Cell Sarcoma of Bone: With Emphasis on Radiation Therapy. *Cancer, 22:*994-998 (November).

1970 Potdar, G. G.: Primary Reticulum-Cell Sarcoma of Bone in Western India. *Br J Cancer, 24:*48-55 (March).

1971 Miller, T. R., and Nicholson, J. T.: End Results in Reticulum Cell Sarcoma of Bone Treated by Bacterial Toxin Therapy Alone of Combined With Surgery and/or Radiotherapy (47 Cases) or With Concurrent Infection (5 Cases). *Cancer, 27:* 524-548 (March).

1971 Shoji, H., and Miller, T. R.: Primary Reticulum Cell Sarcoma of Bone: Significance of Clinical Features Upon the Prognosis. *Cancer, 28:*1234-1244 (November).

1973 Fayemi, A. O., Gerber, M. A., Cohen, I., Davis, S., and Rubin, A. D.: Myeloid Sarcoma: Review of the Literature and Report of a Case. *Cancer, 32:*253-258 (July).

1974 Boston, H. C., Jr., Dahlin, D. C., Ivins, J. C., and Cupps, R. E.: Malignant Lymphoma (So-called Reticulum Cell Sarcoma) of Bone. *Cancer, 34:*1131-1137 (October).

1974 Pear, B. L.: Skeletal Manifestations of the Lymphomas and Leukemias. *Semin Roentgenol, 9:*229-240 (July).

Chapter 17

Chondrosarcoma (Primary, Secondary, Dedifferentiated, and Clear Cell)

Primary Chondrosarcoma

CHONDROSARCOMA should be separated from osteosarcoma because of basic pathologic differences that are reflected in vastly differing clinical, therapeutic, and prognostic features. The exact origin of chondrosarcomas is obscure, but the salient pathologic fact is that their basic proliferating tissue is cartilaginous throughout. Large portions of these tumors may become myxomatous, or calcified or even ossified. Sometimes, fibrosarcomalike splindling of the cells is seen at the peripheries of the lobules of the tumor. Osseous trabeculae, when present, result from differentiation of chondroid substance. When, however, the malignant cells produce an osteoid lacework or osteoid trabeculae directly, even in small foci, the neoplasm has the clinical characteristics of osteosarcoma and belongs in that category.

Chondrosarcoma usually has a slow clinical evolution. Metastasis is relatively rare and often late in appearance. Therefore, unlike that of osteosarcoma, in which prompt ablative surgical treatment is imperative because of early hematogenous dissemination, the basic therapeutic problem is prevention of recurrence by adeuate control of the lesion locally. Attainment of this goal demands adequate, frequently radical, early surgical treatment.

Chondrosarcomas can arise de novo in extraskeletal tissues or in teratomas and other mixed tumors. Their general characteristics are like those of the skeletal examples.

Secondary Chondrosarcoma

Secondary chondrosarcomas most commonly arise in osteochondromas (osteocartilaginous exostoses), especially in the multiple, familial type. In my experience it is extremely unusual to have a chondrosarcoma develop from an enchondroma that was originally clearly benign on critical analysis. In the Mayo Clinic series of fifty-four definite secondary chondrosarcomas, twenty-four occurred in patients with multiple osteochondromas, twenty-two arose in solitary osteochondromas, and eight developed in patients with multiple chondromas. Some of the details concerning these secondary chondrosarcomas are given in Chapters 2 and 3.

Dedifferentiated Chondrosarcoma

In addition to the 419 primary, secondary, and clear cell chondrosarcomas, there are 51 that had given rise to more highly malignant tumors, either fibrosarcomas or osteosarcomas.

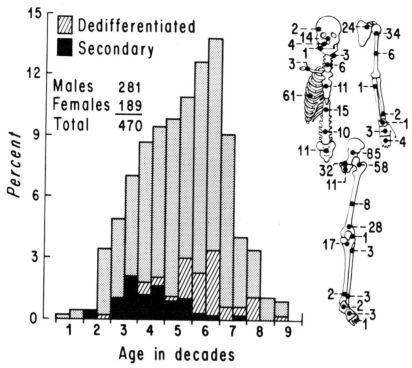

Figure 17-1. Skeletal, age, and sex distribution of chondrosarcomas.

Clear Cell Chondrosarcomas

Among the chondrosarcomas were nine of this special type. Data on them and an additional seven from our consultation files are provided later in this chapter.

Incidence

Chondrosarcoma constituted 10 percent of the malignant tumors in this series, and 76 percent were of the primary type. Dedifferentiation has occurred in both primary and secondary chondrosarcoma. Osteosarcoma was more than twice as common.

Sex

Slightly less than 60 percent were males.

Age

This tumor is primarily one of adulthood and old age. Secondary chondrosarcomas occurred in a younger group on the average. The second decade of life, in which the peak incidence of osteosarcoma occurs, contributed only 3.8 percent of the total. Three patients were less than ten years old, and the youngest was three years old. Any series that has a relatively large number of patients in the first two decades of life probably includes patients with chondroblastic osteosarcoma, a tumor with biologic capability similar to that of the overall osteosarcoma group.

Localization

More than three fourths of the tumors were in the trunk (including the shoulder girdle) and the upper ends of the femora and humeri. The majority in the maxillary region seemed to arise from the cartilage of the walls of the nasal cavity. Three developed from the hyoid bone. One was primary in the synovium and capsule of the knee joint; there was no histologic evidence of pre-existing benign synovial chondromatosis. The remarkable rarity of chondrosarcoma in the distal portions of the extremities, with only fourteen of them occurring distal to the ankle and wrist joints, is noteworthy. Four of those previously called chondrosarcomas of the sphenoid are now considered to be chondroid chordomas at the spheno-occipital synchondrosis. Some of the few reported as periosteal chondrosarcomas in the literature are classed with our chondroblastic osteosarcomas because component malignant cells produce osteoid; these will be described later as periosteal osteosarcoma.

Localization data concerning the secondary chondrosarcomas are given in Table 4.

TABLE 4

LOCATION OF 59 SARCOMAS
ACCORDING TO BENIGN CONDITION

	Multiple Exostoses	Solitary Exostosis	Multiple Chondromas
Innominate bone	13*	11	1
Femur	1	4†	3‡
Tibia		1	3*
Fibula	1	3	
Metatarsal			1
Humerus	1	2	1
Scapula	3	1	
Clavicle	1		
Vertebrae	3		
Sacrum	1	1	
Rib		1	
Skull	1‡		1§
Total	25	24	10

* Dedifferentiated chondrosarcoma in 1.
† Osteosarcoma in 2.
‡ Osteosarcoma in 1.
§ Chondroid chordoma.

As indicated previously, the twenty-four patients with chondrosarcomas complicating multiple exostoses derived from a total of eighty-eight patients who required operation for the latter condition. Of 540 patients requiring operation for solitary exostoses, only 22 had complicating chondrosarcomas. Ten of thirty-six patients operated upon for multiple chondromas of the skeleton had secondary malignant tumor. Two of these ten had chondromas in only one bone, the femur. These data should not be construed to represent the expected incidence of sarcomatous degeneration in the three conditions. Continued follow-up of the total groups will alter the data, and factors of selection probably increase the likelihood that the patient with sarcoma will gravitate to a large medical center. Figure 17-1 shows that patients with secondary chondrosarcoma tend to be younger than the average patient with chondrosarcoma.

Symptoms (All Chondrosarcomas)

Local swelling and pain, alone or in combination, are the significant presenting symptoms. Pain strongly suggests active growth of a central cartilaginous tumor. Except for some of the tumors of the pelvic girdle or spinal column, where referred pain may precede local pain or discernible physical or roentgenographic findings, localization of these tumors is easy. As in other tumors of bone, the characteristics of the pain or swelling offer little differential diagnostic aid. The prolonged clinical course so often observed affords a clue. A gradually enlarging tumor for periods ranging from one to two decades, or even more, may have been noted by those patients who have had an osteochondroma that undergoes malignant transformation. Such transformation often produces pain and rapid increase in size of a tumor of long duration. Patients with primary chondrosarcoma also may have had symptoms for several years before coming to definitive therapy. Inadequately treated tumors produce a typical history of many recurrences and, finally, of inoperable extension or metastasis that leads to death of the host. A few chondrosarcomas run a rapid clinical course because of a higher degree of malignancy initially or because of increased activity with recurrence.

The slow clinical evolution of chondrosarcoma is emphasized by the fact that approximately 10 percent of those that produced recurrence in this series had intervals of from five to ten years between treatment and recurrence. Recurrence may become manifest even more than ten years after first treatment. Since recurrence may be so delayed, it is obvious that conclusions regarding efficacy of any form of treatment must be based not only on a sizable series of cases, but also on such a series followed for a period of at least ten years.

Physical Findings

Many chondrosarcomas produce a mass that can be palpated, but a sizable number of those affecting the trunk, or even the long bones of the extremities if they have not breached the cortex, will cause pain alone to indicate the presence of a lesion. When a mass is palpable, it is characteristically hard and may be painful. When no mass can be palpated, the diagnosis may be difficult. This is especially true of chondrosarcomas of the innominate bone that have not produced definite roentgenologic changes. The region of the acetabulum, where many of the chondrosarcomas originate, is notorious for such "hidden" malignant tumors. One chondrosarcoma of the hyoid bone was associated with Gardner's syndrome.

Roentgenologic Features

The roentgenogram is nearly always helpful and often affords almost pathognomonic evidence of chondrosarcoma. Osseous destruction in the lesional area combined with mottled densities owing to calcification and ossification is the usual finding. Central chondrosarcomas of long bones often produce fusiform expansion of the shaft associated with thickening of the cortex. Cortical destruction allows extraosseous extension of lesions that begin in the medulla. Those that do not involve the medullary cavity may show little or no cortical destruction, but they usually contain minute or massive telltale calcific masses. None of the chondrosarcomas in this series was associated with Paget's disease.

Chondrosarcoma of the innominate bone, especially near the acetabulum, may produce no discernible roentgenographic findings early. This is particularly true of those that are completely lytic. Even large destructive lesions are nonspecific roentgenologically when they do not manifest mottling due to calcification or ossification.

The roentgenogram of an osteochondroma that has undergone malignant transformation may be similar to that of the benign lesion from which it originated, but the surface ordinarily will be indistinct and fuzzy, and the clear demarcation from the adjacent soft tissue may be lost. A large mass, if associated with irregular shadows of bone or calcification, is especially characteristic. Sometimes the chondrosarcoma destroys and obscures the exostosis from which it arose. In the Mayo Clinic series, twenty-four of fifty-four patients with secondary chondrosarcoma had multiple exostoses, and the genesis of the malignant tumor from a benign osteochondroma could logically be assumed in these persons despite obscure evidence in the region of the chondrosarcoma. One of the twenty-four patients had areas of dedifferentiation into a more anaplastic type of sarcoma.

The roentgenogram is so characteristic as to be considered diagnostic in perhaps one third of all cases of chondrosarcoma.

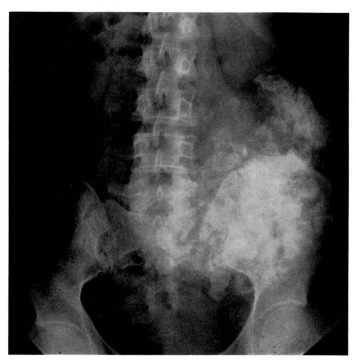

Figure 17-2. Heavily calcified chondrosarcoma of innominate bone of thirty-eight-year-old woman. This tumor had produced pain for four years. In spite of four attempts at radical removal, tumor produced death seventy-six months after its diagnosis. (Reproduced with permission from: Dahlin, D. C., and Henderson, E. D.: *J Bone Joint Surg, 38A:*1025-1038, 1956.)

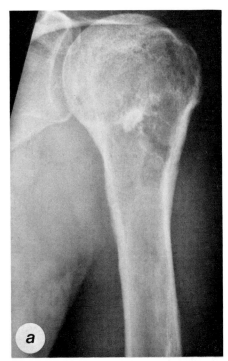 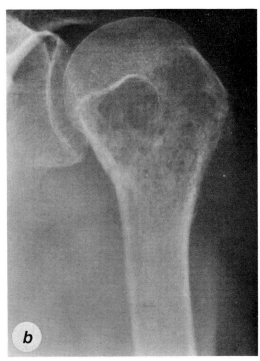

Figure 17-3. *a*. Chondrosarcoma, grade 1, in forty-eight-year-old man who had had pain for eighteen months. Tumor filled upper 11.5 cm of humerus and had perforated cortex. Central calcification is characteristic of cartilaginous tumor. *b*. Grade 2 chondrosarcoma in sixty-two-year-old man. Mass extended nearly to distal end of humerus, but that area had appeared roentgenologically "normal." Soft-tissue extension was present near humeral head. Inoperable pulmonary metastasis was found sixteen months after humeral resection, and death occurred twenty months after that.

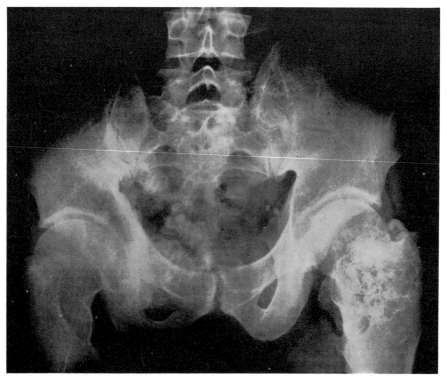

Figure 17-4. Chondrosarcoma of right innominate bone in thirty-six-year-old man who, as is seen in roentgenogram, had multiple osteochondromas.

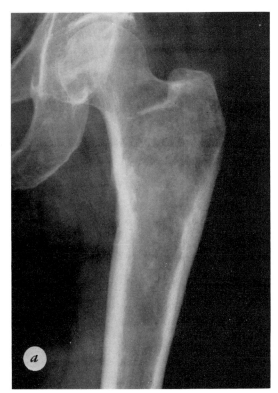
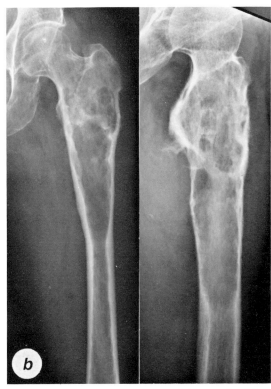

Figure 17-5. *a.* Grade 2 chondrosarcoma (11 by 4 by 4 cm) of upper third of femur in fifty-eight-year-old woman. Mass produced slight expansion of shaft and thickening of cortex. A small amount of calcification is present in tumor. Disarticulation was followed by recurrence at the hip eleven months later, having histologic features of grade 3 fibroblastic osteosarcoma. In spite of hemipelvectomy for this recurrence, death with generalized metastasis occurred fourteen months after first major amputation. *b.* Huge grade 2 chondrosarcoma in fifty-two-year-old man who had had pain for three years. Lesion had perforated cortex. (Case contributed by Doctors D. R. Olson, James Haven, and P. Lynch of Yakima, Washington.)

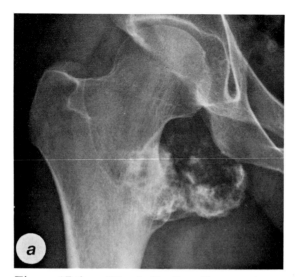
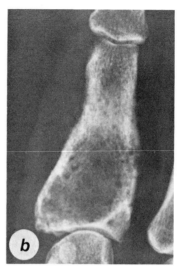

Figure 17-6. *a.* "Borderline" malignant chondroid masses aggregating 7 by 4 by 4 cm in thick irregular cap of osteochondroma in thirty-four-year-old man. *b.* Chondrosarcoma of proximal phalanx of second finger of forty-nine-year-old man. This lesion is more aggressive and permeative than the usual chondrosarcoma. This photograph illustrates importance of roentgenography in assessing malignancy in such lesions. (Figure 17-6*b* reproduced with permission from: Dahlin, D. C., and Salvador, A. H.: *Cancer, 34:*755-760, 1974.)

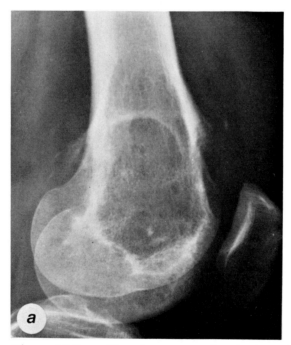
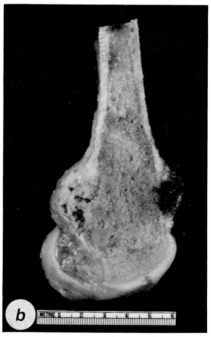

Figure 17-7. *a.* Chondrosarcoma that had produced local pain for three years in fifty-five-year-old woman. Pain had increased recently. Rarefied zone is associated with cortical destruction both anteriorly and posteriorly. *b.* Gross specimen after amputation. Basically, central grade 1 sarcoma, 6 by 5 by 5 cm, extends through cortex behind and in front of bone. Dark zone is site of biopsy.

Gross Pathology

Chondrosarcomas may be divided into central and peripheral types. In the examples in long bones, such a separation is usually obvious, with the rare peripheral sarcoma arising either on an osteochondroma or directly from the surface of a bone. If exostosis is present, a cartilaginous cap, irregularly thickened to more than 1 cm, must be viewed with suspicion; cartilaginous masses of 3 to 4 cm usually indicate chondrosarcoma. In thin or flat bones, such as in the pelvic girdle or thoracic cage, landmarks are so destroyed by the time the average tumor comes to attention that the exact site of origin can only be surmised, but most of them apparently begin centrally. As seen roentgenographically, central chondrosarcomas often produce expansion and concomitant thickening of the cortex of long bones. In such cases,

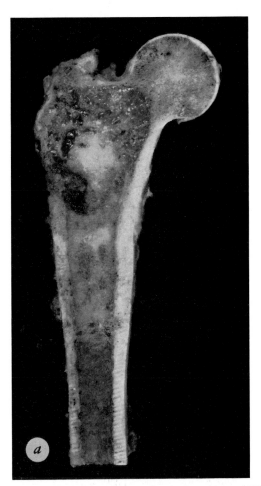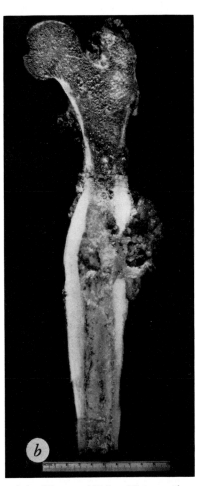

Figure 17-8. *a.* Gross specimen of case illustrated in Figure 17-5*a.* Note rather sharply defined margins of this tumor, which extends into femoral neck and has produced thickening of expanded cortex, especially on medial side. *b.* Chondrosarcoma of midfemur that has broken into periosseous tissues after having produced expansion of bone and thickening of cortex. (Reproduced with permission from: Dahlin, D. C., and Henderson, E. D.: *J Bone Joint Surg, 38A:* 1025-1038, 1956.)

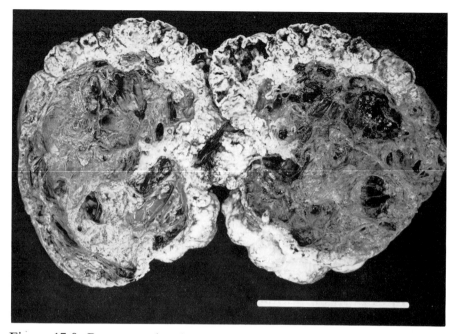

Figure 17-9. Recurrent chondrosarcomatous implant in peritoneal cavity. Primary tumor involved right ilium. Note lobulation, cyst formation, and extensive central zone of necrosis. Scale in lower right corner is 15 cm long. This tumor developed eleven years after first excision of iliac primary grade 1 chondrosarcoma and nearly four years after excision of first recurrent lesion.

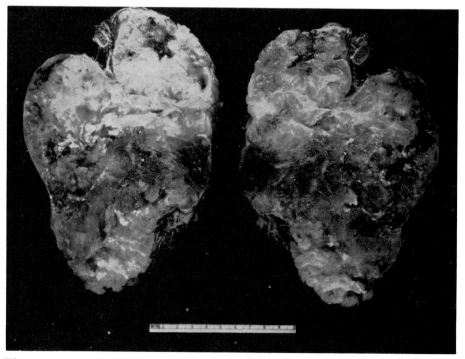

Figure 17-10. Chondrosarcoma of rib of sixty-four-year-old man who had noted swelling for eighteen months. Although this grade 2 chondrosarcoma was 17 by 15 by 13 cm, it was widely resected. Patient remained well for ten years and then developed signs of recurrence and metastasis.

the region of involved marrow is distinctly demarcated. The thickened cortex is invaded by tumor, and eventually breakthrough occurs.

These tumors are characteristically composed of lobules that vary from a few millimeters to several centimeters in diameter. Except at the tumor's periphery, these lobules are usually completely coalesced. The centers of the lobules often become necrotic, liquefied, and cystic. Necrotic foci often calcify in an irregular fashion. Some of the calcific zones observed grossly are actually osseous masses.

Chondrosarcomas produce a matrix substance that varies in consistency from that of firm hyaline cartilage to that of mucus. A myxoid quality is an ominous sign, strongly suggestive of malignancy. Sometimes the periphery or the recurrent form of a cartilaginous tumor is opaque and fibrous, resembling a fibrosarcoma or even as osteosarcoma grossly and microscopically.

Metastasis to regional nodes is distinctly rare. Hematogenous dissemination to the lungs and elsewhere is uncommon when one compares chondrosarcoma with osteosarcoma or fibrosarcoma.

Chondrosarcoma has a marked propensity for local recurrence even when the surgeon "has gotten well around" the tumor.

Histopathology

Without question, chondrosarcoma is the most difficult of the malignant tumors of bone from the standpoint of the histopathologist. The highly malignant ones with numerous normal and pathologic mitotic figures and obvious anaplasia offer no problem. The criteria that separate a low-grade chondrosarcoma from a chondroma, however, are very subtle, and experience with these tumors is necessary for accurate appraisal. Cellularity correlates poorly with malignant potential, as emphasized by the highly cellular but benign chondromas of the hand. The features proposed by Lichtenstein and Jaffe are very helpful. These include, when one studies viable fields, (1) many cells with plump nuclei, (2) more than an occasional cell with two such nuclei, and especially (3) giant cartilage cells with large single or multiple nuclei or with clumps of chromatin. Correct diagnosis depends upon accurate interpretation of these subtle qualitative characteristics. When one remembers, furthermore, that manifestly malignant foci may be overshadowed by regions that are necrotic or by zones with insufficient cytologic evidence for diagnosis of sarcoma, the pathologist's task is placed in proper perspective.

It is obvious that generous material for biopsy is mandatory and that the crutches of clinical and roentgenologic evidence are extremely helpful. One cannot make a microscopic diagnosis on the basis of the clinical and roentgenologic evidence, but such evidence will guide one in the search for pathognomonic microscopic fields.

By Broders' method of numerical grading, in which 1 signifies the least and 4 the most undifferentiated, no tumor in the Mayo Clinic series seemed to qualify for grade 4. The distribution showed that nearly 90 percent of the tumors were grades 1 and 2. During the past four years, approximately 10 percent of these sarcomas

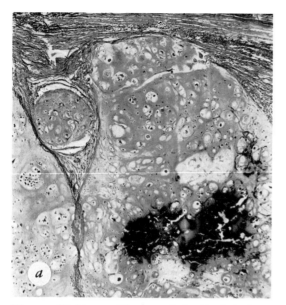
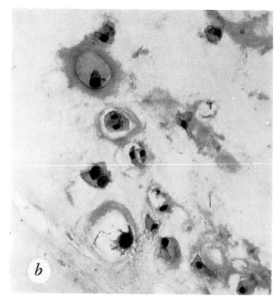

Figure 17-11. *a*. Characteristically lobulated periphery of chondrosarcoma, in this instance a grade 1 lesion. Black zones represent calcification secondary to necrosis. (×40) *b*. Definite cytologic evidence of malignancy includes cells with large, dark, and sometimes multiple nuclei. (×300) (Reproduced with permission from: Dahlin, D. C., and Henderson, E. D.: *J Bone Joint Surg, 38A:*1025-1038, 1956.)

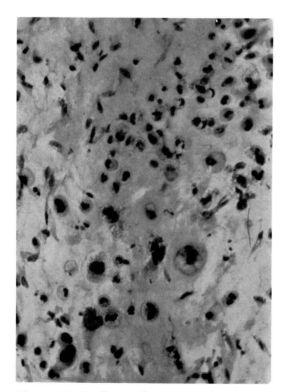
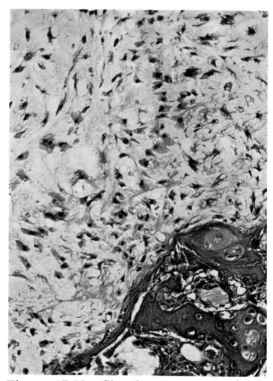

Figure 17-12. Zone of grade 3 chondrosarcoma. Here nuclear abnormalities and mitotic activity make diagnosis of sarcoma obvious. (×195)

Figure 17-13. Chondrosarcoma, grade 1. Fair numbers of binucleated cells are present, and ground substance is myxomatous. Cartilage is differentiating into mature bone. (×180)

have been considered "borderline" or equivocal for evidence of malignancy. This judgment was based on histologic study biased by clinical, roentgenographic, and gross pathological features.

As indicated previously, chondrosarcoma secondary to proved solitary benign enchondroma was not found in this series. In recurrent disease, study of the original specimens, which included all those that had been removed at the Mayo Clinic and many of those that had been removed elsewhere, revealed cytologic evidence sufficient for the prediction of a malignant clinical course in each case. Retrospection makes analysis easier, and, with due allowance for this fact, it must be admitted that in a few instances the primary tissue was sufficiently "borderline" that one might well have hesitated to recommend extensive ablative surgical treatment.

The older literature is replete with descriptions of chondrosarcomas that were presumably secondary to benign central cartilaginous tumors, and many early cases in the present series had been similarly interpreted. Misinterpretation of the original tissue sections, insufficient microscopic sampling of the surgical material, or incomplete removal of the primary tumor can lead to underdiagnosis and the erroneous impression that malignant transformation caused the subsequent recurrence. Calcification results from degeneration of these tumors, but mature bone appears to develop by ossification of the hyaline cartilage.

An additional histopathologic feature of chondrosarcoma requires comment. In approximately 10 percent of these tumors that are allowed to recur, there is an increase in degree of malignancy. Sometimes this is in the form of a more active pure chondrosarcoma; at other times the recurrence is in the form of highly malignant

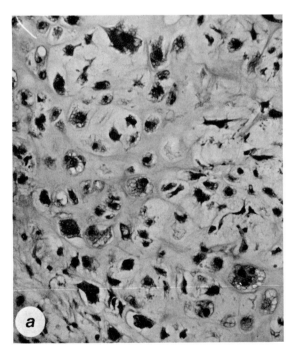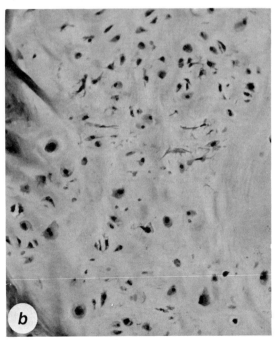

Figure 17-14. *a.* Chondrosarcoma, grade 2, of proximal phalanx, fourth finger. Nuclear atypia alone is enough for diagnosis of malignancy, but roentgenologic correlation is especially necessary for interpretation of such tumors in hands and feet. (×250) *b.* Chondrosarcoma of ilium with relatively sparse but numerous binucleate cells. (×160)

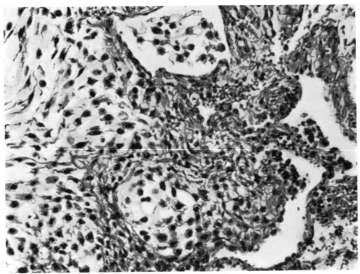

Figure 17-15. Myxomatous grade 2 chondrosarcoma. (×200) This is from pulmonary nodule removed by segmental excision sixteen months after leg had been amputated for primary tumor. Patient was alive and well twelve years after excision of metastatic nodule.

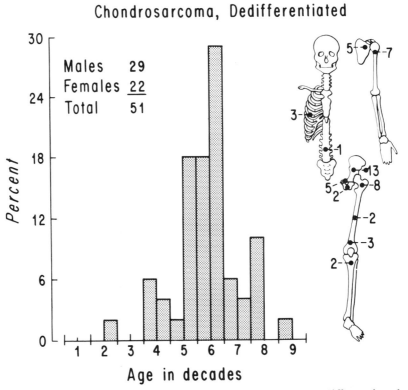

Figure 17-16. Skeletal, age, and sex distribution of dedifferentiated chondrosarcomas.

fibrosarcoma or osteosarcoma. I have seen several instances of similar transformation of chondrosarcomas in the absence of surgical intervention. Dedifferentiation of chondrosarcoma will be considered in detail later in this chapter.

The histopathologist should employ ancillary evidences to support the diagnosis of chondrosarcoma. These include large size, pain, invasiveness, extraosseous extension, myxoid quality, roentgenographic signs of aggressiveness, and rapid growth. Cartilaginous tumors in the distal parts of the skeleton, in a circumscribed subperiosteal location, or in the lining or capsule of joints are almost certain to be clinically benign.

Dedifferentiated Chondrosarcoma

INCIDENCE: Of the 470 patients with chondrosarcoma, 51 showed regions, usually larger than those of the underlying cartilaginous tissue, of significantly more anaplastic sarcoma (usually Broders' grade 3 or 4). In twenty-eight of these fifty-one, the dedifferentiated portion had the spindle-cell quality of fibrosarcoma; the remainder showed osteoid production by malignant cells, and these anaplastic zones were judged to be osteosarcomas. In a few instances, the chondroid precursor was so well differentiated as to be considered "borderline" for malignancy. The problem of dedifferentiation of chondrosarcoma has been alluded to in several publications on chondrosarcoma. Recent papers have accepted this entity. Dedifferentiation can occur in either primary or secondary chondrosarcoma.

Figure 17-16 indicates the distribution of these dedifferentiated tumors.

SYMPTOMS: Clinically, these sarcomas were like the remainder of the chondrosarcomas; in a few instances, there was evidence of a long-standing indolent tumor that had changed to a lesion with aggressive quality. Occasionally, recurrence was the first indication of this increased malignancy.

ROENTGENOLOGIC FEATURES: There were usually calcific foci in the tumor, or sometimes, it had produced remodeling expansion of the involved bone; both of these features were indicative of the cartilaginous precursor. Areas of cortical lysis and extraosseous extension, usually present, were not significantly different from such changes produced by an aggressive chondrosarcoma.

GROSS PATHOLOGY: The cartilaginous precursor was classically centrally located. It was often so small as to be easily overlooked. Sometimes there was evidence that the more anaplastic lesion had destroyed some of the chondroid lesion of origin. The characteristic semitranslucent, sometimes calcified and lobulated, cartilaginous tumor abutted the grayer, fleshy anaplastic tumor. Cortical destruction and extraosseous extension were by this latter component. The anaplastic tumor nearly always dominated the lesion grossly.

HISTOPATHOLOGY: There was typically an abrupt zone where low-grade chondrosarcoma gave way to highly anaplastic tumor. In a few instances, the spindle-cell component at the edges of chondrosarcoma lobules merged into the anaplastic sarcoma. This pattern is distinctly unlike that of the more active ordinary chondrosarcoma that shows a slight spindling quality of cells near the periphery of some of its lobules. Material for biopsy from the peripheral part of a dedifferentiated chondrosarcoma may not indicate the presence of the underlying lesion. Metastasis from such sarcomas is typically only the fibrosarcomatous or osteosarcomatous elements.

TREATMENT: Treatment must be radical and should be dictated by the dedifferentiated portion.

PROGNOSIS: Prognosis for such lesions has been poor. In our earlier study, approximately 80 percent of the patients died of their tumors, usually with known metastasis.

Of more importance is the implication of the possibility of dedifferentiation when one is considering treatment of a cartilaginous tumor. The magnitude of this risk is probably small, but it must be taken into account when one is considering conservative management of a possibly chondroid lesion found on the roentgenogram. Sometimes dedifferentiation accounts for aggressive recurrence of a chondrosarcoma.

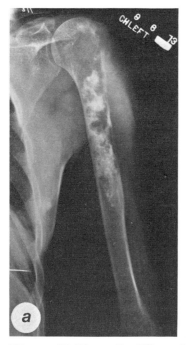
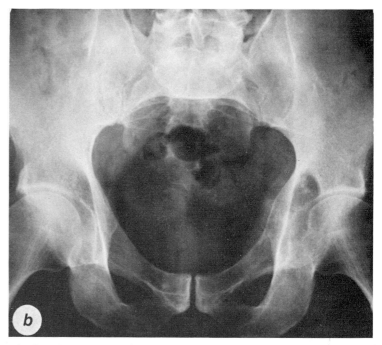

Figure 17-17. *a.* Dedifferentiated chondrosarcoma in seventy-one-year-old man. Protruding through cortex from this extensive grade 1 chondrosarcoma was 10 by 6 by 7 cm mass of grade 3 osteosarcoma, a nodule of which was highly anaplastic and had the pattern of malignant fibrous histiocytoma. *b.* Grade 1 chondrosarcoma at acetabulum of fifty-eight-year-old man with 6 by 5 by 3 cm intrapelvic extension of grade 3 fibroblastic osteosarcoma. Pain had been present four years before diagnosis. Despite hemipelvectomy, death with metastasis occurred in less than five months.

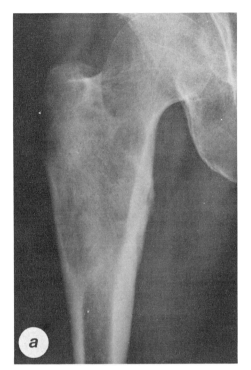 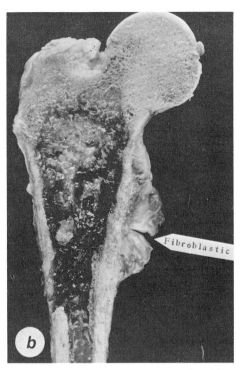

Figure 17-18. *a*. Chondrosarcoma that had produced pain for two years in fifty-three-year-old man. *b*. Central part of this tumor was hemorrhagic owing to extensive curettage for biopsy and showed only grade 1 chondrosarcoma. Dedifferentiated zone of grade 3 fibrosarcoma extended medial to tumor. Patient died with generalized metastasis eleven months after hemipelvectomy.

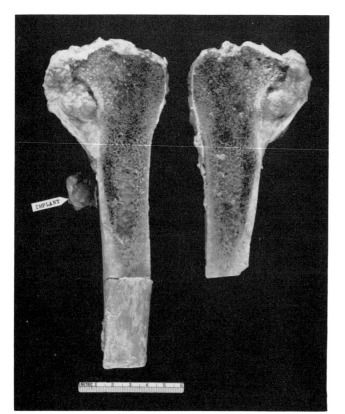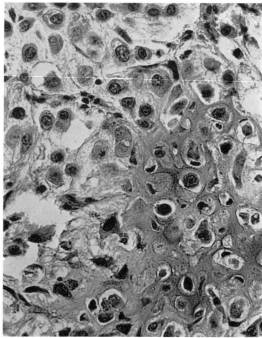

Figure 17-19. *Left.* Recurrence and implant near upper end of tibia one year after curettage for grade 1 chondrosarcoma. *Right.* This tumor was much more anaplastic than original, now having features of osteosarcoma. Death with pulmonary metastasis occurred less than one year after amputation for this dedifferentiated chondrosarcoma. (×300) (Figure 17-19 *left* reproduced with permission from: Dahlin, D. C., and Henderson, E. D.: *J Bone Joint Surg, 38A:* 1025-1038, 1956.)

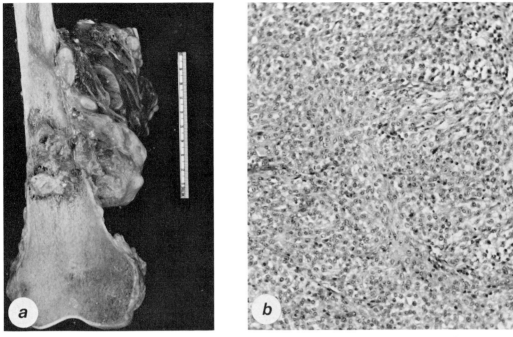

Figure 17-20. *a.* "Borderline" malignant central cartilage lesion in fifty-five-year-old man with extraosseous mass of highly malignant tumor. *b.* This dedifferentiated portion of tumor shown in *a* is coded as fibrosarcoma even though many of the cells have malignant histiocytic quality. (×160) Patient died less than four months after amputation.

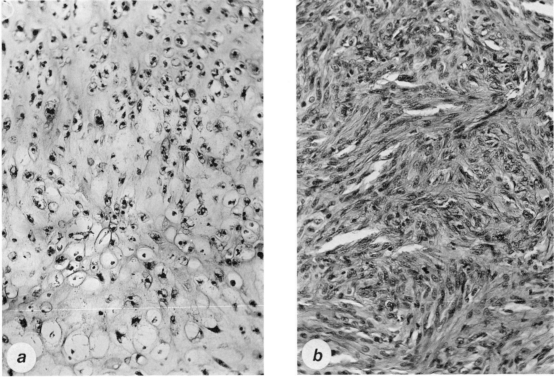

Figure 17-21. *a.* Grade 1 chondrosarcoma 6 by 4 by 3 cm treated by scapulectomy in fifty-three-year-old woman. (×200) *b.* Nineteen months later, recurrence was classic grade 3 fibrosarcoma. (×200) Patient died twenty-one months after forequarter amputation for this recurrent tumor.

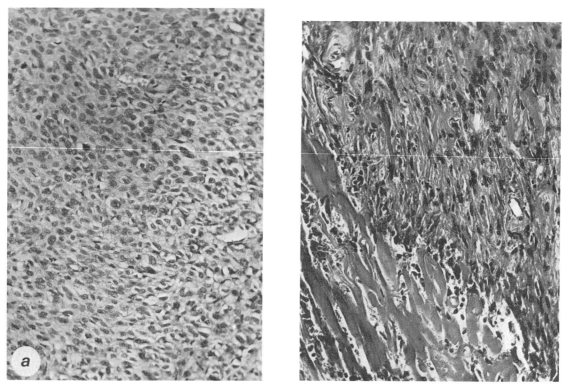

Figure 17-22. *a.* Grade 3 fibrosarcoma extending outward from grade 1 chondrosarcoma of ilium at acetabulum of fifty-two-year-old man. (×200) Patient died two months after hemipelvectomy. *b.* Grade 3 fibroblastic osteosarcoma. Dense strands are considered to be osteoid. This highly malignant tumor developed in scar after amputation for central grade 2 chondrosarcoma of upper femoral shaft of fifty-eight-year-old woman. Patient died with generalized metastasis three months after hemipelvectomy for this recurrence that followed eleven months after disarticulation. (×160) (Reproduced with permission from: Dahlin, D. C., and Henderson, E. D.: *J Bone Joint Surg, 38A*:1025-1038, 1956.)

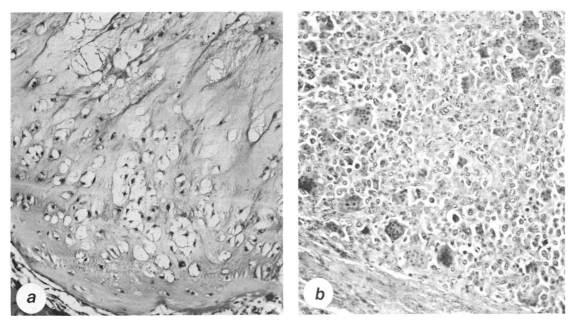

Figure 17-23. *a*. Central grade 1 (borderline for malignant) chondrosarcoma shown in Figure 17-17*a*. There is only slight nuclear enlargement; a few cells are binucleated. (×160) *b*. Highly anaplastic extraosseous mass simulating so-called malignant giant cell tumor of soft parts. Part of dedifferentiated neoplasm extending from this central chondrosarcoma had features of grade 3 osteoblastic osteosarcoma. (×160)

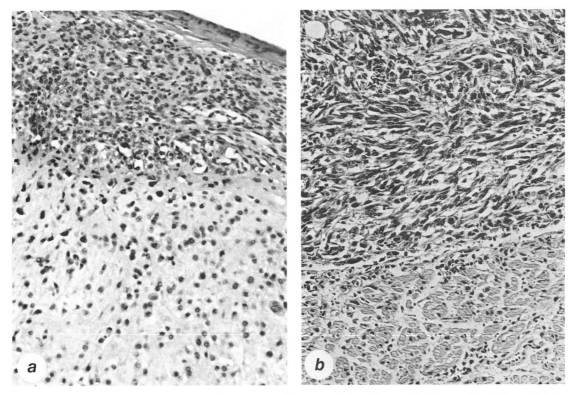

Figure 17-24. Photomicrographs from case illustrated in Figure 3-18. *a*. Dedifferentiated, highly malignant spindling area at periphery of lobule of chondrosarcoma of tibia of forty-seven-year-old man with skeletal chondromatosis. (×250) *b*. Patient died fifty-eight months after amputation, with generalized metastasis having pattern of grade 3 fibrosarcoma only. This is a nodule in myocardium. (×175)

Clear Cell Chondrosarcoma

Data on nine of the chondrosarcomas in this series and on seven additional tumors of this type sent in for consultation formed the basis for a recent study. The importance of this histologic type is that the tumors have frequently been mistaken in the past for osteoblastoma or chondroblastoma. They were usually, however, considered to be atypical examples of these benign conditions.

INCIDENCE: The incidence of this condition is low. Only 9 such tumors were recognized among our total of 470 chondrosarcomas.

SEX: Distribution, although not significantly indicated by this small sample, revealed that ten of the sixteen patients were men.

AGE: The ages of affected patients ranged from nineteen to sixty-eight years. Only one patient was less than twenty years old. There were four in the third, two in the fourth, five in the fifth, one in the sixth, and two in the seventh decade of life. The age of one patient was unknown.

LOCALIZATION: Data showed that the femur was involved in nine cases: its head and neck in three; the neck and trochanteric region in two; the head, neck, and trochanteric region in one; the neck only in one; the head only in one, and the "proximal part" of the femur in one. The humerus was involved in four cases: its head in three, and its head and neck in one. The upper metaphyseal region of the ulna, a vertebral lamina, and the pubic ramus were unusual primary sites.

SYMPTOMS: Clinically, these tumors produced lesions of slow growth. Symptoms were of less than one year's duration in two cases and varied from one to five years in seven cases, from six to ten years in four cases, and were of more than ten years' duration in three cases. Six patients had been told that they had cystic lesions seen on roentgenogram from nineteen months to twenty-two years before their first surgical procedure. Nine had had symptoms referable to a joint, and six had had pathologic fracture. One tumor produced cord compression. Only three had palpable swellings.

ROENTGENOLOGIC FEATURES: These tumors typically produced osteolytic expansion at the end of a long bone. The cortex was usually intact but frequently "expanded." The margins of the lesion were usually sharp and sometimes showed sclerosis. Calcification within the tumor was unusual. Smaller tumors could not be differentiated with assurance from chondroblastoma.

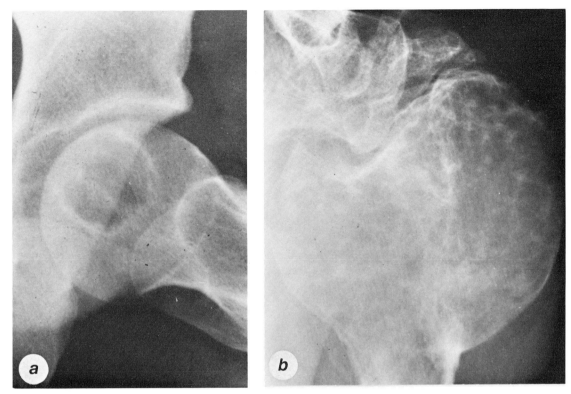

Figure 17-25. *a.* Clear cell chondrosarcoma producing osteolytic lesion in femoral head, with slightly lobulated, sharp sclerotic margin. This is very much like the roentgenogram of benign chondroblastoma. *b.* Clear cell chondrosarcoma of humeral head of more than ten years' duration. There is marked expansion of proximal part of humerus, with mottled mineralization within tumor. Cortex is intact but thinned. (Reproduced with permission from: Unni, K. K., Dahlin, D. C., Beabout, J. W., and Sim, F. H.: *J Bone Joint Surg, 58A:*676-683, 1976.)

GROSS PATHOLOGY: The tumors were often not recognizable as cartilaginous. Minute cystic spaces were sometimes present; one tumor showed prominent cystic change and had been mistaken for aneurysmal bone cyst even after pathologic study.

HISTOPATHOLOGY: These tumors were different from the average chondrosarcoma, which contains no benign giant cells, except perhaps in reactive zones adjacent to the tumor. Benign giant cells were usually found, either in small clusters or singly, throughout these tumors. This feature helps explain why several of these tumors had been considered to be "atypical" chondroblastoma or benign osteoblastoma. Some of the tumors showed fine lines of calcification between tumor cells, as are found in foci of many chondroblastomas. More often, fine or prominent trabeculae of osteoid or bone were present, either near the centers of lobules of tumor or scattered between sheets of tumor cells. The tumor tissue adjacent to trabeculae of bone was sometimes vascular. Lobulation was less prominent than in ordinary chondrosarcoma; lobules tended to be smaller and less distinct. The characteristic feature was the relatively abundant clear cytoplasm of the tumor cells; cell boundaries were usually distinct.

Seven of the sixteen tumors contained areas of conventional low-grade chondrosarcoma. Benign giant cells were not observed in such zones.

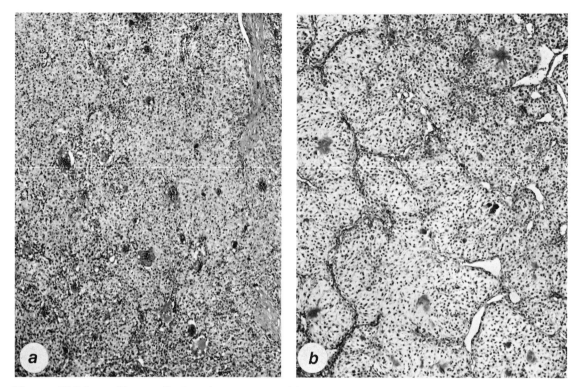

Figure 17-26. *a.* Clear cell chondrosarcoma with sheetlike arrangement of tumor cells, with scattered osteoclastlike giant cells. (×64) *b.* Low-power appearance of clear cell chondrosarcoma showing distinct lobularity. Centers of some lobules contain osteoid. (×64) (Reproduced with permission from: Unni, K. K., Dahlin, D. C., Beabout, J. W., and Sim, F. H.: *J Bone Joint Surg, 58A:*676-683, 1976.)

TREATMENT: Treatment for these lesions has been generally too conservative, partly because of their having been mistaken for benign conditions. The evidence indicates that complete total resection is necessary for hope of cure. Radiation therapy has not been efficacious.

PROGNOSIS: Prognosis has been worse than it probably ought to be because many tumors had been treated by less than early radical resection. Five of the sixteen patients we studied have died, three with metastasis, one from the effects of cord compression, and one of unrelated disease.

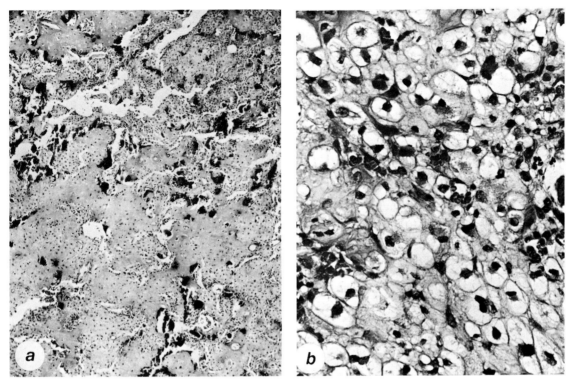

Figure 17-27. *a.* Osteoid formation which simulates that of osteoblastoma. There are fairly heavy deposits of calcium. (×64) *b.* Under high-power magnification, distinct cytoplasmic boundaries of cells are seen. Nuclei are dark, but there is not much atypia. (×400) The various features depicted are seen in clear cell chrondrosarcoma. (Reproduced with permission from: Unni, K. K., Dahlin, D. C., Beabout, J. W., and Sim, F. H.: *J Bone Joint Surg, 58A:* 676-683, 1976.)

Treatment of Ordinary Chondrosarcoma

Surgery is the mainstay in therapy of this radioresistant tumor. Irradiation will serve, at best, as palliation for those tumors not amenable to surgical removal. Surgeons with wide experience in the treatment of bone tumors have learned that the optimal treatment for chondrosarcoma is early radical removal with as wide a margin of uninvolved tissue as possible. Certain of these tumors in the region of the iliac crests can be radically excised with preservation of the lower extremity. Most chondrosarcomas that involve the innominate bone or the upper end of the femur require hindquarter amputation for adequate removal. Those that are in the thoracic cage should be excised widely with an adequate margin of uninvolved tissue. Chondrosarcoma of the clavicle or scapula often can be treated by wide local removal, but a similar tumor in the upper end of the humerus, unless small and confined to the bone, is often best treated by forequarter amputation. For chondrosarcomas of the major tubular bones that are away from the trunk, wide local excision with bone grafting as necessary is sometimes feasible. In such instances, recurrent tumors are often amenable to more radical treatment. Our experience indicates that wide local excision is likely to succeed for chondrosarcomas secondary to exostoses. Equivocal pathologic or roentgenographic evidence is indication for a conservative attitude.

Ideally, as with any of the surgical malignant tumors of bone, the definitive treatment should be carried out at the time of biopsy, but delay is doubtless of less importance in therapy of chondrosarcoma than of more anaplastic sarcomas. The roentgenogram may indicate the most aggressive and infiltrative portion of the tumor, which is the best region for biopsy. The biopsy wound should be planned so that the definitive operation can include it as part of the tissue to be completely removed or ablated because of the notorious capability of chondrosarcomas to produce recurrence by implantation. The tumor itself should be completely excised with an adequate zone of surrounding tissue so that the surgeon does not break into or see the tumor at any time. An occasional recurrent lesion is much more anaplastic than the original tumor and may have features of osteosarcoma or fibrosarcoma, which is another reason for adequate primary surgical treatment. Ideally, the first operation should completely encompass the tumor, be designed to prevent the threat of implantation, and preclude the hazards of recurrence.

As Barnes and Catto indicated, treatment should be predicated on the most ominous feature of the tumor, whether it be clinical, roentgenologic, or pathologic.

Prognosis of Chondrosarcoma

The fact that recurrences of chondrosarcoma are not uncommon after five years and sometimes are encountered even after ten years makes it obvious that five-year survival is not very significant as a criterion of cure. Actually, because of the common error of underdiagnosis and consequent inadequate treatment in the earlier part of the present series, the overall rate of cure for chondrosarcoma was less than for osteosarcoma in those years. Thoracic surgeons learned five decades ago that wide local excision was mandatory if one were to expect cure in the treatment of malignant cartilaginous tumors in the thoracic cage. Accordingly, many of the long-term survivors in the Mayo Clinic series are patients who had chondrosarcoma in this location. But during the last thirty-five years, when radical amputation has become common therapy for tumors in the pelvic and shoulder girdles, the upper part of the humerus, and the upper part of the femur, an increasing number of patients with chondrosarcoma in these locations are being cured. Long-term survival can be obtained in more than half the cases if adequate surgery is employed.

Lindbom, Söderberg, and Spjut reported a 21 percent incidence of distant metastasis in a thorough study of thirty-nine cases of chondrosarcoma.

Lesion with the histologic appearance of chondrosarcoma but in unusual sites such as the larynx or nasal cavities have a different biologic behavior than that of the typical skeletal examples. Those in the larynx metastasize only very rarely; those in the nasal cavities, probably arising from cartilage of the upper respiratory tract, have a relatively slow clinical evolution.

Bibliography

1927 Harrington, S. W.: Surgical Treatment of Intrathoracic Tumors and Tumors of the Chest Wall. *Arch Surg, 14*:406-431.

1943 Lichtenstein, L., and Jaffe, H. L.: Chondrosarcoma of Bone. *Am J Pathol, 19:*553-589.

1952 O'Neal, L. W., and Ackerman, L. V.: Chondrosarcoma of Bone. *Cancer, 5:*551-577.

1960 Kragh, L. V., Dahlin, D. C., and Erich, J. B.: Cartilaginous Tumors of the Jaws and Facial Regions. *Am J Surg, 99:*852-856.

1961 Lindbom, A., Söderberg, G., and Spjut, H. J.: Primary Chondrosarcoma of Bone. *Acta Radiol, 55:*81-96.

1962 Murphy, F. P., Dahlin, D. C., and Sullivan, C. R.: Articular Synovial Chondromatosis. *J Bone Joint Surg, 44A:*77-86.

1963 Goethals, P. L., Dahlin, D. C., and Devine, K. D.: Cartilaginous Tumors of the Larynx. *Surg Gynecol Obstet, 117:*77-82.

1963 Henderson, E. D., and Dahlin, D. C.: Chondrosarcoma of Bone—A Study of Two Hundred and Eighty-eight Cases. *J Bone Joint Surg, 45A:*1450-1458.

1963 Gilmer, W. S., Jr., Higley, G. B., and Kilgore, W. E.: *Atlas of Bone Tumors.* Saint Louis, Mosby, pp. 84-93.

1966 Barnes, R., and Catto, M.: Chondrosarcoma of Bone. *J Bone Joint Surg, 48B:*729-764 (November).

1967 Daniels, A. C., Conner, G. H., and Straus, F. H.: Primary Chondrosarcoma of the Tracheobronchial Tree: Report of a Unique Case and Brief Review. *Arch Pathol, 84:*615-624 (December).

1971 Dahlin, D. C., and Beabout, J. W.: Dedifferentiation of Low-Grade Chondrosarcomas. *Cancer, 28:*461-466 (August).

1972 Reiter, F. B., Ackerman, L. V., and Staple, T. W.: Central Chondrosarcoma of the Appendicular Skeleton. *Radiology, 105:*525-530 (December).

1973 Spjut, H. J.: Cartilaginous Malignant Tumors Arising in the Skeleton. *Proc Natl Cancer Conf, 7:*921-924.

1974 Dahlin, D. C., and Salvador, A. H.: Chondrosarcomas of Bones of the Hands and Feet: A Study of 30 Cases. *Cancer, 34:*755-760 (September).

1974 Fu, Y.-S., and Perzin, K. H.: Non-epithelial Tumors of the Nasal Cavity, Paranasal Sinuses, and Nasopharynx: A Clinicopathologic Study. III. Cartilaginous Tumors (Chondroma, Chondrosarcoma). *Cancer, 34:*453-463 (August).

1974 Mirra, J. M., and Marcove, R. C.: Fibrosarcomatous Dedifferentiation of Primary and Secondary Chondrosarcoma: Review of Five Cases. *J Bone Joint Surg, 56A:*285-296 (March).

1974 Schajowicz, F., Cabrini, R. L., Simes, R. J., and Klein-Szanto, A. I. P.: Ultrastructure of Chondrosarcoma. *Clin Orthop, 100:*378-386 (May).

1975 Campanacci, M., Guernelli, N., Leonessa, C., and Boni, A.: Chondrosarcoma: A Study of 133 Cases, 80 With Long Term Follow Up. *Ital J Orthop Traumatol, 1:*387-414 (December).

1976 Chambers, R. G., and Friedel, W.: Chondrosarcoma of the Larynx. *Laryngoscope, 86:*713-717 (May).

1976 Unni, K. K., Dahlin, D. C., Beabout, J. W., and Sim, J. H.: Chondrosarcoma: Clear-Cell Variant: A Report of Sixteen Cases. *J Bone Joint Surg, 58A:*676-683 (July).

1976 Dahlin, D. C.: Chondrosarcoma and Its "Variants." In Abell, M. R. (Ed.): *Bones and Joints,* IAP Monography No. 17. Baltimore, Waverly Pr, pp. 300-311.

Chapter 18

Mesenchymal Chondrosarcoma

THIS IS A CHARACTERISTIC malignant tumor recognized by the World Health Organization (WHO) as an entity in the 1972 Histologic Typing of Bone Tumours. The lesion is characterized by a basically bimorphic pattern consisting of sheets or clusters of highly undifferentiated small round cells, which may have a slight spindling quality and small or larger chondroid islands. The cartilaginous component is paradoxically well differentiated or even benign in appearance.

About one third of the tumors of this character have arisen in somatic soft tissues.

This malignant tumor is nearly always distinctly different from a high-grade or a dedifferentiated chondrosarcoma, the more malignant spindle-shaped or osteoid-producing cells of which are considerably larger.

The evidence suggests this is a relatively radioresistant tumor that is best treated by radical resection.

This lesion was described by Lichtenstein and Bernstein in 1959. At that time, I had tentatively labeled as mesenchymomas a group of ten strikingly similar tu-

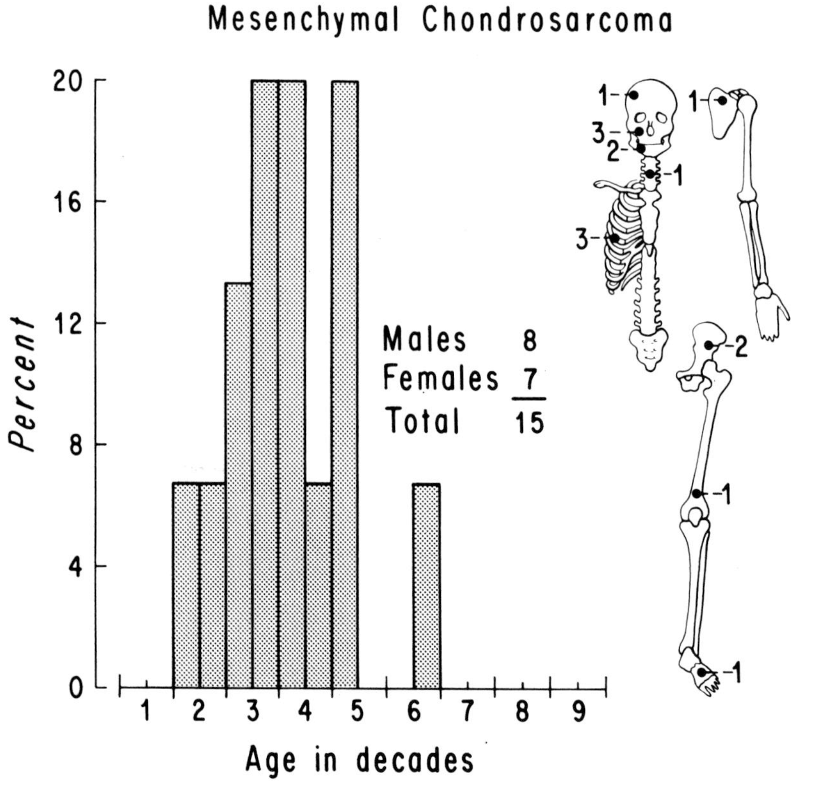

Figure 18-1. Skeletal, age, and sex distribution of mesenchymal chondrosarcomas.

218

mors that fit their description exactly. Other cases have been documented by Benedetti (1961), Gilmer and associates (1963), and Dowling and others (1964). The other unusual chondroid tumors described by Lichtenstein and Bernstein do not have counterparts I have recognized in the material available for study. If any are present, they have been classed with chondrosarcoma, chondromyxoid fibroma, and chondroblastoma.

Primitive multipotential primary sarcoma of bone, as described in 1965, includes cases that fit this description of mesenchymal chondrosarcoma. "Polyhistioma of bone and soft tissue" is a more recently suggested term for malignant tumors that have areas of small, round to oval cells. In such zones, the tumors bear a striking similarity to Ewing's sarcoma, but they differ from Ewing's tumor in that other areas show various types of differentiation, especially chondroid, osteoid, or fibromatoid, and with corresponding matrix. Hence, mesenchymal chondrosarcoma may artificially exclude some related tumors. Unfortunately, the exact delimitations of these other varieties of so-called polyhistioma are not yet well defined.

Incidence

The total of fifteen mesenchymal chondrosarcomas of bone in the Mayo Clinic cases indicates the rarity of this lesion. They comprised only one third of 1 percent of malignant tumors. Two identical tumors of soft-tissue origin have been found in our material.

Sex

Slightly more than half of reported cases have involved females.

Age

Only two patients were less than twenty years old: One was fourteen and the other was sixteen years of age, and both had mandibular tumors.

Localization

These skeletal tumors occurred in a wide variety of bones, but the jaws provided five of them. The predilection for jawbones is seen also in our material sent in for consultation. This tumor rarely involves major tubular bones, although it has shown a widespread skeletal distribution. Approximately one third of fifty-one such tumors that we studied in 1971 had arisen in nonskeletal tissue. In 1974, Sevel described the sixth case with orbital involvement.

Symptoms

Pain and sometimes swelling are the usual symptoms and are not unlike those of any malignant tumor. Approximately one third of patients have had symptoms for more than one year.

Physical Findings

No specific findings are produced by this lesion. Sometimes mass relates to its being a soft-tissue tumor.

Roentgenologic Features

In bones, the lesions are primarily lytic. Some are sharply defined, and others fade gradually into normal bone, but none in our series presented with a complete sclerotic margin. Calcification was present in three fourths of those of bony origin. Sometimes this calcification was pronounced. Although each lesion that was primary in bone had the appearance of a malignant neoplasm, it did not differ significantly from chondrosarcoma of the ordinary type. Mesenchymal chondrosarcomas of soft-tissue origin typically contain stippled or large areas of calcification.

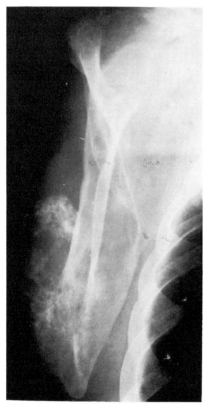 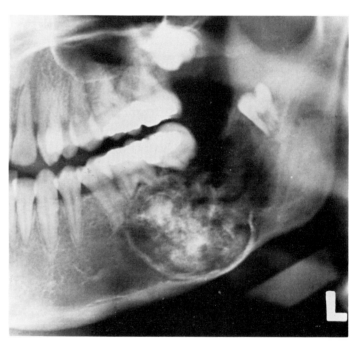

Figure 18-2. *Left.* Mesenchymal chondrosarcoma of scapula of fifty-eight-year-old man. Patient died with generalized bony and soft-tissue metastasis eight years after scapulectomy, having had left pneumonectomy for metastasis in the interim. *Right.* Mesenchymal chondrosarcoma in sixteen-year-old girl. She had noted tumefaction for six years, but with increased growth for one year. Patient was well 3.5 years after hemimandibulectomy. (Figure 18-2 *left* reproduced with permission from: Dahlin, D. C., and Henderson, E. D.: *Cancer, 15*:410-417, 1962.)

Gross Pathology

The tumors are typically gray-to-pink, firm or soft, and usually well defined. In rare instances, they appear to be lobulated. They vary in size to 14 cm in diameter. Most of the tumors contain hard, mineralized material that varies in amount from scattered foci to prominent zones. Some have a cartilaginous appearance, at least in part. Zones of necrosis and hemorrhage may be seen. Multicentric skeletal lesions have been described.

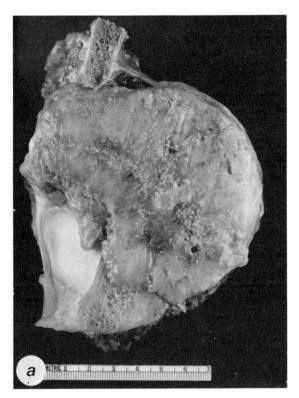 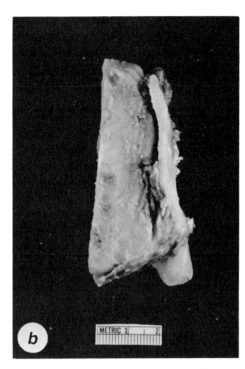

Figure 18-3. *a.* Mesenchymal chondrosarcoma of ilium and acetabular region of twenty-one-year-old man who had had pain for three months. Tumor was moderately calcified near its center. Patient was well two years after hemipelvectomy. *b.* Juxtamandibular example. This tumor probably began in soft tissues adjacent to mandible of twenty-three-year-old man. He had local recurrence and subcutaneous metastasis to his back thirty-eight months after hemimandibulectomy.

Histopathology

Mesenchymal chondrosarcoma shows the paradoxical histologic combination of highly cellular zones composed of anaplastic small cells and islands of relatively benign-appearing chondroid substance, which may be calcified and even ossified. The chondroid islands vary in size and number from one tumor to another and even in different regions within a neoplasm. The small cells that shade into the cells of the chondroid islands are usually somewhat spindle-shaped, but they may simulate reticulum cells and are sometimes related to blood vessels, reminding one of hemangiopericytoma.

Tumors of this type have been mistaken for Ewing's sarcoma. Confusion with this or some other small, round cell malignant tumor is avoided by studying multiple sections, but especially by being assured that the histologic material represents the mineralized portion of the tumor. Reference to the roentgenogram may be necessary for such correlation.

Chondrosarcoma of ordinary type but showing spindling of cells at the periphery of lobules or zones of highly malignant tumor as a result of dedifferentiation should not be mistaken for mesenchymal chondrosarcoma. The malignant small cells of the anaplastic part of mesenchymal chondrosarcoma are distinctly different from the larger ones of those in such zones of the former lesions.

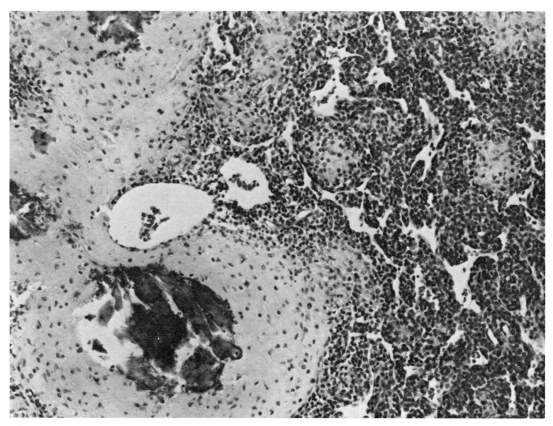

Figure 18-4. Classic appearance of mesenchymal chondrosarcoma with highly undifferentiated small round cells, here in a hemangiopericytoma pattern and abutting chondroid islands with central calcification. (×200) (Reproduced with permission from: Salvador, A. H., Beabout, J. W., and Dahlin, D. C.: *Cancer, 28:*605-615, 1971.)

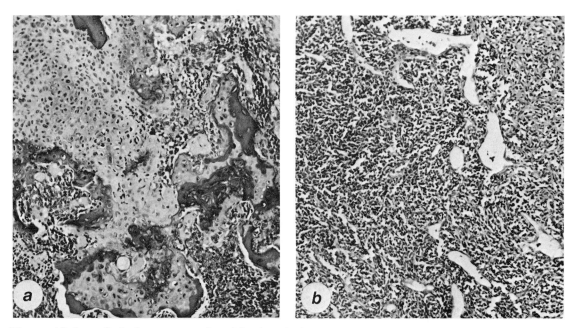

Figure 18-5. *a.* Soft-tissue example with chondroid zone, partially calcified and even ossified. Tumor had produced moderate mineralization visible by roentgenogram of this thirty-five-year-old man's thigh. (×160) *b.* Cellular area of mesenchymal chondrosarcoma with hemangio-pericytoma-like arrangement and slight spindling of small cells. (×160)

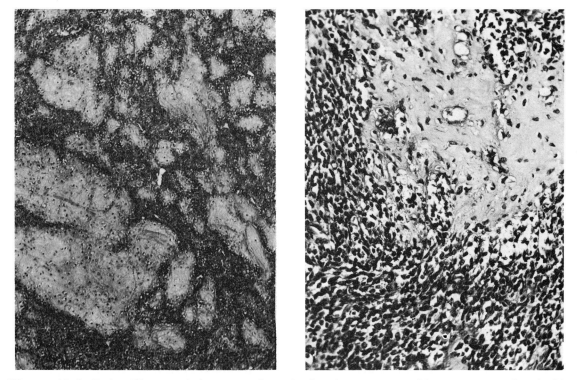

Figure 18-6. *Left.* Characteristic mesenchymal chondrosarcoma with numerous chondroid islands of varying size and a stroma of small cells with spindling nuclei. Note small size of nuclei within lacunae. (×95) *Right.* A characteristic zone in tumor of this group. Matrix has osteoid aura, and cells are somewhat more spindling than usual. (×200) (Reproduced with permission from: Dahlin, D. C., and Henderson, E. D.: *Cancer, 15:*410-417, 1962.)

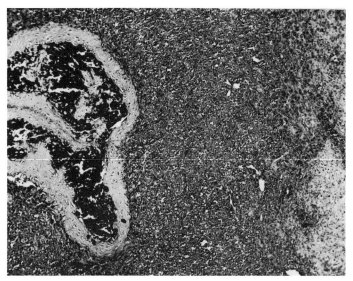

Figure 18-7. Commonly observed calcification within chondroid island. Sometimes ossification occurs in such zones. (×90) (Reproduced with permission from: Dahlin, D. C., and Henderson, E. D.: *Cancer, 15:*410-417, 1962.)

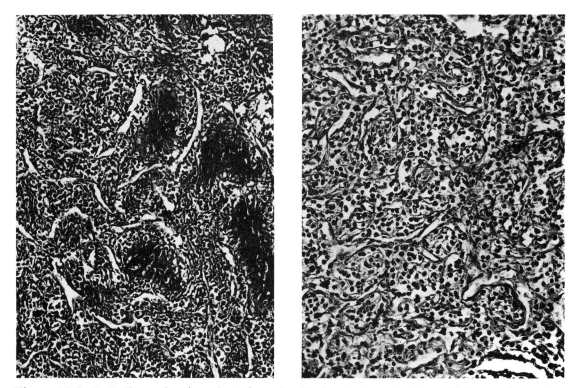

Figure 18-8. *Left.* Zone showing clustering of cells in relation to thin-walled vessels, pattern reminiscent of hemangiopericytoma. Note mineralization of chondroid foci. (×170) *Right.* Another instance of clustering of cells of mesenchymal chondrosarcoma. Note some resemblance to both reticulum cell sarcoma and hemangiopericytoma. (×245) (Reproduced with permission from: Dahlin, D. C., and Henderson, E. D.: *Cancer, 15:*410-417, 1962.)

Treatment

Mesenchymal chondrosarcoma is probably best treated by radical surgery, with the goal of completely removing the tumor from the host. There is some evidence that the Ewing-like small cell component of the tumor is responsive to radiation therapy.

Prognosis

Too few cases have been followed for a sufficient time to provide completely convincing data. The available evidence indicates that this is a highly malignant tumor with a strong capability of producing metastasis. Twelve of our fifteen patients with skeletal tumors of this type have died of their tumors, usually with metastasis. Six of these twelve survived from five to ten years inclusive and then died either of multiple metastases to lungs and bones or of local recurrences. In one patient, pulmonary metastasis developed twelve years after diagnosis of her maxillary tumor. In another, pulmonary metastasis developed that was histologically identical to the primary lesion that had been diagnosed twenty-two years before.

Three patients have survived twenty-three months, thirty-five months, and thirty-eight months after radical removal. The first of these, however, was lost to follow-up at twenty-three months.

Bibliography

1959 Lichtenstein, L., and Bernstein, D.: Unusual Benign and Malignant Chondroid Tumors of Bone. *Cancer, 12:*1142-1157.

1961 Benedetti, G. B.: Tumor Condroblastico Della Mandibola A Caratteri Istologici Peculiari. *Chir Organi Mov, 50:*135-144.

1962 Dahlin, D. C., and Henderson, E. D.: Mesenchymal Chondrosarcoma: Further Observations on a New Entity. *Cancer, 15:*410-417.

1966 Hutter, R. V. P., Foote, F. W., Jr., Francis, K. C., and Sherman, R. S.: Primitive Multipotential Primary Sarcoma of Bone. *Cancer, 19:*1-25 (January).

1967 Goldman, R. L.: "Mesenchymal" Chondrosarcoma, a Rare Malignant Chondroid Tumor Usually Primary in Bone: Report of a Case Arising in Extraskeletal Soft Tissue. *Cancer, 20:*1494-1498 (September).

1971 Salvador, A. H., Beabout, J. W., and Dahlin, D. C.: Mesenchymal Chondrosarcoma: Observations on 30 New Cases. *Cancer, 28:*605-615 (September).

1973 Guccion, J. G., Font, R. L., Enzinger, F. M., and Zimmerman, L. E.: Extraskeletal Mesenchymal Chondrosarcoma. *Arch Pathol, 95:*336-340 (May).

1973 Steiner, G. C., Mirra, J. M., and Bullough, P. G.: Mesenchymal Chondrosarcoma: A Study of the Ultrastructure. *Cancer, 32:*926-939 (October).

1974 Mazabraud, A.: Le Chondrosarcome Mésenchymateux: A Propos de Six Observations. *Rev Chir Orthop, 60:*197-203 (April-May).

1974 Sevel, D.: Mesenchymal Chondrosarcoma of the Orbit. *Br J Ophthalmol, 58:*882-887 (October).

1975 Jacobson, S. A.: Polyhistioma: A Pluripotential Small Round Cell Sarcoma of Bone and Soft Tissue (Abstract). *Am J Pathol, 78:*41a (March).

Chapter 19

Osteosarcoma

To QUALIFY in this category, the proliferating malignant cells of the neoplasm must produce osteoid substance or material histologically indistinguishable from it in at least small foci. A qualifying tumor, when sampled throughout, may show a predominance of elements with osteoid, chondroid, or fibromatoid differentiation. Accordingly, this series of osteosarcomas is divided into osteoblastic, chondroblastic, and fibroblastic types, depending on the dominating element. This classification may be confusing until one realizes that its function is merely to indicate that wide variation is seen in the histopathology of osteosarcoma. All of these tumors, however, have similar characteristics regarding bones of predilection, age of affected patients, pronounced tendency to early hematogenous dissemination, and necessity for prompt ablative surgical therapy. Malignant fibroblastic tumors with no definite osteoid production by neoplastic cells, regardless of their degree of anaplasia, are classed as fibrosarcomas. Similarly, those chondroblastic malignant tumors with no definite direct production of osteoid are designated as chondrosarcomas. Sometimes exact designation is difficult and must be arbitrary, since there is no special stain for osteoid and its qualities merge with those of collagen and cartilaginous matrix.

It has not seemed practical to divide the osteosarcomas into "sclerotic" and "lytic" subtypes, but some special types such as "periosteal," "telangiectatic," and "low-grade central" have shown special features that will be elaborated.

Although the great majority of these tumors are of unknown cause, Paget's disease is a precursor of some sarcomas, especially in older people. Of the 962 osteosarcomas in the present series, 30 arose in Paget's bone, as did 5 fibrosarcomas and 1 giant cell tumor.

An increasing number of sarcomas occurring after radiation therapy to bone are being recorded. There were thirty-five postradiation osteosarcomas in this series, twenty-nine fibrosarcomas, three chondrosarcomas, one Ewing's tumor, one malignant lymphoma, and one clinically malignant chondroblastoma.

Dedifferentiated chondrosarcomas with foci of osteosarcoma are described in Chapter 17, and osteosarcoma of the jaws has special features to be described.

A special type of osteosarcoma which grows slowly, metastasizes late if at all, and is characteristically juxtacortical or parosteal in location is known as parosteal osteosarcoma. This is discussed in the next chapter.

The rare extraskeletal osteosarcomas are very likely to metastasize and require aggressive therapy, but they must be carefully differentiated from benign heterotopic ossification.

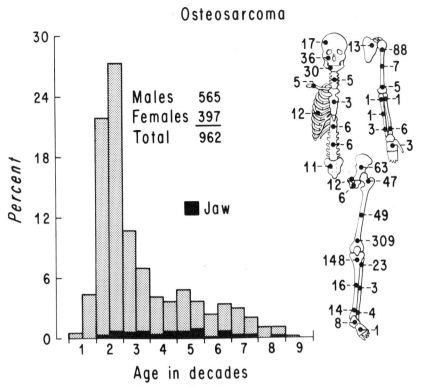

Figure 19-1. Skeletal, age, and sex distribution of osteosarcomas. (Reproduced with permission from: Dahlin, D. C., and Unni, K. K.: *Am J Surg Pathol, 1:*61-72, 1977.)

Incidence

The 962 osteosarcomas (excluding the parosteal variety) comprised 20.2 percent of the total sarcomas in this series. Except for myeloma it was the most common primary bone tumor.

Sex

Males contributed nearly 59 percent of all osteosarcomas and 62 percent of those in the jawbones.

Age

Although there are a few osteosarcomas in the first decade of life, the peak incidence is in the second decade, and there is a steady, gradual decrease thereafter. The youngest of the 962 patients with osteosarcoma was 2.9 years old. Osteosarcomas of the jaws occur in an older age-group on the average; this is not related to the fact that eight of the sixty-six were postradiation sarcomas.

Localization

The metaphyseal part of the long bones is the site of predilection, and the region of the knee accounted for half of the total number of osteosarcomas in this series. Of the total number of osteosarcomas, only twelve were distal to the ankle and wrist joints. Those sarcomas that did not extend to within 5 cm of an articular surface of a long bone are indicated as being in its midportion in Figure 19-1.

Excluding osteosarcomas of the jaws, 75 percent of the overall group arose in long tubular bones. In patients more than twenty-four years old, only 59 percent occurred in such bones. Paget's disease, postradiation sarcomas, the higher incidence of osteosarcoma in flat bones, and other factors probably influenced this difference.

Skeletal, Age, and Sex Distribution

Earlier studies of our material, as illustrated in Figure 19-2, emphasize the basic kinship of the osteoblastic, chondroblastic, and fibroblastic types of osteosarcoma. Males predominate in all types. All three types have a predilection for the metaphyseal region of the long tubular bones, but chondroblastic osteosarcoma has a greater tendency to involve the trunk than do the other two types.

The age distributions were similar for all three types, and contrary to some observations in the literature, no secondary peak was found in the older age groups. This secondary peak of incidence has been blamed on the influx of sarcomas secondary to Paget's disease in older people.

Data compiled on our first 469 osteosarcomas and 218 chondrosarcomas are

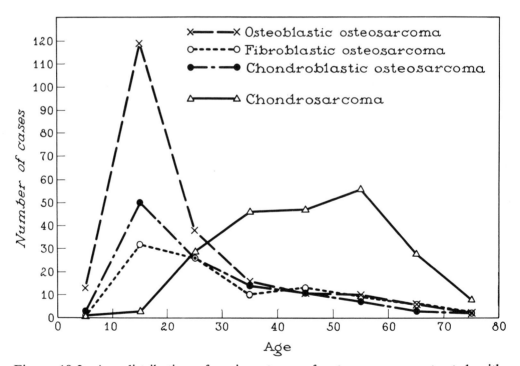

Figure 19-2. Age distribution of various types of osteosarcoma contrasted with that of chondrosarcoma. If the data for osteosarcoma had been expressed in percentages rather than in numbers of cases, the lines representing the three types would have been practically superimposed. Note that there are practically no chondrosarcomas in the second decade, the age of peak incidence of all histologic types of osteosarcoma. In middle and old age, when chondrosarcoma is common, the osteosarcomas become increasingly rare.

shown in Figure 19-2. They indicate the similarity of the distribution by age of the osteogenic sarcomas and its contrast with that of chondrosarcoma.

The term "osteosarcoma" for osteogenic sarcoma has been employed in this third edition because osteogenic sarcoma implies, for some, a wider variety of primary sarcomas in bone.

Symptoms

Pain, which may be intermittent at first, and swelling are again the cardinal symptoms. They are obviously nonspecific, and for this reason one should not ignore the possibly serious nature of these complaints, especially when they occur in childhood, adolescence, or young adulthood. Pathologic fracture is uncommon. One fibroblastic osteosarcoma of the femur occurred in an old infarct, and one developed in chronic osteomyelitis of the tibia.

The duration of symptoms prior to definitive therapy varies from a few weeks to several months. A history of trouble for more than one year is uncommon in patients with ordinary osteosarcoma. Increasing pain or swelling is suggestive of malignant change in Paget's disease. Likewise, a flare-up of symptoms in a patient who has had irradiation for a benign condition of bone should arouse suspicion. Similarly, a rapid increase in progression of disease is an ominous sign in patients with known or suspected cartilaginous tumors.

Elevation of alkaline phosphatase level, occurring in about half of the patients, is a reflection of osteoblastic activity.

Physical Findings

A painful mass in the affected region is usually apparent. Sometimes the mass is very large, and then it may be associated with overlying engorged veins and even edema distal to the lesion. Physical examination is noncontributory in some of the tumors that are covered by a thick layer of tissues. Evidence of pathologic fracture is distinctly uncommon.

Some osteosarcomas are familial, and some are associated with generalized skeletal diseases such as osteogenesis imperfecta.

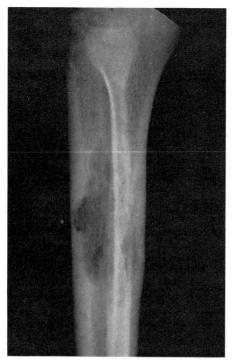

Figure 19-3. Almost completely lytic, fibroblastic osteosarcoma of upper, central portion of tibia.

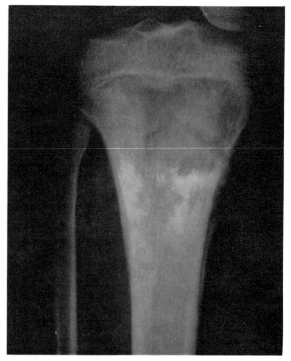

Figure 19-4. Lytic and sclerotic sarcoma of upper part of metaphysis of tibia, the second most common site of origin of osteosarcoma.

Roentgenologic Features

Depending on the amount of ossification and calcification found in osteosarcoma, there is great variation in the roentgenographic shadows produced. Tumors may be completely lytic or predominantly sclerotic, but they usually exhibit a combination of these features. The destructive process may be limited to the medulla but usually involves the cortex as well, since it is nearly always perforated by the growing tumor. There is a gradual transition from zones of marked lysis to zones of uninvolved bone, making the borders of the lesion indistinct. Non-neoplastic bone is deposited, sometimes in layers, when the periosteum is elevated by the perforating tumor. With continued development of the neoplasm, one frequently sees a large soft-tissue mass contiguous to the bone.

Varying degrees of density are seen within the affected portion of bone when the osteosarcoma produces calcifying and ossifying osteoid substance. These densities often extend into the contiguous soft tissues. The proliferated bone produced by the neoplastic cells characteristically has a streaked texture and ill-defined margins. The roentgenologic diagnosis is usually easily made in those tumors that show a combination of destruction of bone and proliferation of new bone, but definitive therapy should never be recommended without confirmation by biopsy. These sarcomas may be deceptively benign-appearing; some even resemble cysts of bone.

Osteoid substance, even if present in large amounts in an osteoblastic osteosarcoma, produces no radiopacity if it is completely uncalcified.

Pulmonary metastasis is sometimes demonstrable when the patient first seeks medical advice.

Skeletal survey may provide important information and is necessary before deciding appropriate therapy. Computerized tomograph and isotope bone scans are often valuable.

So-called myositis ossificans, a soft-tissue lesion, characteristically shows a delimiting peripheral shell of ossification, unless it is very early.

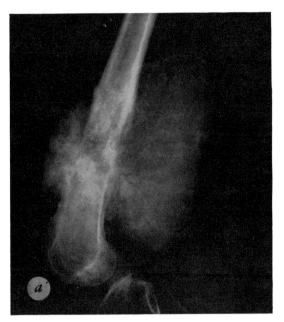 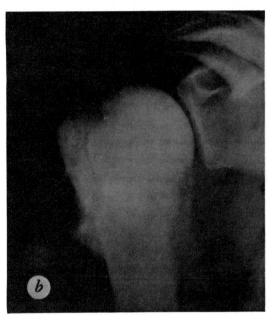

Figure 19-5. *a*. Osteosarcoma of distal part of femur with cortical destruction sufficient to produce pathologic fracture. *b*. Sclerosing osteosarcoma of upper part of humerus, one of the more common sites for this tumor. Note "sunburst" effect.

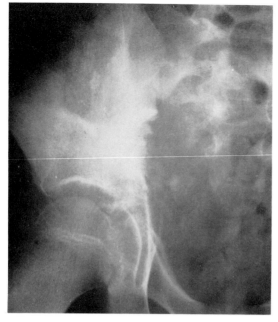

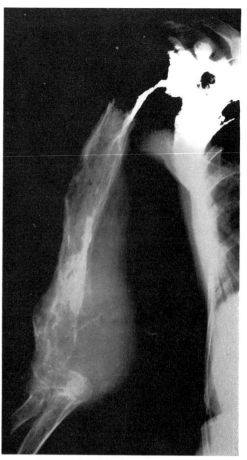

Figure 19-6. *Above*. Chondroblastic osteosarcoma of right ilium causing sclerosis. Note intrapelvic extension.

Figure 19-7. *Right*. Lytic but osteoblastic osteosarcoma of distal portion of right humerus. Entire bone shows severe changes of Paget's disease.

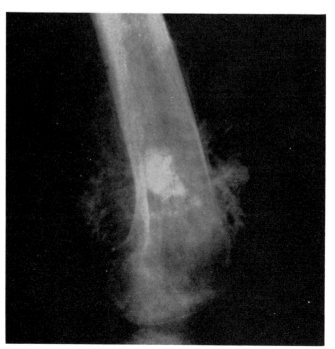

Figure 19-8. Osteosarcoma of distal portion of femur. Note destruction, sclerosis, and "sunburst" effect.

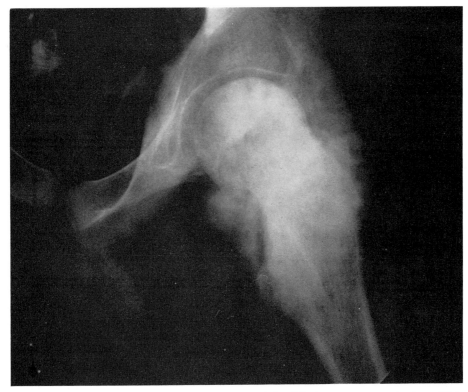

Figure 19-9. Grade 4 osteosarcoma treated by hindquarter amputation. This operation has effected a survival of more than eighteen years to the present time. (Reproduced with permission from: Coventry, M. B., and Dahlin, D. C.: *J Bone Joint Surg, 39A*:741-757, 1957.)

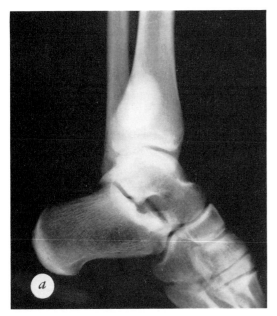

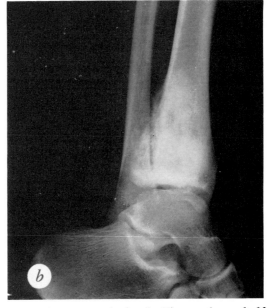

Figure 19-10. *a.* Early osteosarcoma inadvertently treated conservatively. *b.* Five and one-half months later, tumor has produced obvious cortical perforation and other signs indicative of malignancy. In spite of delay in therapy, patient has survived ten years since amputation.

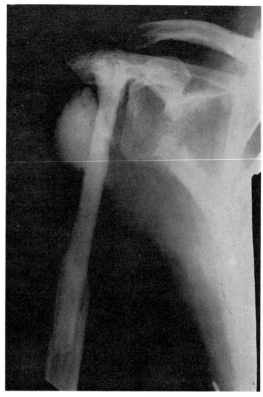

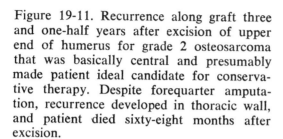

Figure 19-11. Recurrence along graft three and one-half years after excision of upper end of humerus for grade 2 osteosarcoma that was basically central and presumably made patient ideal candidate for conservative therapy. Despite forequarter amputation, recurrence developed in thoracic wall, and patient died sixty-eight months after excision.

Gross Pathology

By the time an osteosarcoma receives definitive therapy, it has generally breached the cortex. The extraosseous mass may even completely encircle the bone. The periosteum presents a barrier that often becomes greatly distended before it is perforated. Slight to complete cortical destruction is found in the site of perforation.

Some of these tumors spread in the marrow cavity for surprisingly great distances, not infrequently beyond that visible in the roentgenogram, and this must be reckoned with during therapy. In nearly all instances, the extent of the marrow involvement is readily apparent grossly when the bone is sawed longitudinally, and most tumors do not spread in the marrow beyond their gross extraosseous limits. Skip areas of medullary involvement are extremely rare in my experience, but Enneking has stressed their importance in his material.

Nearly all osteosarcomas have such a prominent central component that a central origin is logically assumed. Rarely, however, a highly malignant one is outside the bone and involves only the outer portion of the cortex, suggesting a periosteal origin.

As suggested by the roentgenogram, these tumors vary from extremely soft, friable, and granular masses, through a variety that is firm and fibrous with foci of irregular ossification and variable amounts of chondroid material, to the densely sclerotic ones. Sclerosis, when present, is invariably most pronounced in the central regions. Nearly all osteosarcomas, however sclerotic, have soft peripheral zones that can be sectioned without preliminary decalcification. Areas of necrosis, cyst formation, telangiectasis, and hemorrhage are most likely to occur in the soft tumors.

Metastasis is predominantly hematogenous, with the production of pulmonary deposits. Metastasis to other bones may be early and widespread, suggesting multifocal origin of sarcoma, or delayed and localized, suggesting that a new tumor has developed. Twelve patients in this series had at least two major amputations because such presumably new osteosarcomas appeared. One patient survived twenty-six years after the first and twelve years after the second amputation. The other

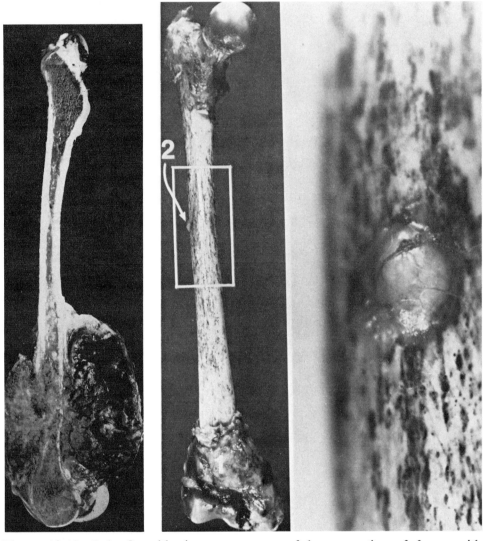

Figure 19-12. *Left.* Osteoblastic osteosarcoma of lower portion of femur with large "telangiectatic" area. Hemorrhage and degeneration but practically no intramedullary spread are seen. Roentgenogram of this tumor is shown in Figure 19-5a. *Right.* Osteosarcoma of distal femur with an unsuspected proximal "skip" metastasis. Primary lesion was anatomically remote from the more proximal "skip" (2) shown in more detail in the close-up photograph on right. (Reproduced with permission from: Enneking, W. F., and Kagan, A.: *Cancer, 36:*2192-2205, 1975.)

long-term survivor was alive and free of sarcoma twelve years after the appearance of the first tumor and seven years after treatment of the fourth. Lymphatic metastasis was rare in our material, but the vast majority of patients died at home and autopsy was not done.

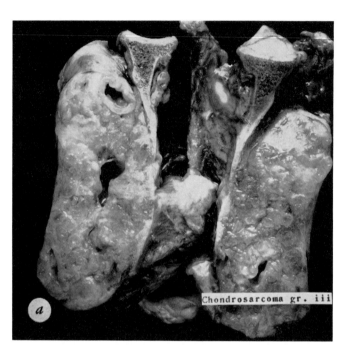
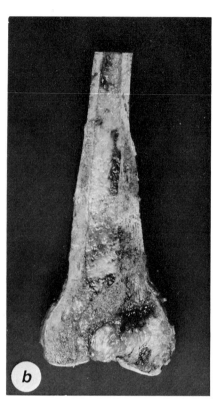

Figure 19-13. *a.* Chondroblastic osteosarcoma with areas of practically pure chondrosarcoma. This scapular tumor occurred in fifty-one-year-old woman. *b.* Paget's disease of lower third of femur has produced thickening of cortex and widening of shaft. There is secondary grade 4 fibroblastic osteosarcoma in medial condyle. This fifty-seven-year-old man died ten months after disarticulation for the sarcoma.

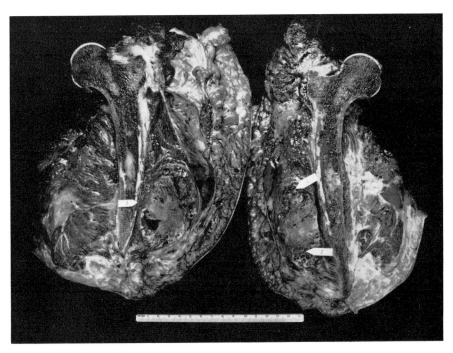

Figure 19-14. An unusual finding—recurrence in the stump after high amputation through the thigh for osteosarcoma of lower end of femur. This may have been the result of implantation of tumor cells, if proper precautions were not observed, since the biopsy immediately preceded amputation. Primary tumor, in this case, was in distal 8 cm of femur, and there was no medullary spread.

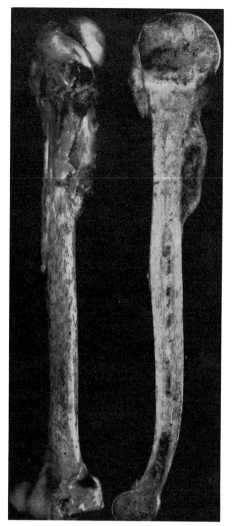
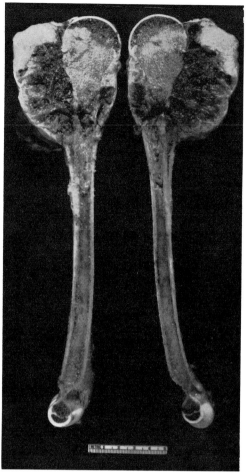

Figure 19-15. *Left.* Densely sclerotic osteosarcoma of upper part of humerus. Intramedullary spread nearly to elbow has occurred. *Right.* Predominantly cartilaginous (chondroblastic) osteosarcoma of upper end of humerus of eleven-year-old girl. Medullary spread extends 5 cm below external bulge of tumor but not beyond "Codman's angle," which has been produced by elevation of periosteum.

Histopathology

A great variability in the histopathology of osteosarcoma exists, as previously indicated. Lichtenstein has tersely stated the essential criteria as: "(1) the presence of a frankly sarcomatous stroma, and (2) the direct formation of tumor osteoid and bone by this malignant connective tissue."

Although these sarcomas rather conveniently fall into the osteoblastic, chondroblastic, and fibroblastic groups, depending on the dominating histologic pattern, it is necessary to be arbitrary in some cases. One occasionally encounters a highly anaplastic tumor that contains no osteoid but is otherwise so similar in histologic appearance to osteoid-producing tumors that it logically must be classified as osteoblastic sarcoma. Some such tumors have features that qualify them as malignant (fibrous) histiocytomas. Some tumors that appear as nearly pure fibrosarcomas contain foci of homogeneous, afibrillar, eosinophilic material that resembles hyalinized collagen. When such foci cannot be differentiated with certainty from osteoid tissue, tumors containing them are best classed as fibroblastic osteosarcoma. An occasional fibroblastic tumor, with only questionable osteoid production, produces very sclerotic metastasis. The usual member of this group, however, contains obvious osteoid material. One must be similarly arbitrary in the case of occasional chondroblastic osteosarcomas, in which osteoid production directly by malignant cells is debatable. But, with few exceptions, it is possible to make a clear-cut differentiation of these lesions from chondrosarcoma.

According to the predominant differentiation, more than half (343) of 650 osteosarcomas were osteoblastic, 155 chondroblastic, and 152 fibroblastic. Grading osteosarcomas by the method of Broders is difficult, and most of them are in the anaplastic high grades. Nuclear abnormalities are most important in judging anaplasia. Many anaplastic tumors contain much osteoid and even bone. In this series, approximately 85 percent were of grades 3 and 4, and only 1 percent were grade 1. These latter sarcomas are differentiated from benign conditions such as fibrous dysplasia with difficulty. Mitotic activity is typically most pronounced in the cellular peripheral portions of these tumors. The roentgenogram, or as a last resort the clinical course, may resolve the problem.

The original osseous trabeculae are destroyed to a variable extent in the lesional zone. Frequently, however, especially in the more sclerotic tumors, residual trabeculae are seen being enveloped by the advancing neoplasm. The central portions of osteoblastic tumors are routinely the most sclerotic, and in practically every case, there are peripheral lobules that are nonossified. The latter zones are the most satisfactory for histologic diagnosis because of the tendency for the cells to become small and less ominous in appearance when surrounded by sclerosing matrix. Some of the highly malignant, cellular tumors contain extensive zones of necrosis and hemorrhage.

Benign multinucleated cells in variable numbers are seen in a few osteosarcomas, thus introducing the possibility of confusion with benign giant cell tumor of bone. The problem is especially difficult in the case of sarcomas with relatively small cells. In these, the subtle evidences of nuclear anaplasia are fortified by a malignant appearance in the roentgenogram, which also usually reveals a metaphyseal epicenter for the tumor. Jacobson introduced the term "polyhistioma," and it apparently includes the extremely rare "small cell" osteosarcomas that we recognize.

Difficulty in diagnosis is caused by some osteosarcomas when they occur in unusual sites, in patients in the older age-group, and when the roentgenologic features of the lesions are not characteristic. Osteoid or chondroid substance in them may be of questionable quality, and osteosarcoma cells may be disposed in a glandlike fashion similar to those of metastatic carcinoma. The problem is aggravated because the osteoid and bone produced by the non-neoplastic cells in some metastatic osteoblastic carcinomas may rather closely mimic those of osteosarcoma.

Malignant fibrous histiocytoma as described in Chapter 24 is a tumor with a histiocytic quality and zones of fibrogenesis exhibiting a storiform pattern. Eighteen of the tumors in this osteosarcoma series are included also as malignant fibrous histiocytomas because zones were compatible with the latter diagnosis.

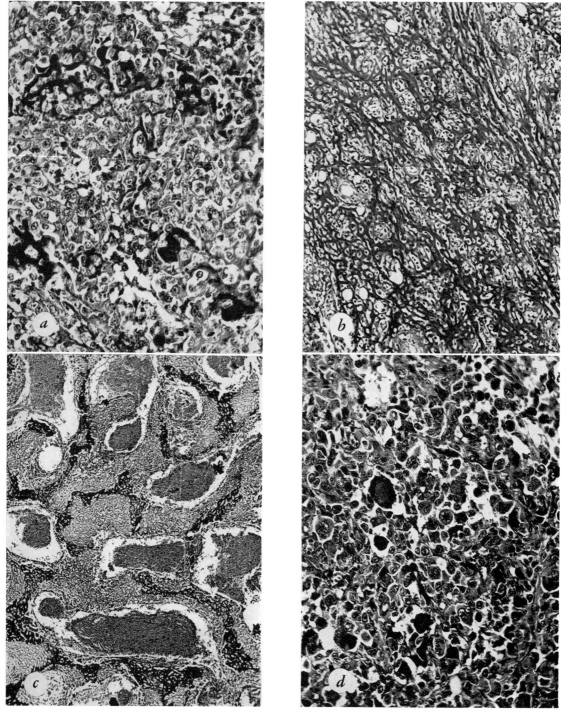

Figure 19-16. Osteoblastic osteosarcomas. *a.* Typical lacelike pattern of uncalcified and (dark) calcified osteoid being produced by highly anaplastic cells. (×200) *b.* Densely sclerotic zone with shriveled cells compressed by osteoid. (×100) *c.* Large pools of blood in hemorrhagic "telangiectatic" lesion. (×35) *d.* Extremely anaplastic osteosarcoma with no osteoid production in this field. (×165) (Figure 19-16*a* reproduced with permission from: Coventry, M. B., and Dahlin, D. C.: *J Bone Joint Surg, 39A:741-757, 1957.*)

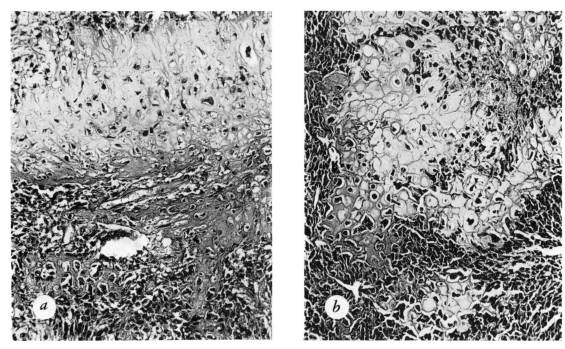

Figure 19-17. *a* and *b*. Sections from two chondroblastic osteosarcomas, both of which contain dominating chondroid substance. But both also contain distinct, fine, darker-staining osteoid trabeculae that are derived from neoplastic cells near the bottom of each photograph. (*a*, ×110; *b*, ×115) (Figure 19-17*a* reproduced with permission from: Coventry, M. B., and Dahlin, D. C.: *J Bone Joint Surg, 39A:*741-757, 1957.)

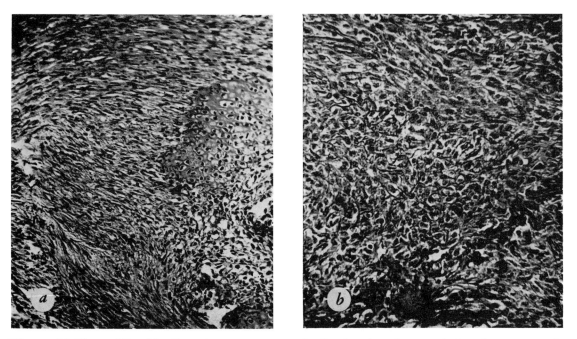

Figure 19-18. *a*. Fibroblastic osteosarcoma, grade 2, showing focus of chondrosarcoma in this field. (×100) *b*. Another basically fibroblastic tumor, however, that is producing "tumor" osteoid in the lower portion of photograph. (×185) (Figure 19-18*b* reproduced with permission from: Coventry, M. B., and Dahlin, D. C.: *J Bone Joint Surg, 39A:*741-757, 1957.)

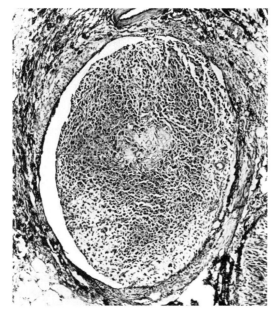

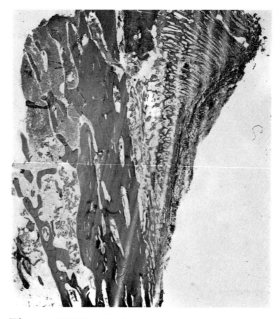

Figure 19-19. Grade 3 chondroblastic osteo-sarcoma of upper end of humerus, shown here in lumen of small regional vein. (×70)

Figure 19-20. Codman's reactive "angle." Striae of non-neoplastic bone are seen at right angles to the almost vertical, broad trabeculae of invaded cortical bone. (×5)

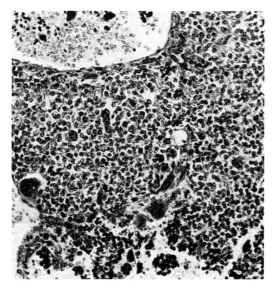

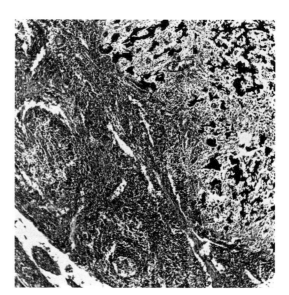

Figure 19-21. *Left*. Grade 4 osteosarcoma in Paget's disease of humerus. In this zone, cells are so small that they resemble those of Ewing's tumor, and benign giant cells are present to confuse the issue further. (×150) *Right*. Osteosarcoma producing irregular black masses of osteoid in lymph node. Lymph-nodal metastasis was conspicuously rare in our material. (×65)

Exuberant callus, especially in some patients with fractures secondary to osteo-genesis imperfecta, has been mistaken for sarcoma. This error can be avoided if one insists on cytologic evidence of malignancy in the diagnosis of sarcoma. It should be remembered, also, that the reactive subperiosteal new bone in "Codman's angle" is non-neoplastic and worthless for biopsy. The cells in pseudosarcomatous "myositis ossificans" lack anaplasia even in the zones where mitotic figures are numerous; the rather orderly production of bone in these lesions, especially periph-erally, as they become more mature also helps in recognition of the benign process. The same is true of callus.

Osteosarcoma is often considered to be a diagnosis that indicates a stereotyped and standard type of disease with relatively predictable clinical behavior. Any sizeable series, to the contrary, contains a wide variety of subtypes, each of which has its own, and often significantly differing, clinical features and prognostic impli-cations. Table 5 indicates the varieties that we have recognized. Some of the fea-tures of each type will be indicated in the subsequent remarks.

TABLE 5

TYPES OF OSTEOSARCOMA

Type		Number of Cases
"Usual" osteosarcoma*		962
In jaws	66	
In Paget's disease	30	
Telangiectatic	25	
Malignant fibrous histiocytoma?	18	
Periosteal	14	
In other benign lesions	8	
Multicentric	3	
Low-grade central	10	
Parosteal osteosarcoma		36
Postradiation osteosarcoma		35
Dedifferentiated chondrosarcoma		23

* May mimic osteoblastoma.

Osteogenic Sarcoma of the Jaws

Several peculiarities of osteosarcoma of jawbones deserve special comment. The average age of the patients is significantly greater than that of patients with tumors in conventional sites. This is true regardless of the dominant histologic pattern. Chondroid differentiation is more common; nearly half of the tumors were chon-droblastic, while the osteoblastic and fibroblastic varieties comprised the remainder. Osteoid production may be minimal and difficult to recognize. In fact, some ob-servers believe that some members of the chondroblastic group in this series should be called "chondrosarcomas." This is a disagreement of academic interest primarily, as evidenced by observations of Scofield and Garrington, who obviously regarded them as chondrosarcomas and found that osteosarcomas and chondrosarcomas of jaws affected patients of the same ages and gave practically identical five-year survival rates. Long-term survival was poorer in their chondrosarcoma group. Chondrosarcoma of classic type, as seen in other portions of the skeleton, has been extremely uncommon in my experience.

Grading by the Broders' method indicates an appreciably smaller amount of anaplasia in the osteosarcomas of the jaws. One result is that occasional tumors are differentiated from benign processes with difficulty. Regardless of relatively little anaplasia, chondroid differentiation in a lesion of the jaws should be viewed with alarm, because it is almost never found in a benign process, exclusive of callus, in these bones.

Hematogenous metastasis is much less frequently observed from osteosarcoma of the jaws than from those in more usual sites. Accordingly, wide resection provides a reasonable chance of curing patients with these tumors, and the prognosis has been better than that for osteosarcoma in the usual sites.

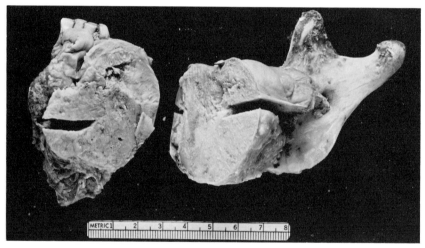

Figure 19-22. Grade 3 chondroblastic osteosarcoma of mandible of forty-four-year-old man. Patient has survived more than ten years after right hemimandibulectomy.

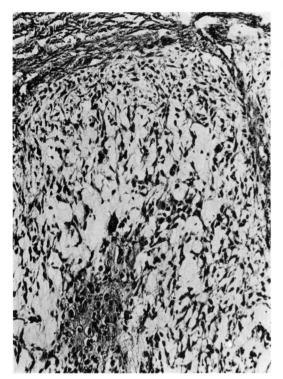 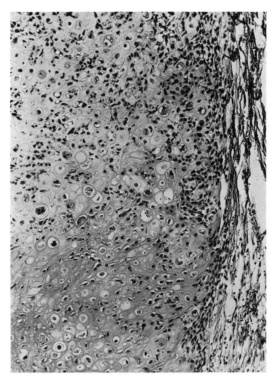

Figure 19-23. Two common patterns in chondroblastic osteosarcoma of jaws. Some prefer to class such tumors with chondrosarcomas. *Left.* Most of this tumor shows chondromyxoid differentiation, but near lower center, homogeneous acidophilic osteoid tissue is seen. (×100) *Right.* Despite predominant chondroblastic differentiation, tumors like this produce osteoid in their peripheral portions, such as that along right side. Regardless of how these tumors are classified, they behave like the more conventional osteosarcomas of jaws.

Osteogenic Sarcoma in Paget's Disease

Thirty (3.1%) of the 962 osteosarcomas were complications of Paget's disease. The humerus appears to have a predilection for this problem, and in this series, five of twelve osteosarcomas of the middle and lower portions of the humerus arose at sites of Paget's disease. The ilium contributed twelve cases, the pubis two, the femur seven, and various parts of the skeleton the remainder. Two were in the skull and one in a jaw. Twenty of the patients were in the seventh decade of life or older. Long-term survival for this type of sarcoma is rare, but one patient in this series with sarcoma of the femoral head was alive twelve years after hindquarter amputation, another with sarcoma of the lower part of the humerus was alive seven years after disarticulation at the shoulder, and a third was alive seven years after biopsy and cobalt-60 irradiation for an 8 by 6 cm lytic sarcoma in an ilium affected by Paget's disease. This last case is one of three osteosarcomas complicating Paget's disease with features suggestive of malignant fibrous histiocytoma, as described in Chapter 24, which may be an appropriate designation for them.

Although in patients with severe osteitis deformans, there is perhaps a 10 percent chance of sarcoma developing, the figure for all patients with Paget's disease is only about 1 percent. Fibrosarcoma, chondrosarcoma, and even giant cell tumor can complicate Paget's disease, and our series included five fibrosarcomas and one giant cell tumor, plus the thirty osteosarcomas.

Telangiectatic Osteosarcoma

Until recently, we have considered telangiectatic osteosarcoma to be an ordinary subtype of osteosarcoma. The twenty-five cases of this disease that we have recently segregated from the overall group make its recognition seem important. Twenty-three of the patients have died of their tumors, one has had two pulmonary metastatic lesions resected recently, six months after amputation for her femoral tumor, and the last patient was alive seventy-six months after amputation. A few patients in this group had delay in appropriate surgery because erroneous diagnoses, such as aneurysmal bone cyst and giant cell tumor, had been made initially. Nevertheless, most of the patients had appropriate early surgery, and still their prognosis has been poor.

Clinically, these patients did not differ significantly from the "average" with osteosarcoma. The tumors were lytic throughout, and the roentgenographic findings nearly always indicated that the disease was malignant. Six patients had sustained pathologic fracture. Grossly, the tumors appeared to be "cystic." They often were filled with clotted blood and necrotic debris. Viable tumor was often small in amount and confined to small zones at the periphery of the sarcoma. Care was taken to exclude from this group the fairly common osteosarcoma that has telangiectatic areas. Reference to sclerosis in the roentgenogram and significantly large microscopic regions of ordinary osteosarcoma helped exclude those that were telangiectatic only in part.

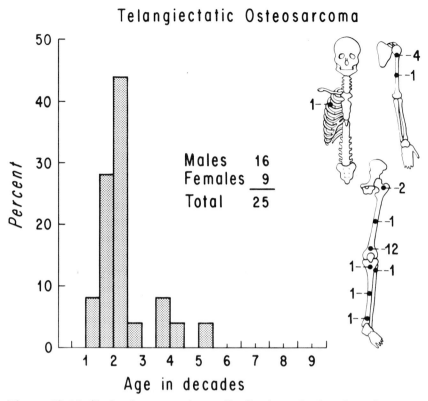

Figure 19-24. Skeletal, age, and sex distribution of telangiectatic osteosarcoma.

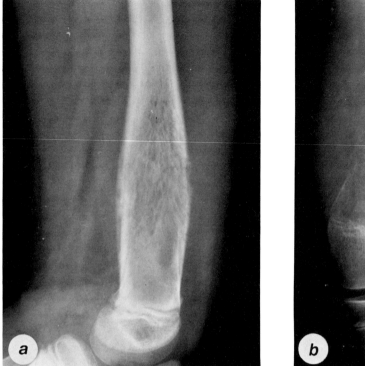 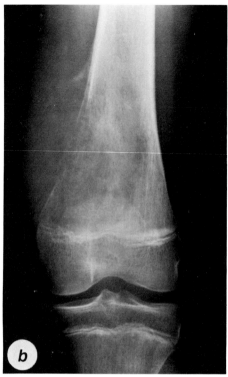

Figure 19-25. *a.* Telangiectatic osteosarcoma of femur in six-year-old girl. Note apparent expansion of shaft and resemblance to other lytic tumors such as Ewing's sarcoma. *b.* Telangiectatic osteosarcoma of sixteen-year-old boy who had had pain for three weeks.

Microscopic recognition that these were sarcomas depended on assessment of the nuclei of the mononuclear cells. Hyperchromasia and irregularities in nuclear size and shape were critical. Low-power histologic appearance often suggested the erroneous diagnosis of aneurysmal bone cyst. Benign giant cells were commonly found in these tumors. In many, the osteoid appeared to be typically like that of the ordinary osteosarcoma; but in a few cases, it was debatably present, sometimes resembling fibrinous deposits.

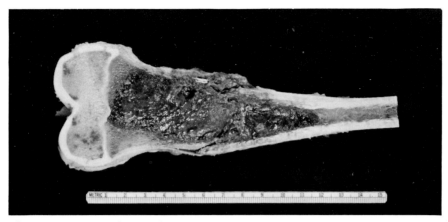

Figure 19-26. Specimen after amputation of sarcoma illustrated in Figure 19-25*a*. Sarcoma has nearly been replaced by blood and necrotic debris.

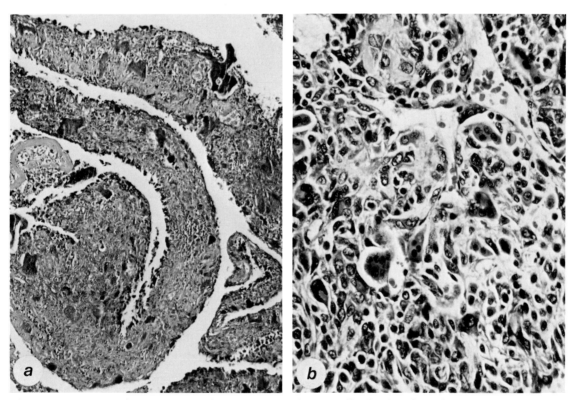

Figure 19-27. *a*. Thin strands of tissue curetted from wall of telangiectatic osteosarcoma producing pattern, at low magnification, of aneurysmal bone cyst. (×100) *b*. At high magnification, anaplasia indicative of malignancy is obvious in mononuclear cells. (×400)

In very rare sarcomas of bone, a benign aneurysmal-bone-cyst-like component is engrafted on the malignant tumor. In such cases, reference to the roentgenogram aids in assuring the pathologist that he has sampled the most significant part of the lesion.

Malignant (Fibrous) Histiocytoma

The details of thirty-five cases in this series that fit the description for this disease are given in Chapter 24. Eighteen of the tumors in that chapter had been coded as osteosarcoma and seventeen as fibrosarcoma primarily. They have been retained in our statistics relating to these two types of tumors because the long-term validity of this new designation is still uncertain.

Periosteal Osteosarcoma

Eleven tumors among these 962 fulfilled the criteria for what we have designated periosteal osteosarcoma. These have been called "chondrosarcoma" by some observers, and Jaffe referred to them as cortical osteosarcomas. Most observers have ignored this disease. Although chondroid differentiation usually dominates the histologic pattern of these lesions, near the centers of the neoplastic lobules, there is a condensation of pink matrix that has the quality of osteoid. Furthermore, typical spicules of new bone, sometimes numerous, are nearly always found near the underlying cortex. When a tumor of this type involves cancellous bone beneath the extraosseous mass, we have excluded it because of its similarity to the remainder of the chondroblastic osteosarcomas; it then merges into the overall spectrum of that disease. Whether these tumors begin in the periosteum or in the outer portion of the cortex is not known, but their appearance made the term "periosteal osteosarcoma" seem appropriate.

The only slightly greater than 1 percent incidence of this tumor type indicates its rarity in our experience. Our study of twenty-three examples included twelve sent for consultation. Fourteen of the twenty-three patients had tumors of the tibia, seven of the femur, one the humerus, and one the mandible. The tumors of the long bones were often at or near the midshaft. Thirteen patients were males. Only four of the twenty-three patients have died of metastatic disease. The evidence suggest that wide local resection—resection well around the tumor when possible—is acceptable therapy.

These tumors were higher grade (Broders) than the average parosteal osteosarcoma but were not as malignant at the conventional osteosarcoma. Although rare tumors exist in which differentiation of periosteal from parosteal osteosarcoma is difficult, they are usually clearly different. Details of parosteal osteosarcoma, a rare tumor itself but one which is much more common than periosteal osteosarcoma, are given in Chapter 20.

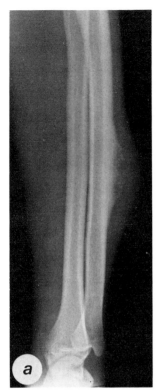
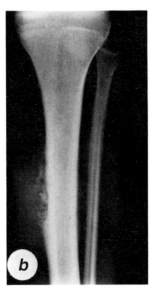
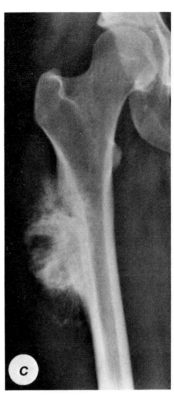

Figure 19-28. *a*. Periosteal grade 3 chondroblastic osteosarcoma of midportion of ulna of eighteen-year-old man. Patient was well nine years after amputation. This lesion was not in our series. *b*. Grade 2 periosteal chondroblastic osteosarcoma in fifteen-year-old girl. Patient had noted increasing swelling for one year. *c*. Grade 3 periosteal chondroblastic osteosarcoma near midshaft of femur of fifteen-year-old girl. This was largest tumor in our series, measuring 10.5 by 8 by 7 cm. Underlying marrow was not involved.

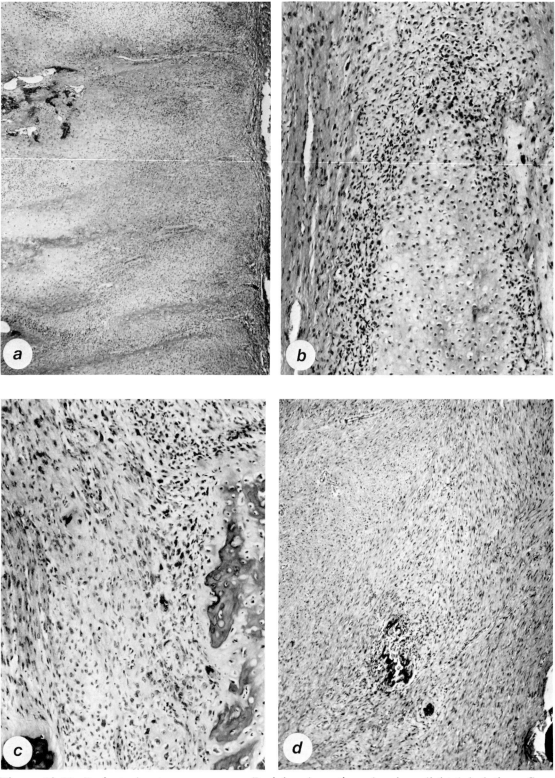

Figure 19-29. Periosteal osteosarcomas. *a.* Peripheral portion showing slight lobulation. Centers of lobules often ossify, giving rise to feathery appearance on roentgenogram. Cortex is at left of photomicrograph (×40) *b.* Spindling cells at periphery of lobule. (×100) *c.* Ossification and nuclear anaplasia. (×100) *d.* Faint osteoid seen among spindle cells. (×64) (Reproduced with permission from: Unni, K. K., Dahlin, D. C., and Beabout, J. W.: *Cancer, 37:*2476-2485, 1976.)

Osteosarcoma in Other Benign Lesions

The importance of these cases relative to the 962 osteosarcomas is unknown, but it should be noted that 2 osteosarcomas arose in solitary osteochondromas (exostoses), 1 in an exostosis of a patient with multiple exostoses, 1 in a patient with multiple chondromas, 1 in an old infarct of bone, 1 in a chronic osteomyelitic sinus tract, 1 in fibrous dysplasis, and 1 in a typical benign osteoblastoma. Details regarding this last case are given in Chapter 8.

Multicentric Osteosarcoma

Only 3 of these 962 osteosarcomas were multicentric when the patients were first seen. This is exclusive of those with the usual metastatic deposits when first studied. It is impossible to know whether such apparent multicentricity is produced by metastasis from one of the lesions. The involvement of more than one bone naturally compounds the therapist's problems. Metachronous multicentric osteosarcomas are described on page 235.

Low-grade Central (Intramedullary) Osteosarcoma

Of the 962 osteosarcomas in this series, 10 were very difficult to diagnose because they were so well differentiated. We have collected 15 additional cases from the files of problems sent in for consultation and 2 cases seen at the Mayo Clinic in 1976. The sexes were equally affected. The ages of the patients ranged from ten to sixty-five years, but most of the patients were in the second to fourth decades of life. The long bones were the sites of most of the tumors, but the mandible and the os calcis hosted one each. Roentgenograms helped differentiate these lesions from fibrous dysplasia, which it mimicked most closely. Roentgenographic examination betrayed that the average lesion was more poorly marginated than is fibrous dysplasia. The overlying cortex was sometimes destroyed and breached. In patients with mature bone growth, the lesion often extended to the end of the bone.

The pattern of fibrous dysplasia often was simulated by these tumors, but the pattern of new bone, variable in amount, was even more disorderly than that of fibrous dysplasia. The most striking difference was that the fibroblastic nuclei were more hyperchromatic than are those of fibrous dysplasia; many were long and spindly, and there was a tendency for them to be irregular in size and shape. These fibroblastic cells, even though bone is produced much as in parosteal osteosarcoma, provided the nuclear atypia which, along with the roentgenologic findings, allowed the pathologist to judge that the tumors were malignant. Many patients had protracted histories, often with several futile attempts to control their tumors by local removal. In only four of the patients has metastasis developed, but one patient showed implantation along with local recurrence after curettage and iliac bone grafting for a tibial tumor. Three of the tumors had become conventional high-grade osteosarcomas with recurrence. The evidence is that wide local resection is the treatment of choice for these lesions unless their size makes amputation more advisable. Osteoid production, even in small foci by the tumor, differentiates the very fibrogenic examples from so-called desmoplastic fibroma of bone.

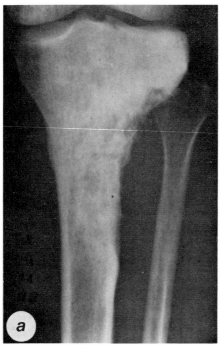
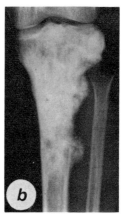
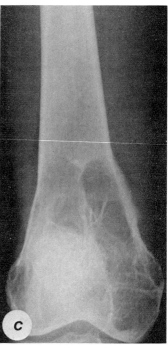

Figure 19-30. *a.* Low-grade central osteosarcoma in fifty-four-year-old woman. She had had tumor excised from this area two years previously. *b.* Nine years later, this slowly growing tumor had extended in- and outside bone. Amputation was performed one year after this roentgenogram was made. *c.* Low-grade, central, predominantly fibroblastic osteosarcoma in twenty-nine-year-old woman. Recurrent tumor, then with areas of grade 3 sarcoma, necessitated amputation eleven years four months after lesion shown had been treated by "enucleation" and radiotherapy. Patient died of unrelated disease thirty-six years after amputation.

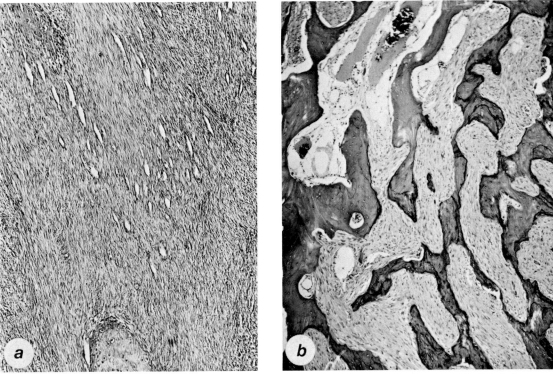

Figure 19-31. *a.* Grade 1, central, predominantly fibroblastic osteosarcoma of distal femoral shaft. (×50) Seventy-six months later, recurrence, then grade 3, had developed at site and necessitated amputation. *b.* Another intramedullary tumor whose nuclear pleomorphism betrays its malignancy and difference from fibrous dysplasia. (×64)

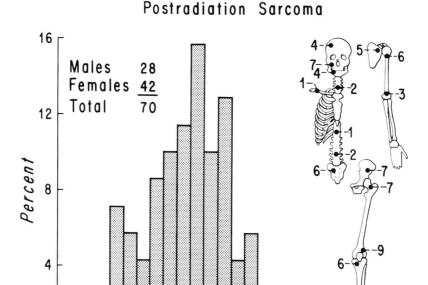

Figure 19-32. Skeletal, age, and sex distribution for postradiation sarcomas.

Parosteal Osteosarcoma

(This subject will be elaborated in Chapter 20.)

Postradiation Osteosarcoma

Thirty-five of the osteosarcomas in this series developed in bones that had been subjected to ionizing radiation. The total of seventy postradiation sarcomas of bone includes twenty-nine fibrosarcomas, three chondrosarcomas, one Ewing's sarcoma, one malignant lymphoma, and one metastasizing chondroblastoma. The interval between radiation and the diagnosis of sarcoma varied from 2.75 to 42 years. In sixty-one cases, the interval was at least 5 years, and the average of all was 13.4 years.

The groups of conditions for which radiation had been employed is indicated in Table 6. The sarcomas that developed were at least as lethal as similar malignant tumors that occurred in nonradiated bones.

This group of cases emphasizes the folly of using radiation therapy in benign conditions for which it has no proved value. A cause-and-effect relationship cannot be established unequivocally in any of these seventy cases, but overwhelming experimental and clinical evidence indicates that one exists. When osteosarcoma or

TABLE 6

INDICATIONS FOR RADIATION

Condition	Number of Cases*
Unverified osseous lesion	13
Giant cell tumor of bone	13
Carcinoma of uterus	11
Fibrous dysplasia	7
Carcinoma of breast	6
Aneurysmal bone cyst	3
Unverified brain tumor	2
Miscellaneous benign bone tumors	3
Miscellaneous soft-tissue tumors	8
Miscellaneous soft-tissue lesions	4
Total	70

* Through 1975.

fibrosarcoma develops in a patient in the older age group, he should be suspected of having precursors such as Paget's disease or prior irradiation.

These postradiation sarcomas were characteristically highly anaplastic sarcomas so not of debatable malignancy.

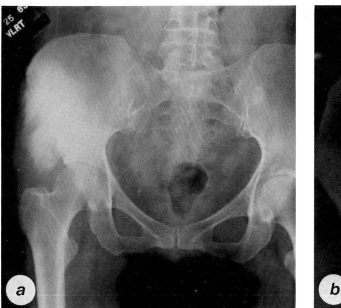 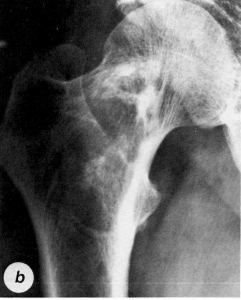

Figure 19-33. *a.* Osteoblastic osteosarcoma of right ilium of sixty-one-year-old woman who had had hysterectomy and radiation for adenocarcinoma of the endometrium sixty-two months previously. She died eight months after hemipelvectomy for this sarcoma. *b.* Grade 2 fibroblastic osteosarcoma of femoral neck and shaft of seventy-nine-year-old man who had had bone infarct in area for at least sixteen years. Patient died with metastasis twenty months after resection of this neoplasm.

Dedifferentiated Chondrosarcoma

The twenty-three osteosarcomas and twenty-eight fibrosarcomas that complicated low-grade cartilaginous tumors have been described in Chapter 17.

Treatment (All Osteosarcomas)

Because osteosarcoma is a radioresistant neoplasm, ablative surgical treatment is the procedure of choice. Surgical treatment of cancer aimed at cure is based on the premise that the tumor should be removed from the patient before metastasis becomes established. Metastasis obviously must occur at some specific time in the evolution of a given sarcoma. Accordingly, some patients will pay with their lives when treatment is delayed unnecessarily. One must, of course, examine the patient as well as roentgenograms of his chest, and the remainder of his skeleton for evidence of metastasis before instituting therapy.

Nearly all osteosarcomas contain small or large foci that require no decalcification prior to sectioning, and these foci routinely have the best cytologic details for diagnosis. Good fresh-frozen sections are adequate for definitive diagnosis by one familiar with the pathology of bone. Extreme care should be employed to prevent implantation of tumor cells at the definitive amputation level. Those averse to diagnosis by fresh-frozen sections should have permanent sections of nearly all osteosarcomas ready for diagnosis in one day's time. Delayed study of heavily ossified portions of the tumor or adjacent cortical bone is not necessary in establishing the correct diagnosis.

A good rule is to amputate through the bone above the affected bone, but it requires modification in the treatment of the common sarcomas of the distal portion of the femur. Data have not yet proved whether disarticulation at the hip is preferable to amputation through the upper part of the femur for these. Since a small percentage of osteosarcomas show pronounced spread in the marrow, the level of transection must be checked to determine the adequacy of any amputation through the affected bone. "Skip" areas as described by Enneking require consideration. They did not pose a significant problem in our material. Hindquarter amputations are necessary for most tumors of the upper end of the femur and for some of those in the innominate bone, and forequarter amputations are necessary for most of those of the upper part of the humerus. Lymph nodes are so rarely involved that dissection of nodes is probably not indicated unless they are enlarged.

Radical local resection with preservation of the limb should be employed for many of the smaller sarcomas, especially if they are relatively low grade. Radical local removal should be accomplished whenever possible for those tumors not in the extremities.

Radiation therapy is indicated for those tumors not amenable to ablative surgical treatment. Its value as early treatment for patients later to be amputated is questionable.

A growing number of patients in whom a localized pulmonary metastatic growth develops after the primary one has been controlled have had pulmonary resection.

The overall value of such resections for metastatic osteosarcoma is as yet unknown, but many long-term "cures" have been effected, and this modality of treatment is to be encouraged for properly selected patients.

Many therapeutic regimens adjunctive to surgical ablation have been employed in recent years. Chemotherapeutic agents, transfer factor, other immunologic manipulations, and interferon have their proponents. The final value of any of these agents awaits further analysis.

Prognosis

The five-year survival rate for 408 eligible patients we studied in 1967 was 20.3 percent, and the ten-year rate for 359 patients was 17.3 percent. More than 99 percent of patients in these groups had been traced. All patients who had no known metastasis and who had their definitive treatment at the Mayo Clinic are included in these survival data. Seven were known to have died of their sarcomas more than five years after therapy. For reasons unknown, tumors of the tibia were more favorable than those of the femur, the five-year survival rates being 36.6 and 18.6 percent respectively. The five-year survival rates for the osteoblastic, chondroblastic, and fibroblastic types were 17.1, 22.3, and 25.5 percent respectively. The highly undifferentiated sarcomas had but a slightly poorer prognosis than the better differentiated minority. Age did not have a significant bearing on prognosis. Three patients with sarcomas complicating Paget's disease survived, as did a few who had radiation alone, for at least five years.

These relatively favorable data on a large series of patients should help dispel the unfounded notion held by some that the prognosis of osteosarcoma is so poor that prompt and proper therapy is useless.

Bibliography

1955 Cade, S.: Osteogenic Sarcoma: A Study Based on 133 Patients. *J R Coll Surg Edinb,* *1:*79-111.

1956 Sabanas, A. O., Dahlin, D. C., Childs, D. S., Jr., and Ivins, J. C.: Postradiation Sarcoma of Bone. *Cancer, 9:*528-542.

1956 Fine, G., and Stout, A. P.: Osteogenic Sarcoma of the Extraskeletal Soft Tissues. *Cancer, 9:*1027-1043.

1957 Coventry, M. B., and Dahlin, D. C.: Osteogenic Sarcoma: Critical Analysis of 430 Cases. *J Bone Joint Surg, 39A:*741-757.

1957 Porretta, C. A., Dahlin, D. C., and Janes, J. M.: Sarcoma in Paget's Disease of Bone. *J Bone Joint Surg, 39A:*1314-1329.

1958 Kragh, L. V., Dahlin, D. C., and Erich, J. B.: Osteogenic Sarcoma of the Jaws and Facial Bones. *Am J Surg, 96:*496-505.

1961 Bacon, G. A., and Moe, J. H.: Primary Bone Tumor Study 1940-1956. *Univ Minnesota M Bull, 32:*312-319.

1961 Tanner, H. C., Dahlin, D. C., and Childs, D. S.: Sarcoma Complicating Fibrous Dysplasia. *Oral Surg, 14:*837-846.

1961 Lindbom, A., Söderberg, G., and Spjut, H. J.: Osteosarcoma. A Review of 96 Cases. *Acta Radiol, 56:*1-19.

1962 Platt, Sir H.: Survival in Bone Sarcoma. *Acta Orthop Scand, 32:*267-280.

1962 Wende, S.: Sarkom der Schädelkalotte nach Röntgentherapie. *Fortschr Geb Roentgenstr, 96:*278-282.

1963   Brody, G. L., and Fry, L. R.: Osteogenic Sarcoma: Experience at The University of Michigan. *Univ Michigan M Bull, 29:*80-87.

1964   McKenna, R. J., Schwinn, C. P., Soong, K. Y., and Higinbotham, N. L.: Osteogenic Sarcoma Arising in Paget's Disease. *Cancer, 17:*42-66.

1964   Lee, E. S., and MacKenzie, D. H.: Osteosarcoma: A Study of the Value of Pre-operative Megavoltage Radiotherapy. *Br J Surg, 51:*252-274.

1965   Steiner, G. C.: Postradiation Sarcoma of Bone. *Cancer, 18:*603-612.

1965   Scofield, H. H., and Garrington, G. E.: *Osteogenic Sarcoma and Chondrosarcoma of the Jaws.* Exhibit at the annual Meeting of the American Society of Clinical Pathologists, October.

1966   McKenna, R. J., Schwinn, C. P., Soong, K. Y., and Higinbotham, N. L.: Sarcomata of the Osteogenic Series (Osteosarcoma, Fibrosarcoma, Chondrosarcoma, Parosteal Osteogenic Sarcoma, and Sarcomata Arising in Abnormal Bone): An Analysis of 552 Cases. *J Bone Joint Surg, 48A:*1-26.

1967   Dahlin, D. C., and Coventry, M. B.: Osteogenic Sarcoma: A Study of Six Hundred Cases. *J Bone Joint Surg, 49A:*101-110 (January).

1968   Lowbeer, L.: Multifocal Osteosarcomatosis, a Rare Entity. *Bull Pathol, 9:*52-53 (March).

1969   Amstutz, H. C.: Multiple Osteogenic Sarcomata—Metastatic or Multicentric? Report of Two Cases and Review of Literaure. *Cancer, 24:*923-931 (November).

1971   Allan, C. J., and Soule, E. H.: Osteogenic Sarcomata of the Somatic Soft Tissues: Clinicopathologic Study of 26 Cases and Review of Literature. *Cancer, 27:*1121-1133 (May).

1971   Campanacci, M., and Pizzoferrato, A.: Osteosarcoma Emorragico. *Chir Organi Mov, 60:*409-421.

1972   Sim, F. H., Cupps, R. E., Dahlin, D. C., and Ivins, J. C.: Postradiation Sarcoma of Bone. *J Bone Joint Surg, 54A:*1479-1489 (October).

1973   Fitzgerald, R. H., Jr., Dahlin, D. C., and Sim, F. H.: Multiple Metachronous Osteogenic Sarcoma: Report of Twelve Cases With Two Long-Term Survivors. *J Bone Joint Surg, 55A:*595-605 (April).

1974   Lewis, R. J., and Lotz, M. J.: Medullary Extension of Osteosarcoma: Implications for Rational Therapy. *Cancer, 33:*371-375 (February).

1975   Campanacci, M., and Cervellati, G.: Osteosarcoma: A Review of 345 Cases. *Ital J Orthop Traumatol, 1:*5-22 (April).

1975   Dahlin, D. C.: Pathology of Osteosarcoma. *Clin Orthop, 111:*23-32 (September).

1975   Enneking, W. F., and Kagan, A.: "Skip" Metastases in Osteosarcoma. *Cancer, 36:*2192-2205 (December).

1975   Ohno, T., Abe, M., Tateishi, A., Kako, K., Miki, H., Sekine, K., Ueyama, H., Hasegawa, O., and Obara, K.: Osteogenic Sarcoma: A Study of One Hundred and Thirty Cases. *J Bone Joint Surg, 57A:*397-404 (April).

1975   Pritchard, D. J., Finkel, M. P., and Reilly, C. A., Jr.: The Etiology of Osteosarcoma: A Review of Current Considerations. *Clin Orthop, 111:*14-22 (September).

1976   Matsuno, T., Unni, K. K., McLeod, R. A., and Dahlin, D. C.: Telangiectatic Osteogenic Sarcoma. *Cancer, 38:*2538-2547 (December).

1976   Spanos, P. K., Payne, W. S., Ivins, J. C., and Pritchard, D. J.: Pulmonary Resection for Metastatic Osteogenic Sarcoma. *J Bone Joint Surg, 58A:*624-628 (July).

1976   Unni, K. K., Dahlin, D. C., and Beabout, J. W.: Periosteal Osteogenic Sarcoma. *Cancer, 37:*2476-2485 (May).

1976   Williams, A. H., Schwinn, C. P., and Parker, J. W.: The Ultrastructure of Osteosarcoma: A Review of Twenty Cases. *Cancer, 37:*1293-1301 (March).

1977   Dahlin, D. C., Unni, K. K., and Matsuno, T.: Malignant (Fibrous) Histiocytoma of Bone—Fact or Fancy? *Cancer, 39:*1508-1516 (April).

Chapter 20

Parosteal Osteosarcoma (Juxtacortical Osteosarcoma)

THIS TUMOR is considered separately from the remainder of the osteosarcomas because it is distinctly less malignant, and therefore, has a vastly different clinical behavior. As the name implies, this tumor is on the outer surface of the cortex of a bone, and some prefer to call it a juxtacortical osteosarcoma. The validity of the concept of parosteal osteosarcoma as a distinct clinicopathologic entity demands that the tumor be well differentiated (low-grade by Broders' method) and that it arise on the surface of a bone.

The rarity of this lesion, comprising less than 4 percent of osteosarcomas, has delayed its general recognition. Although occasional typical cases were documented in the literature, it was not until the description of a collected series by Geschickter and Copeland in 1951 that the entity was established. There are gradations from the even more uncommon, completely benign parosteal osteoma through the lesion with minimal evidence of malignancy to the frankly malignant but fairly well differentiated parosteal tumor. It is obvious that when the diagnosis of sarcoma depends on such subtle changes as are found in some of these tumors, the problem is often a difficult one.

Osteogenic tumors of a high degree of malignancy histologically (that is, of high grade by the method of Broders) are occasionally seen predominantly on the surface of a bone, but they do not belong in the category under discussion. Inclusion of tumors that are histologically like the ordinary osteosarcoma or fibrosarcoma will decrease the usefulness of the term "parosteal osteosarcoma." Periosteal osteosarcoma as described in Chapter 19 is usually distinctly different from a parosteal osteosarcoma.

Although there is a rare benign counterpart of parosteal osteosarcoma (Figs. 6-4, 6-5, and 6-6), our series suggests that the usual tumor of this type is an indolent malignant growth from its inception, and the dense basal region of the tumor results from progressive ossification of this older portion.

There are very rare, extremely well differentiated osteosarcomas that begin within bone. These low-grade central (intramedullary) osteosarcomas are described in Chapter 19. Reference to the roentgenogram or to the gross specimen is required in differentiating them from parosteal osteosarcoma. Correct diagnosis and proper management of patients with these tumors is heavily dependent on judgment based on experience with them.

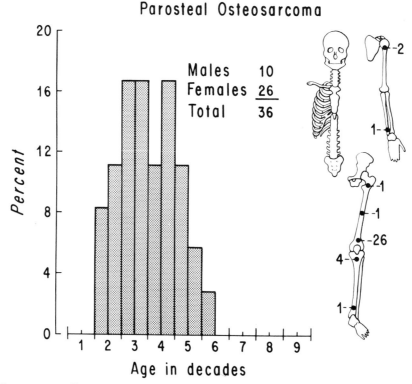

Figure 20-1. Skeletal, age, and sex distribution of parosteal osteosarcomas.

Incidence

Parosteal osteosarcoma is a distinctly rare neoplasm. It comprised less than 1 percent of the Mayo Clinic series of malignant tumors primary in bone.

Sex

Females constituted 72 percent of the patients in this series, but males have predominated in some series. Two tumors of the humerus in males from our earlier group have been deleted, one because it contained no definitely malignant zones, and the other because it is now considered to be an ossified subperiosteal hematoma. Of the 962 osteosarcomas in Chapter 19, 59 percent were in males.

Age

The average age of patients with this tumor is greater than that of those with ordinary osteosarcoma, a difference that can be explained at least in part by its slow growth.

Localization

Practically all of the recorded parosteal osteosarcomas have involved the femur, humerus, and tibia. Other bones, however, may be affected. By far the most common site for its development is the posterior distal portion of the shaft of the femur. In common with the ordinary osteosarcoma, this lesion most often affects the metaphyseal region.

Symptoms

Swelling is the most important symptom. Because of the inherent slow growth of the tumor, the swelling is often of several years' duration. Sometimes the patient has noted swelling for only a few days or weeks when it is obvious from the roentgenograms and pathologic characteristics that the lesion has been present for much longer. The tumor may be painful or may interfere with function of the adjacent joint.

A common and practically pathognomonic history is as follows: Several years previously the patient underwent excision of a tumor that had been considered roentgenologically to be an atypical osteochondroma. The pathologist regarded it as an unusual osteochondroma and perhaps described it as cellular. In the interim, the tumor may or may not have required repeated excision because of recurrence. When seen now, there is a recurrent, ossified juxtacortical mass in one of the sites of predilection.

Physical Findings

A mass at the lesional site, which is sometimes painful to pressure, is the only significant physical finding. The mass may be of enormous size.

Roentgenologic Features

The tumor is seen to be juxtacortical and usually has a remarkable tendency to encircle the shaft. This is best demonstrated by tomography. The lesion is seen to be firmly attached to the cortex along a part of its broad base, but it tends to grow peripherally in mushroom fashion to lie near, but not necessarily attached to, the remainder of the underlying shaft that it encircles. In most cases, therefore, there is a partially free space of varying length and 1 to 3 mm in thickness between the tumor and the underlying bone. Ordinarily the tumor is lobular in outline, but sometimes angular projections extend into the soft tissues. From 75 to 90 percent of the tumor's bulk shows a variable, usually pronounced, degree of ossification. The periphery of the tumor is typically less ossified than its base. Numerous poorly defined and irregular radiolucent defects may be seen in the substance of the tumor because of zones of irregular fibrous or cartilaginous tissue. Ordinarily the osseous mass is amorphous, but occasionally true osseous trabeculation may be observed. Periosteal elevation at the edge of the tumor and consequently Codman's angle are conspicuously absent. Medullary involvement ordinarily does not occur except in extremely long-standing tumors or in tumors that have been previously treated unsuccessfully. Even recurrent tumors, however, are usually juxtacortical.

The roentgenogram is important in the differential diagnosis. The heterotopic bone seen in myositis ossificans usually shows a well-organized and clear-cut trabecular pattern, in contrast to what is seen in parosteal osteosarcoma. Although the lesion of myositis ossificans may abut on a bone and overlap it when seen on only one roentgenographic projection, careful study will show that it does not have the characteristic broad base of parosteal osteosarcoma. Osteochondroma (osteocartilaginous exostosis) can ordinarily be differentiated roentgenographically with assurance from parosteal osteosarcoma from the roentgenographic standpoint. The continuity of the bony cortex with the pedunculated or sessile base of an osteochondroma, as well as the continuity of the cancellous bone with the core of an osteochondroma, is absent in parosteal osteosarcoma. Evidence of cortical destruction, extensive medullary involvement, Codman's reactive angle, and an ill-defined border differentiate ordinary osteosarcoma from parosteal osteosarcoma. Occasional benign parosteal osteomas, which in the author's experience are much less common than the malignant counterpart under discussion, may be impossible to differentiate roentgenographically. This fact is not surprising when one realizes that the differentiation is so subtle that it can sometimes be made with no real assurance even by the histopathologist.

The roentgenogram is usually so characteristic that the correct diagnosis of parosteal osteosarcoma, especially in advanced disease is practically certain on this basis alone.

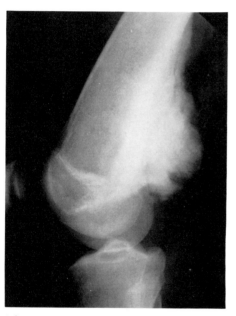 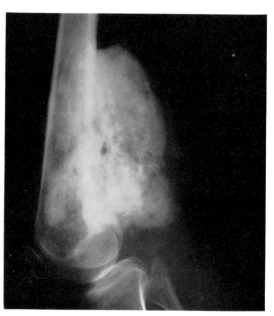

Figure 20-2. *Left.* Parosteal osteosarcoma of lower portion of shaft of femur posteriorly. Without tomography, the absence of medullary involvement is not apparent. This tumor recurred within a year after local excision. *Right.* This tumor of femur had been present for seven years. At time of biopsy and amputation, zones of grade 2 sarcoma were present, but there was still no medullary involvement. Patient died with pulmonary metastasis six years after amputation. (Reproduced with permission from: Dwinnell, L. A., Dahlin, D. C., and Ghormley, R. K.: *J Bone Joint Surg, 36A:*732-744, 1954.)

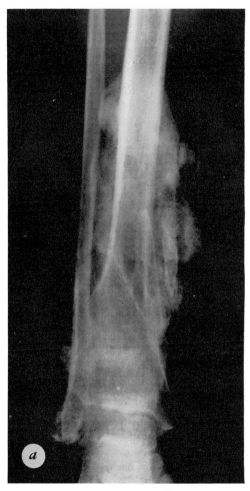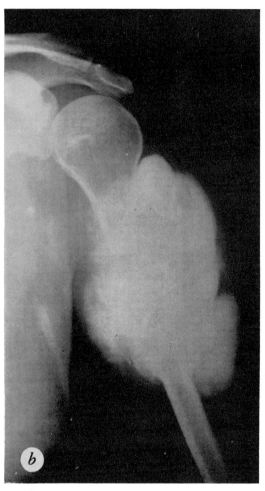

Figure 20-3. *a.* Parosteal osteosarcoma of tibia. Excision was followed by recurrence and eventual death from metastasis. *b.* This parosteal sarcoma encased upper portion of shaft of humerus. Local removal was unsuccessful in controlling lesion. (Reproduced with permission from: Dwinnell, L. A., Dahlin, D. C., and Ghormley, R. K.: *J Bone Joint Surg, 36A:*732-744, 1954.)

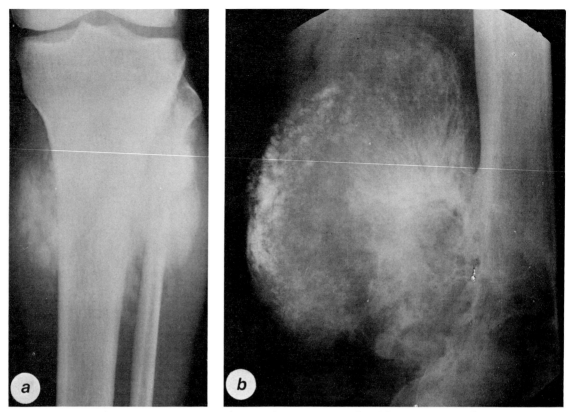

Figure 20-4. *a*. Parosteal osteosarcoma, grades 1 and 2, in thirty-one-year-old woman who had noted increasing swelling for one year. Despite amputation, at which time no tumor was found in marrow, she died with extensive pulmonary and intra-abdominal metastasis six years four months later. *b*. This tumor in twenty-three-year-old man was "shelled" off the femur. Excised specimen was 15 by 10 by 9 cm. Recurrence required amputation twenty-one months later. Apparent intraosseous tumor in this original roentgenogram suggests that this tumor, although of low histologic grade, will behave like ordinary osteosarcoma. Patient died six months after amputation.

Gross Pathology

Although these tumors merge with the cortex of the affected bone, they do not disrupt it until late, and ordinarily only after one or more recurrences following inadequate therapy. Accordingly, medullary involvement is a late phenomenon if it occurs at all.

As indicated by the roentgenograms, these tumors are predominantly ossified. Ordinarily, however, there are softer, fibrous foci, especially near or at the periphery of the neoplasms. These zones are the ones most likely to afford histologic evidence of malignancy. Small or prominent chondroid foci are often found in these lesions.

Recurrent tumors of this type, especially when they show an increased degree of malignancy histologically, may be only slightly sclerotic if at all. In fact, such lesions may simulate closely the appearance of ordinary osteosarcoma.

Myositis ossificans, which must be considered in the differential diagnosis, is often completely separated from the bone. When it does abut on bone, it rarely coapts itself to the cortex so as to produce an extensive broad base such as that

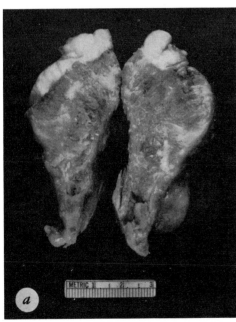
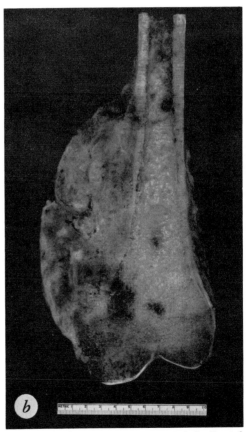

Figure 20-5. *a.* Cut surface of parosteal osteosarcoma illustrated in Figure 20-2 left. Local excision was followed by recurrence within a year and amputation was performed. *b.* Gross specimen of lesion shown in Figure 20-2 right. Although this tumor had been present for seven years, there was no medullary involvement. (Reproduced with permission from: Dwinnell, L. A., Dahlin, D. C., and Ghormley, R. K.: *J Bone Joint Surg, 36A*:732-744, 1954.)

seen in parosteal osteosarcoma. Another important differential feature is the maturation and ossification usually found first in the peripheral portion of a mass of benign heterotopic ossification, whereas the advancing edge of these sarcomas is nearly always the least mature and the least ossified part.

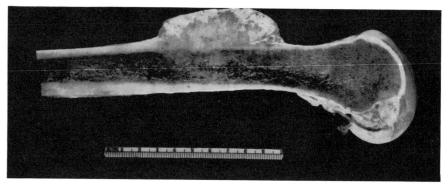

Figure 20-6. Although this tumor resembles a parosteal osteosarcoma of the ordinary type, it is actually a high-grade osteosarcoma and does not belong in the indolent pathologic variety under discussion.

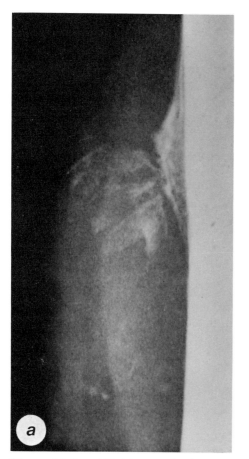
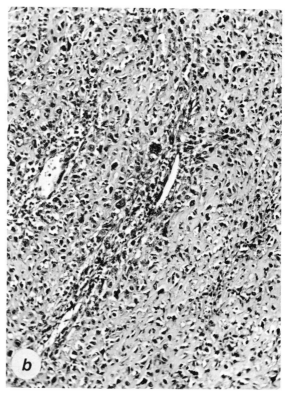

Figure 20-7. *a.* Highly anaplastic (grade 4) osteosarcoma on surface of distal part of humeral shaft of twenty-four-year-old man. Tumor engaged the cortex, but only superficially. Pulmonary metastasis developed and patient died ten months after forequarter amputation. *b.* Grade 4 osteosarcoma throughout lesion shown in left portion of photomicrograph. (×160) (Case contributed by Doctors B. Stener and L. Angervall of Göteborg, Sweden.)

Histopathology

The most prominent feature of parosteal osteosarcoma is its component of rather regularly arranged osseous trabeculae. Apparently the more immature trabeculae undergo maturation in this slowly developing tumor and become "normalized." Between these nearly normal trabeculae are atypical, proliferating, spindle-shaped, or polyhedral cells in which one finds occasional or sometimes fairly numerous mitotic figures. The spaces between the trabeculae are not filled with fat or hematopoietic cells as in osteochondroma. This fact alone serves clearly to differentiate osteocartilaginous exostosis from parosteal osteosarcoma. The same atypical spindle cell elements alluded to comprise the purely fibrous zones of these tumors. Evidence of malignancy may be found only in small foci, making it necessary to study multiple sections for accurate appraisal. Variable amounts of osteoid may be found in the proliferating spindle cell stroma, apparently owing to metaplasia of the basically fibroblastic cells into a type capable of producing osteoid. This osteoid matures into the bony trabeculae. Islands of chondrosarcoma are commonly seen in these tumors. Although a poorly formed cartilaginous "cap" may be seen, it tends to be irregular and its cells show the features of chondrosarcoma. Foci that contain benign giant cells have been found in these tumors.

Occasional tumors in this group show an increase in histologic activity with recurrence. Such malignant zones have the quality of ordinary fibrosarcoma, chondrosarcoma, or osteosarcoma.

Most parosteal osteosarcomas reveal, at their peripheries, an intermixing with muscle and fat cells. This finding has added to the confusion that exists in the dif-

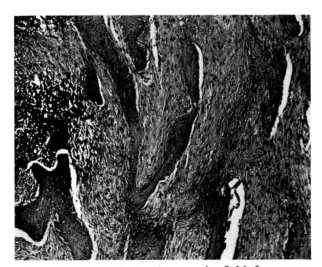

Figure 20-8. Typical microscopic field from parosteal osteosarcoma. Note well-formed osseous trabeculae separated by actively proliferating fibroblastic tissue that is undergoing metaplasia to a type capable of producing osteoid substance and bone. (×100)

ferentiation of this malignant tumor from myositis ossificans and pathologically suggests a kinship with desmoid tumors of the soft tissues of the extremities.

Differentiation of this malignant tumor from myositis ossificans histologically depends on the lack of true anaplasia in the proliferating cells of the latter lesion. Gross and roentgenographic guidance should direct one's suspicion, as previously indicated. Similar criteria aid in the recognition of benign heterotopic ossification of other kinds, including that resulting from avulsion of periosteum from any cause. Cytologic evidences of activity, including numerous mitotic figures, may be found in these benign conditions.

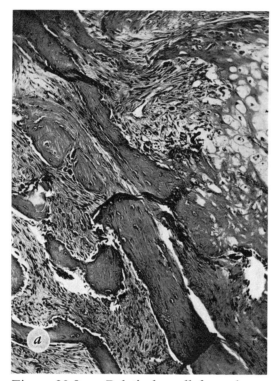 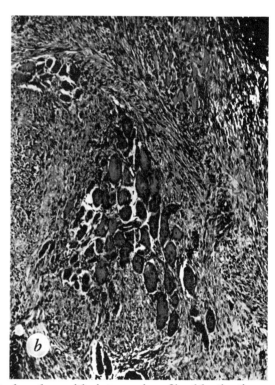

Figure 20-9. *a.* Relatively well formed osseous trabeculae with intervening fibroblastic tissue and chondroid zone. (×100) *b.* Periphery of parosteal osteosarcoma showing invasion of striated muscle, large fibers of which are shown in cross-section. (×80) (Reproduced with permission from: Dwinnell, L. A., Dahlin, D. C., and Ghormley, R. K.: *J Bone Joint Surg, 36A:* 732-744, 1954.)

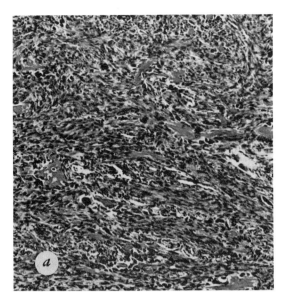
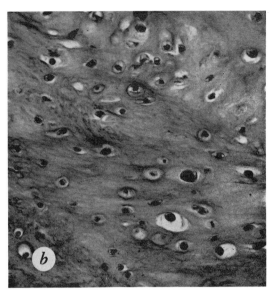

Figure 20-10. *a*. Peripheral zone of grade 2 fibrosarcoma in tumor illustrated in Figures 20-2*b* and 20-5*b*. *b*. Island of chondrosarcoma from one of these tumors. (×200) (Reproduced with permission from: Dwinnell, L. A., Dahlin, D. C., and Ghormley, R. K.: *J Bone Joint Surg, 36A*:732-744, 1954.)

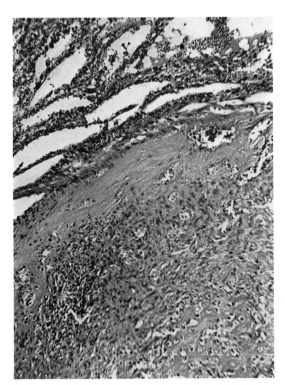
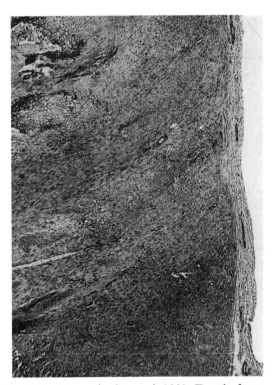

Figure 20-11. *Left*. Nodule of metastatic parosteal osteosarcoma in lung. (×100) Death from metastasis occurred twenty years after first surgical treatment for lesion of distal portion of femur and six years after amputation. *Right*. Typical cellular fibroblastic advancing edge of parosteal osteosarcoma. (×35)

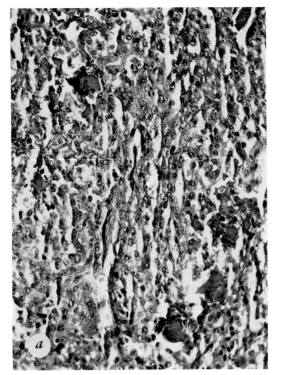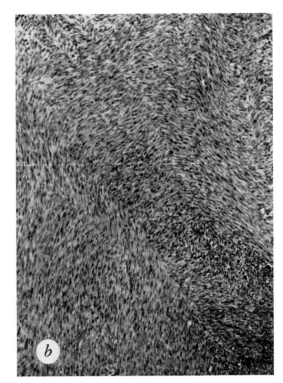

Figure 20-12. *a.* High-grade osteoblastic osteosarcoma. (×200) *b.* High-grade fibroblastic osteosarcoma. (×80) Both of these were found in recurrent tumors that followed local excision for
parosteal osteosarcoma. (Figure 20-12*b* reproduced with permission from: Dwinnell, L. A.,
Dahlin, D. C., and Ghormley, R. K.: *J Bone Joint Surg, 36A:*732-744, 1954.)

Treatment

Studies of several series now reported support the following conclusions. Simple
excision inevitably leads to recurrence. If the tumor has indisputable, albeit minimal, histologic evidence of malignancy, amputation is the treatment of choice for
those tumors that are large or recurrent. For small, nonrecurrent parosteal osteosarcomas, it may be feasible to employ resection, but the surgeon must be able to
encompass the tumor widely, getting well into normal bone and uninvolved soft tissues. Segmental resection and arthrodesis or prosthetic replacement at the first operation is logical therapy for many of these tumors.

If critical analysis, which may require study of the entire tumor, fails to uncover
proof that the tumor is malignant, wide local excision and careful follow-up
studies are indicated.

A factor of importance in contemplating conservative management is that these
tumors may increase in histologic activity with recurrence, and some may become
highly malignant, rapidly metastasizing sarcomas.

Prognosis

Several of our thirty-six patients have died with metastases; all but one of these
had local excision as their primary treatment and had at least one recurrence before amputation was performed.

The indolent behavior of parosteal osteosarcoma is emphasized by one of the fatal cases. A recurring tumor of the lower end of the femur was subjected to six excisions during a fourteen-year period. Then amputation was performed but the patient died with proved pulmonary metastasis six years after amputation and twenty years after the first excision.

Early adequate treatment should cure most patients. A long-term survival rate of 80 to 90 percent is to be expected.

Bibliography

1951 Geschickter, C. F., and Copeland, M. M.: Parosteal Osteoma of Bone: A New Entity. *Ann Surg, 133:*790-806.

1954 Dwinnell, L. A., Dahlin, D. C., and Ghormley, R. K.: Parosteal (Juxtacortical) Osteogenic Sarcoma. *J Bone Joint Surg, 36A:*732-744.

1957 Stevens, G. M., Pugh, D. G., and Dahlin, D. C.: Roentgenographic Recognition and Differentiation of Parosteal Osteogenic Sarcoma. *Am J Roentgenol, 78:*1-12.

1959 D'Aubigné, R. M., Meary, R., and Mazabrand, A.: Sarcome Ostéogénique Juxtacortical. *Rev Chir Orthop, 45:*873-884.

1959 Copeland, M. M., and Geschickter, C. F.: The Treatment of Parosteal Osteoma of Bone. *Surg Gynecol Obstet, 108:*537-548.

1962 Scaglietti, O., and Calandriello, B.: Ossifying Parosteal Sarcoma: Parosteal Osteoma or Juxtacortical Osteogenic Sarcoma. *J Bone Joint Surg, 44A:*635-647.

1967 Van Der Heul, R. O., and Von Ronnen, J. R.: Juxtacortical Osteosarcoma: Diagnosis, Differential Diagnosis, Treatment, and an Analysis of Eighty Cases. *J Bone Joint Surg, 49A:*415-439 (April).

1968 Companacci, M., Giunti, A., and Grandesso, F.: Sarcoma Periostale Ossificante (31 Osservazioni). *Chir Organi Mov, 57:*3-28.

1971 Edeiken, J., Farrell, C., Ackerman, L. V., and Spjut, H. J.: Parosteal Sarcoma. *Am J Roentgenol, 111:*579-583 (March).

1976 Unni, K. K., Dahlin, D. C., Beabout, J. W., and Ivins, J. C.: Parosteal Osteogenic Sarcoma. *Cancer, 37:*2466-2475 (May).

1976 Unni, K. K., Dahlin, D. C., and Beabout, J. W.: Periosteal Osteogenic Sarcoma. *Cancer, 37:*2476-2485 (May).

Chapter 21

Ewing's Tumor

EWING'S TUMOR is a distinctive, small round cell sarcoma that is the most lethal of the bone tumors. It is the subject of controversy in the literature because of the somewhat nonspecific histologic characteristics of the tumor, which is composed of solidly packed, small cells. Formerly, some of the small cell osteosarcomas, most of the reticulum cell sarcomas, and even benign conditions such as eosinophilic granuloma were at times classified with Ewing's tumor.

A practical working definition is to regard as Ewing's tumors those highly anaplastic, small round to oval cell sarcomas that have the clinical and roentgenographic characteristics of a primary osseous lesion. Inherent in this concept is the exclusion of cytologically incompatible lesions such as myeloma, malignant lymphoma, and histiocytosis X. Production of a chondroid or osteoid matrix by the neoplastic cells likewise excludes Ewing's sarcoma. It is sometimes impossible to differentiate a biopsy specimen of a metastatic malignant tumor such as neuroblastoma, small cell cancer of the lung, or even leukemic infiltrate from a specimen of Ewing's tumor even after critical histologic study according to modern concepts. Practically, however, when the physician, after careful study of the patient, is confronted with what is clinically a primary lesion in bone that is typical of Ewing's tumor, he is obliged to treat it as such and he will rarely make a significant error. Armchair meditations regarding whether the tumor being appraised may be a metastatic lesion from an undisclosed primary tumor usually can be verified only after studies at autopsy.

Speculation regarding the possible origin of the cells that comprise Ewing's tumor has been fruitless, and it seems best to regard them as arising from undifferentiated mesenchyme.

Although Ewing's tumor and reticulum cell sarcoma can be distinguished histologically in most cases, occasional tumors appear to fall midway between them. In the present series, some tumors contained cells that were larger and somewhat more irregular than those of classic Ewing's tumor. Their clinical characteristics and prognosis made it seem most practical to include them with Ewing's tumors rather than to attempt to segregate a new tumor type.

A soft-tissue counterpart of Ewing's sarcoma is occasionally encountered.

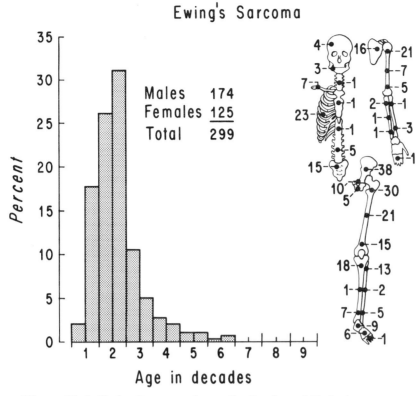

Figure 21-1. Skeletal, age, and sex distribution of Ewing's tumors.

Incidence

Ewing's tumor comprised slightly more than 6 percent of the total malignant tumors in the Mayo Clinic series.

Sex

Ewing's tumor has a distinct predilection for males.

Age

The persons affected by this tumor are, on the average, younger than those affected by any other primary malignant tumor of bone. The youngest patient in the present series was eighteen months of age; five others were less than five years old. When confronted with the problem of Ewing's tumor in patients who are past the third decade of life, one must be especially careful to exclude metastatic carcinoma. In the very young, metastatic neuroblastoma and even acute leukemia must be considered.

Localization

Most Ewing's tumors are in the extremities, but any bone of the body may be involved. Any portion of a long tubular bone may be affected. The lower extremities and pelvic girdle accounted for 60.5 percent of the tumors in this series. Twenty-two involved the spinal column, including the sacrum, and twenty involved the fibula. Many of those in long bones affected nearly all of the shaft.

Symptoms

Pain and swelling are the most common symptoms of Ewing's tumor. Pain is the first symptom in well over half the cases. It may be intermittent at first, and it tends to increase in severity with time. Although swelling in the region of the tumor is common by the time the patient seeks medical advice, it is rarely the first symptom. Pathologic fracture is unusual. The average patient has had symptoms for several months before he seeks medical care.

Patients whose symptoms lasted for six months or longer did not differ in survival from patients who had symptoms of shorter duration.

Physical and Laboratory Findings

Most patients have a palpable tender mass, and some have dilated veins over the tumor. The patient should be thoroughly examined and a search should be made for evidence of a primary tumor or for indications of metastatic disease elsewhere.

Patients with Ewing's tumor sometimes have an elevated temperature and increased sedimentation rate of erythrocytes, often associated with some secondary anemia and sometimes with leukocytosis. These findings may suggest that the osseous lesion is inflammatory in origin. It has been found that Ewing's tumor, when associated with these systemic features, has a prognosis that is even worse than average.

Neuroblastoma with metastasis to bone simulating Ewing's sarcoma can be diagnosed reliably in most cases by qualitative and quantitative determinations of catecholamine metabolites in the urine.

Roentgenologic Features

Ewing's tumor tends to be extensive, sometimes involving the entire shaft of a long bone. Even so, generally more of the bone will be found involved pathologically than was obvious from the roentgenogram. Lytic destruction is the most common finding, but there may be regions of density owing to stimulation of new bone formation. As the tumor bursts through the cortex, which may show only minimal roentgenographic changes, it often elevates the periosteum gradually. This elevation produces the characteristic multiple layers of subperiosteal reactive new bone which gives the "onionskin" appearance of Ewing's tumor. Radiating spicules from the cortex of an affected bone are not uncommon, a fact that complicates the differentiation from osteosarcoma. When the initial roentgenogram shows extensive destruction of bone combined with a large extraosseous mass, the lesion is usually clearly malignant. Occasionally, Ewing's tumor produces an expansion of the affected bone and may even superficially resemble a cyst.

The roentgenographic appearance had no relationship to survival in our series.

Rare examples of Ewing's sarcoma have little or no medullary component. A few are almost completely in a juxtaosseous position and show but little cortical destruction of part of a bone's circumference. Edeiken has stressed that "saucerization" of the exterior surface of the cortex is an early and characteristic sign of those tumors presenting subperiosteally.

Experienced observers have concluded that, although Ewing's tumor can sometimes be diagnosed with a high degree of assurance from its roentgenologic features, and although it very often produces features that are virtually pathognomonic of malignant bone tumor, a number of conditions can produce similar features. Among these conditions are acute or chronic osteomyelitis, eosinophilic granuloma, malignant lymphoma, metastatic malignant tumor, and even osteosarcoma.

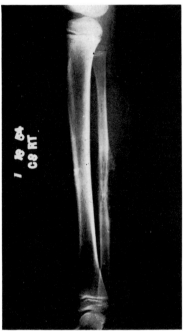

Figure 21-2. Ewing's tumor of fibula. Gross lesion is shown in Figure 21-6; histology is shown in Figure 21-9.

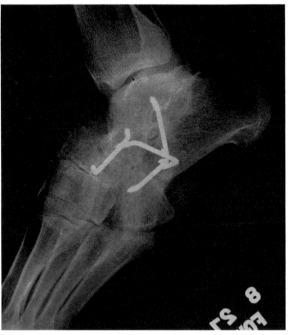

Figure 21-3. Ewing's tumor of tarsal navicular. An attempt had been made to produce arthrodesis pursuant to an erroneous diagnosis. Gross lesion is shown in Figure 21-7.

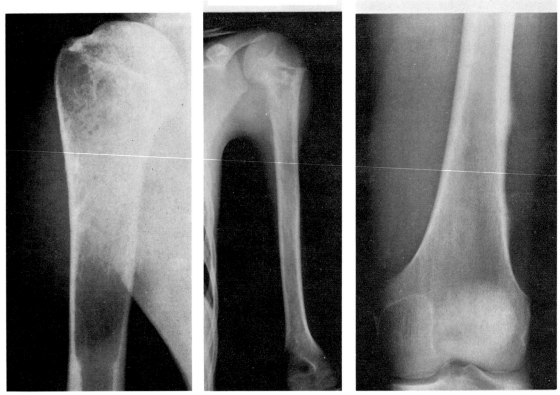

Figure 21-4. *Left.* Ewing's tumor producing cystlike rarefaction of upper third of humerus. There was no definite cortical breakthrough. *Middle.* Ewing's tumor of upper third of humerus of twelve-year-old boy who had noted local pain for nine months. *Right.* Ewing's tumor that had produced pain for only ten days in seventeen-year-old boy. Tumor has "saucerized" outer surface of cortex.

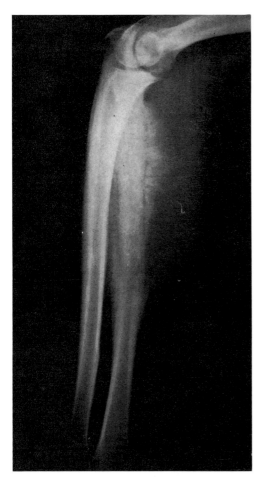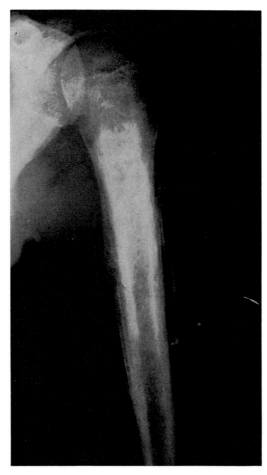

Figure 21-5. *Left.* Ewing's tumor of radius with prominent radial spicules in periosseous tissue. *Right.* Ewing's tumor of humerus showing multiple layers of subperiosteal, reactive, non-neoplastic, new bone. (Reproduced with permission from: McCormack, L. J., Dockerty, M. B., and Ghormley, R. K.: *Cancer, 5:*85-99, 1952.)

Gross Pathology

Solid masses of viable tumor are characteristically gray white, moist, glistening, and somewhat translucent. They may be almost liquid in consistency. Tumor frequently invades bone beyond the limits suggested by the roentgenogram. Zones of necrosis, hemorrhage, and even cyst formation are common. The neoplastic tissue is often admixed with proliferating bony and fibrous tissue in the periosseous regions.

The medullary cavity appears to be the site of origin of nearly all of these tumors. Although the tumors may affect any portion of a long bone and commonly involve a great length of it, the bulk of the tumor is frequently in the metaphyseal region.

Metastasis is characteristically to the lungs and to other bones. The latter feature is so prominent that some have suggested that Ewing's tumor may have a multicentric origin. Lymph-nodal metastasis has been recorded in as high as 20 percent of cases, and viscera other than the lungs may be involved.

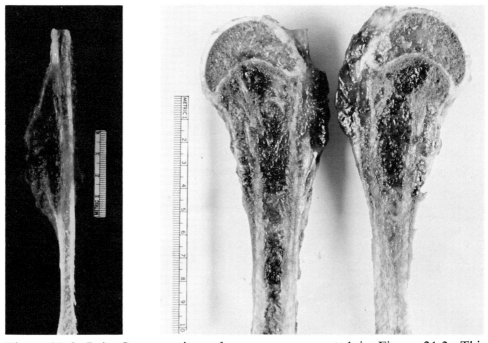

Figure 21-6. *Left.* Gross specimen from case represented in Figure 21-2. This six-year-old girl was treated by above-knee amputation and was well nineteen years later. *Right.* Bivalved humerus after forequarter amputation for lesion shown in Figure 21-4. *Middle.* Solitary pulmonary nodules were removed on three later occasions from fourteen to fifty-six months later. Patient was well seventy-eight months after last resection.

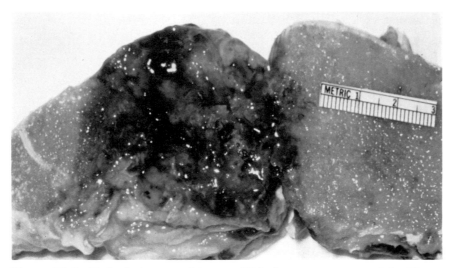

Figure 21-7. Ewing's tumor of tarsus. This is case represented in Figure 21-3. Note gelatinous, almost fluid consistency of tumor. Patient was alive and well ten years after amputation. Histology of this tumor is shown in Figures 21-10*a* and 21-11*a*.

Histopathology

Even with low-power magnification, the microscopist observes that Ewing's tumor is remarkably cellular and that there is little intercellular stroma except for widely separated strands of fibrous tissue. These strands compartmentalize the cellular aggregates into zones that are sometimes larger than the area covered by a high-power microscopic field. The cells that lie in the compartments are noteworthy for their regularity when studied under higher magnification, and they have round to oval nuclei. The cytoplasm surrounding these nuclei is slightly granular, and the cell outlines are indistinct. The nuclei themselves contain a rather finely dispersed chromatin that imparts a "ground-glass" appearance. Nucleoli may be present, but they are inconspicuous. Mitotic figures are rarely numerous.

Special stains disclose that there is little stainable reticulin within the compartments described above. Minor variation in nuclear size from region to region in one of these tumors often occurs because some zones are undergoing necrosis and the nuclei are degenerating. The perithelial pattern that has led to the belief that this tumor arises from blood vascular endothelial cells is sometimes prominent. Collars of viable cells often surround small blood vessels, and beyond these viable collars, the cells are necrotic—a histologic pattern that is best explained on a nutritional basis and one that seems unlikely to be explained on the basis of derivation of the tumor.

Occasionally, one encounters a tumor the cells of which contain nuclei that are somewhat larger and less regular in shape than are those of an average Ewing's tumor. The general histologic structure is otherwise like the remainder of the Ewing group. These larger celled lesions do not have the specific cytologic features of the malignant lymphomas. Their prognosis is very poor, and it seems appropriate to regard them as variants of Ewing's tumor.

The presence of reactive osseous and fibroblastic tissue resulting from periosteal elevation and invasion of soft tissues as well as large zones of necrosis may complicate the histologic pattern.

Schajowicz (1959) advocated the glycogen stain in the differentiation of Ewing's sarcoma from reticulum cell sarcoma, stating that the cells of the former tumor contain glycogen, whereas those of the latter do not. Actually, however, some tumors necessarily called Ewing's sarcoma morphologically contain no recognizable glycogen by special stains, even when fixed in 80% ethanol.

Mesenchymal chondrosarcoma may have large zones with highly malignant small round cells similar to those of Ewing's sarcoma.

Newer methods of study, including detailed electron microscopic observations, have failed to elucidate completely the nature of the cells in these tumors.

"Rosettes" are seen in a small percentage of tumors obviously primary in bone, although such have been used as evidence of neuroblastomatous origin for Ewing's tumor.

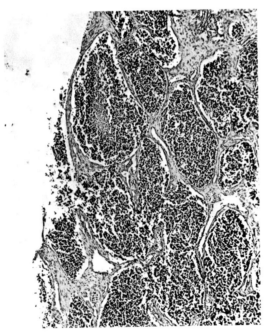

Figure 21-8. Characteristic loculation of Ewing's tumor cells by septa of connective tissue that are widely separated. (×50)

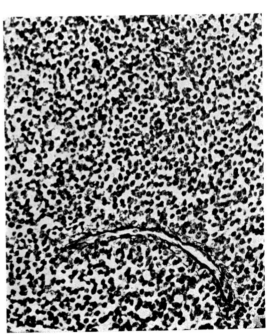

Figure 21-9. Regular round to oval nuclei with little stainable reticulin are characteristic of Ewing's tumor. (Reticulin stain; ×250)

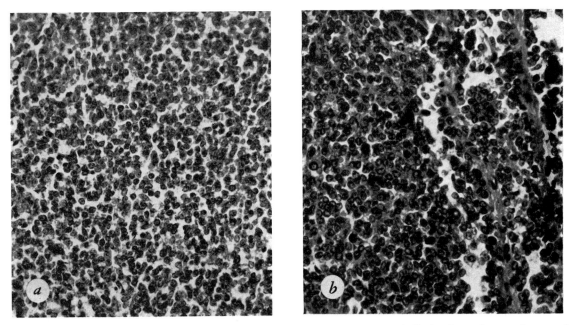

Figure 21-10. *a*. Note remarkable regularity of nuclei and poor delimitation of cytoplasm of cells of these tumors. Practically no ground substance is present. (×265) *b*. Another photomicrograph to emphasize features already described. (×285)

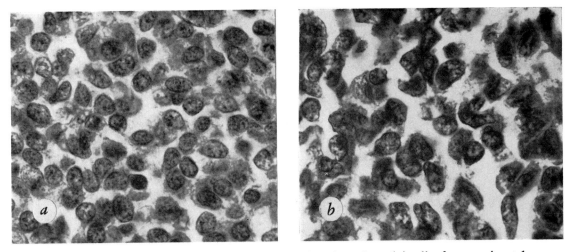

Figure 21-11. *a*. Typical Ewing's tumor with round and oval nuclei, all of approximately same size. (×800) *b*. Larger cell type of Ewing's tumor. Note nuclei are more irregular in shape. (×800)

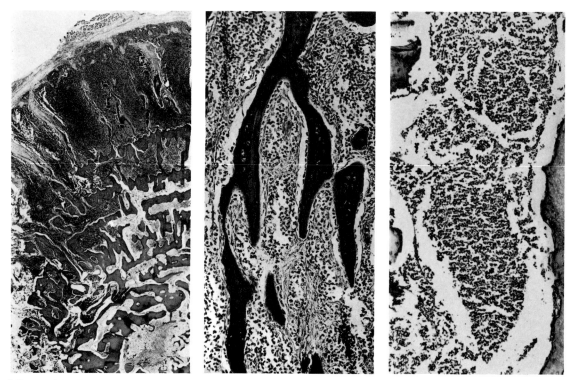

Figure 21-12. *Left.* Ewing's tumor of fibula showing "onionskin" layers and vertical trabeculae of new bone. Central part of tumor, at lower right, is necrotic. (×8) *Middle.* Ewing's tumor cells among trabeculae of new bone. Early reactive osteoid clumps like these may be confused with osteoid produced by malignant cells. (×100) *Right.* Infiltrate of acute leukemia in femur of two-year-old child was erroneously interpreted as Ewing's sarcoma prior to hematologic investigation. (×100)

Treatment

Opinion is divided as to whether irradiation or ablative surgical treatment is best for Ewing's tumor. The rarity of the tumor and the low incidence of cure makes it difficult to procure convincing data on this point. Amputation has the advantage that it assures control of the local lesion. It sometimes becomes necessary as a palliative measure whether the primary tumor has been irradiated or not. Bhansali and Desai (1963) concluded, after reviewing the literature, that "surgery appears to be the superior treatment when feasible." Nevertheless, most authorities consider irradiation the mainstay of therapy for Ewing's tumor. My preference is to amputate for Ewing's sarcomas located below the midfemur. Our recent studies have indicated that surgery provides some advantage in survival. Chemotherapy, adjunctive to control of the primary tumor by radiation or surgical therapy, has given promising improvement in results.

Prognosis

Careful study of the pathologic changes and follow-up data on nearly 98 percent of the patients with Ewing's sarcomas in the present series indicated the serious nature of the tumor, but there were some hopeful aspects. The five-year survival rate was 16.2 percent; tumors from these survivors were not pathologically distinguishable from those of the remainder. The ten-year survival rate was 13.9 percent. Without metastasis demonstrable at the initial visit of the patient, the five– and ten-year survival rates were 19 and 16 percent respectively. In an earlier study, we found that six of the twenty patients who had survived five years subsequently died of their tumors; one patient had survived twelve years after initial treatment. Our experience parallels that of several other series in that a number of the long-term survivors underwent radiation therapy for metastatic disease, most often in the lungs.

Apparently, reliable reports in the literature give five-year survival rates that vary down to 0 percent. Our experience, however, shows that patients with Ewing's tumor have a chance for survival if prompt adequate treatment is employed. We have noted some increased chance for survival in recent years, and chemotherapeutic agents have considerable effectiveness.

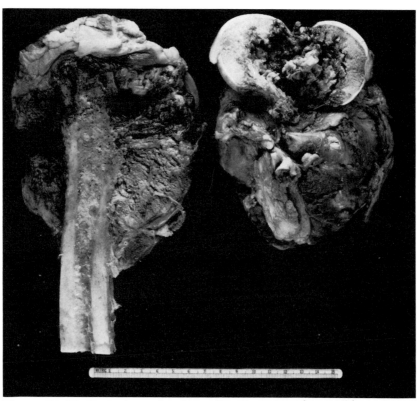

Figure 21-13. Ewing's tumor from long-term survivor. This recurrent lesion, 13 by 12 by 10 cm, of upper portion of femur in twenty-two-year-old man, was removed by hindquarter amputation after several courses of radiation, the first of which had been given four years previously. Pulmonary metastatic lesions were demonstrated by roentgenogram and radiated four months after amputation. Patient was alive and well seventeen years after amputation.

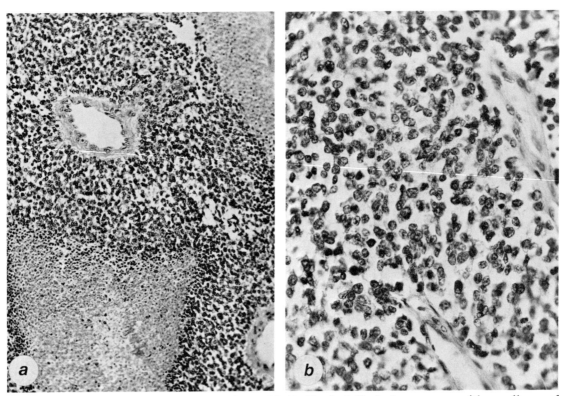

Figure 21-14. *a.* Tumor illustrated in Figure 21-13. Typical Ewing's sarcoma with small round to oval, viable cells, especially near blood vessels. (×200) *b.* Higher magnification to indicate cell detail more clearly. (×425)

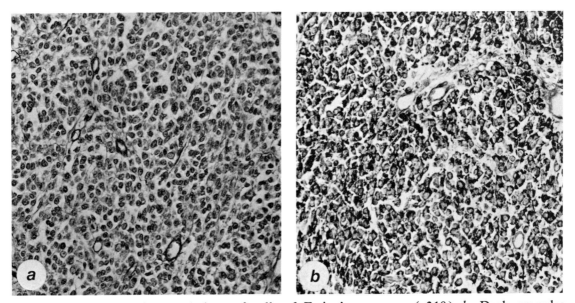

Figure 21-15. *a.* Classic morphology of cells of Ewing's sarcoma. (×310) *b.* Dark granules with periodic acid-Schiff stain indicates glycogen in cytoplasm of this tumor's cells. Diastase removed the material. (×310)

Bibliography

1921 Ewing, J.: Diffuse Endothelioma of Bone. *Proc N Y Pathol Soc ns, 21:*17-24.

1948 Uehlinger, E., Botsztejn, C., and Schinz, H. R.: Ewingsarkom und Knochenretikulosarkom: Klinik, Diagnose und Differentialdiagnose. *Oncologia, 1:*193-245.

1952 McCormack, L. J., Dockerty, M. B., and Ghormley, R. K.: Ewing's Sarcoma. *Cancer, 5:*85-99.

1953 Wang, C. C., and Schulz, M. D.: Ewing's Sarcoma: A Study of Fifty Cases Treated at the Massachusetts General Hospital, 1930-1952 Inclusive. *N Engl J Med, 248:* 571-576.

1955 Bethge, J. F. J.: Die Ewingtumoren oder Omoblastome des Knochens. Differentialdiagnostische und Kritische Eröterungen. *Ergeb Chir Orthop, 39:*327-425.

1956 Lumb, G., and Mackenzie, D. H.: Round-cell Tumours of Bone. *Br J Surg, 43:*380-389.

1959 Schajowicz, F.: Ewing's Sarcoma and Reticulum Cell Sarcoma of Bone: With Special Reference to the Histochemical Demonstration of Glycogen as an Aid to Differential Diagnosis. *J Bone Joint Surg, 41A:*394-356.

1960 Willis, R. A.: *Pathology of Tumors,* ed. 3. Washington, D.C., Butterworth, p. 691.

1961 Dahlin, D. C., Coventry, M. B., and Scanlon, P. W.: Ewing's Sarcoma. A Critical Analysis of 165 Cases. *J Bone Joint Surg, 43A:*185-192.

1963 Baird, R. J., and Krause, V. W.: Ewing's Tumor: A Review of 33 Cases. *Can J Surg, 6:*136-140.

1963 Bhansali, S. K., and Desai, P. B.: Ewing's Sarcoma: Observations on 107 Cases. *J Bone Joint Surg, 45A:*541-553.

1967 Falk, S., and Alpert, M.: Five Year Survival of Patients with Ewing's Sarcoma. *Surg Gynecol Obstet, 124:*319-324 (February).

1973 Dahlin, D. C.: Is It Worthwhile to Differentiate Ewing's Sarcoma and Primary Lymphoma of Bone? *Proc Natl Cancer Conf, 7:*941-945.

1974 Mehta, Y., and Hendrickson, F. R.: CNS Involvement in Ewing's Sarcoma. *Cancer, 33:*859-862 (March).

1975 Angervall, L., and Enzinger, F. M.: Extraskeletal Neoplasm Resembling Ewing's Sarcoma. *Cancer, 36:*240-251 (July).

1975 Imashuku, S., Takada, H., Sawada, T., Nakamura, T., and LaBrosse, E. H.: Studies on Tyrosine Hydroxylase in Neuroblastoma, in Relation to Urinary Levels of Catecholamine Metabolites. *Cancer, 36:*450-457 (August).

1975 Johnson, R. E., and Pomeroy, T. C.: Evaluation of Therapeutic Results in Ewing's Sarcoma. *Am J Roentgenol, 123:*583-587 (March).

1975 Macintosh, D. J., Price, C. H. G., and Jeffree, G. M.: Ewing's Tumour: A Study of Behaviour and Treatment in Forty-Seven Cases. *J Bone Joint Surg, 57B:*331-340 (August).

1975 Pritchard, D. J., Dahlin, D. C., Dauphine, R. T., Taylor, W. F., and Beabout, J. W.: Ewing's Sarcoma: A Clinicopathological and Statistical Analysis of Patients Surviving Five Years or Longer. *J Bone Joint Surg, 57A:*10-16 (January).

Chapter 22

Malignant Giant Cell Tumor

To be certain of the diagnosis of malignant giant cell tumor, the pathologist must be able to demonstrate zones of typical benign giant cell tumor in the malignant neoplasm under appraisal or in previous tissue obtained from the same neoplasm. When confronted with an obviously malignant growth that contains a few or many benign, osteoclastlike giant cells, one can prove a relationship to benign giant cell tumor in no other way. This is true because other neoplasms of bone, including many of the osteosarcomas, contain a scattering or many of these benign giant cells. I have seen classic low-grade parosteal osteosarcoma recur as a highly malignant sarcoma with such an abundance of benign giant cells that, without reference to the original neoplasm, one might make the mistake of regarding it as a malignant giant cell tumor. Some of the osteosarcomas of soft-tissue origin also contain numerous benign giant cells but obviously bear no relationship to giant cell tumor of bone. The stromal cells, not the benign multinucleated cells, in any given neoplasm must determine its classification. Troup and coworkers (1960) have provided clinicopathologic correlations to support this point of view.

With this absolute type of definition of malignant giant cell tumor, fifteen of the twenty such tumors in the present series occurred after treatment for typical benign giant cell tumors—tumors that contain no feature distinguishing them from the remainder of the group of giant cell tumors. Thirteen of the fifteen "secondary" malignant tumors occurred after histologically verified benign giant cell tumors at intervals that averaged 10.8 years from the time of treatment of the benign neoplasm; treatment included radiation in each instance. In these thirteen instances, the malignant tumor completely overran and destroyed any evidence of the original benign tumor. The fourteenth "secondary" malignant tumor developed one and one half years after simple curettage of the benign giant cell tumor, and remnants of it remained at the time of amputation. In the fifteenth case, fibrosarcoma developed at the site of a giant cell tumor that had been treated by curettage and bone grafting twenty-two years and again fifteen years previously, and no radiation had been employed; death with metastasis occurred ten months after amputation for the sarcoma. The remaining five tumors contained foci of sarcoma as indicated in Chapter 9 under Prognosis.

Increasing evidence is being accumulated that radiation may be influential in triggering the malignant transformation of various osseous lesions, especially giant cell tumor. In seven of the twenty cases in this series, however, radiation could not be incriminated.

Analysis of the literature on malignant giant cell tumor is virtually impossible because of lack of strict definition of this entity. The subject is further clouded by the extremely rare "benign metastasizing" giant cell tumor. Two such cases, each with solitary pulmonary deposits, were noted in the series of 264 giant cell tumors.

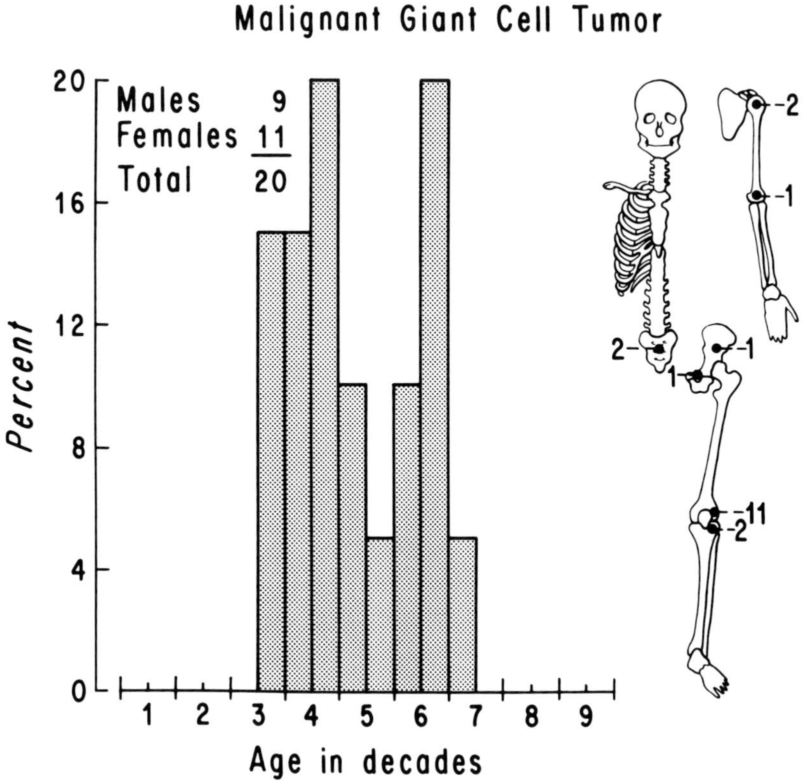

Malignant Giant Cell Tumor

Figure 22-1. Skeletal, age, and sex distribution of malignant giant cell tumors.

Incidence

The malignant giant cell tumors comprised less than 0.5 percent of the total group of malignant tumors and 7.5 percent of the giant cell tumors.

Sex

In this small group, men and women were nearly equally affected, whereas females represented 58 percent of the cases of benign giant cell tumor. The tumor in one of the women in the earlier series has been reclassified.

Age

These patients were somewhat older, on the average, than were those with benign giant cell tumor. This is at least partially explained by the fact that most of the tumors developed several years after treatment of their benign precursors.

Localization

The distribution of these tumors is not significantly different from that of the benign giant cell tumors that do not undergo malignant transformation. As may be seen above, thirteen of them involved the region of the knee, three the humerus, and two each the innominate bone and the sacrum.

Symptoms

Most of these twenty patients had the symptoms of ordinary benign giant cell tumor at the outset. Fifteen of the twenty malignant tumors occurred an average of 10.9 years after the histologic diagnosis of giant cell tumor, and early therapy had included radiation in thirteen of these. The longest interval between the diagnosis of giant cell tumor and the development of sarcoma in the same area was thirty-eight years; the primary therapy in this case had been curettage, bone grafting, and radiation. The five patients whose giant cell tumors contained malignant foci at the original operation had had preoperative pain in the region for three months, one, one, two, and eight years respectively. The last patient had had fracture in the area.

It should be stressed that when the originally benign giant cell tumors became sarcomas, the clinical features changed abruptly from those of slowly progressing or quiescent giant cell tumors to those of the rapidly growing sarcomas they had become.

Physical Findings

The physical examination reveals the evidence likely to be presented by any malignant tumor of bone. Cutaneous changes from prior radiation are common and may alert the physician to elicit the history of such therapy.

Roentgenologic Features

Roentgenologic changes do not differ from those described for fibrosarcoma or osteosarcoma except that in long bones the lesion is almost certain to be in the very end of the bone. The classic features of malignant destruction are present, and usually the process is completely lytic. Earlier roentgenograms of the lesion ordinarily afford evidence of the preexisting benign giant cell tumor. Sometimes the malignant change is reflected in the roentgenogram considerably later than its occurrence had been suggested by the clinical history.

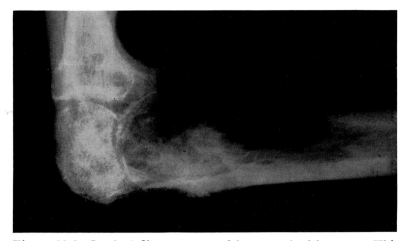

Figure 22-2. Grade 4 fibrosarcoma of lower end of humerus. This tumor arose at site of benign giant cell tumor that had expanded epiphyseal and adjacent metaphyseal region of bone. It had been treated by curettage and radiation eight years before roentgenogram was made. Despite amputation, death occurred within one year.

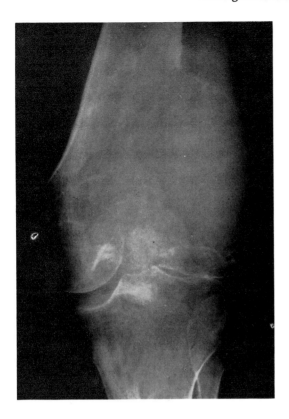

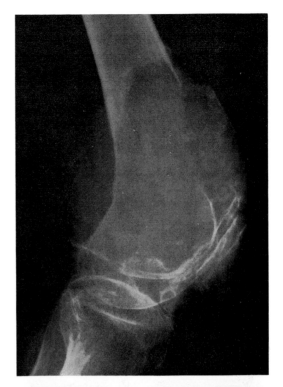

Figure 22-3. *Top left and top right.* Antero-posterior and lateral views of benign giant cell tumor of lower end of femur. Patient was treated by insertion of radium following curettage. *Bottom right.* Same lesion two years after treatment. Two years after this roentgenogram was taken, leg was amputated for grade 3 fibrosarcoma that had completely replaced original benign tumor. Patient was well thirty-five years after amputation.

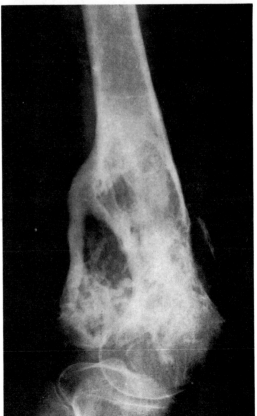

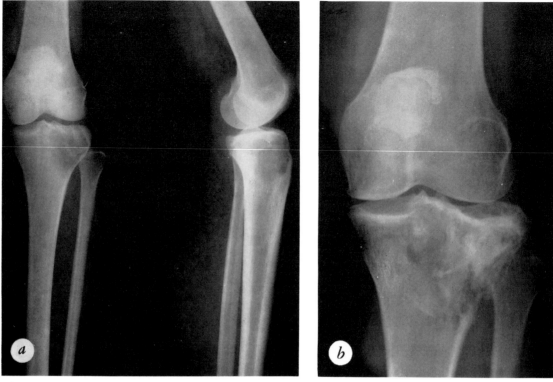

Figure 22-4. *a*. Anteroposterior and lateral views of benign giant cell tumor of upper end of left tibia. Tibia was curetted in 1943 and given roentgen therapy in 1944. *b*. Same lesion in 1948. By this time, grade 3 fibrosarcoma had replaced benign tumor, and despite amputation, patient died with pulmonary metastasis three years later. (Figure 22-4*a* reproduced with permission from: Sabanas, A. O., Dahlin, D. C., Childs, D. S., Jr., and Ivins, J. C.: *Cancer, 9:* 528-542, 1956.)

Gross Pathology

The rare malignant giant cell tumor that shows both benign and sarcomatous zones at the time of the first treatment is grossly indistinguishable from its benign counterpart. The tumor may, however, contain zones of abnormal consistency. It produces variable degrees of expansion of the end of a bone, and it is ordinarily contained by the expanded periosteum. The more common secondarily malignant giant cell tumor exhibits characteristic evidence of sarcoma such as invasion of surrounding osseous and soft tissues, hemorrhage, and necrosis, although the last two of these are by no means uncommon in genuine benign giant cell tumor. The gross appearance of these secondary sarcomas often has been modified by previous treatment, which commonly includes the incorporation of bone grafts into the defect that follows curettage. Such grafts have been partially or completely dissolved.

In general, the gross features of malignant giant cell tumor are not specific, and frequently multiple microscopic sections must be taken to establish that foci of sarcoma are present in a lesion that still contains benign regions. Any grossly unusual-appearing areas must be included in the microscopic assessment.

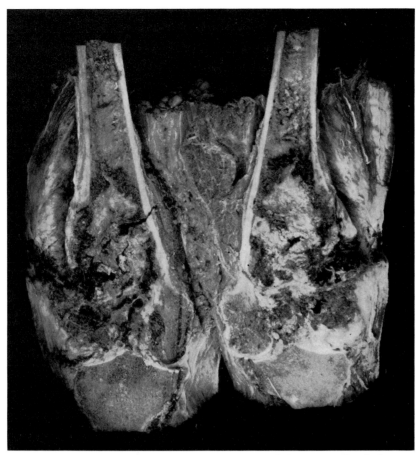

Figure 22-5. Malignant giant cell tumor of lower end of femur. Roentgenograms of this lesion are shown in Figure 22-3.

Histopathology

In most cases, in my experience, when sarcomatous change has occurred, the preexisting benign giant cell tumor is no longer recognizable as such. The sarcoma that replaces it is ordinarily overtly malignant and presents no problem in diagnosis. In fact, in fifteen sarcomas in this series that were originally completely benign, one could not have suspected a relationship to benign giant cell tumor from study of the subsequent sarcoma. Twelve of these secondary tumors were pure fibrosarcomas and three were osteosarcomas. In the five other tumors, one of which had had previous surgical therapy, there were foci of osteosarcoma or fibrosarcoma. These sarcomatous foci contrasted sharply with the zones of residual giant cell tumor. The sarcomas apparently arise from the stomal cells.

Careful review of the numerous tissue sections of the benign tumors in this series that subsequently underwent malignant change offered no histologic clue by which one might differentiate them from those that remained benign. Furthermore, the giant cell tumors that recurred after conventional therapy were not distinguishable from those that did not. Grading of bona fide giant cell tumors on a histologic basis has not been of value in my experience.

The entity of primary diffusely malignant giant cell tumor with a roentgenogram consonant with the diagnosis of giant cell tumor is extremely unusual, and no such case was encountered in this series.

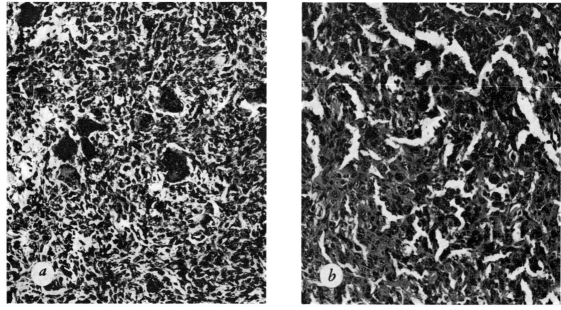

Figure 22-6. *a.* Benign giant cell tumor of distal end of femur. (×175) *b.* Recurrent tumor, one and one-half years later, contain foci of sarcoma like that shown, admixed with typically benign areas of giant cell tumor. (×175) Patient was thirty-seven-year-old man who died with metastasis eight months after amputation for sarcoma.

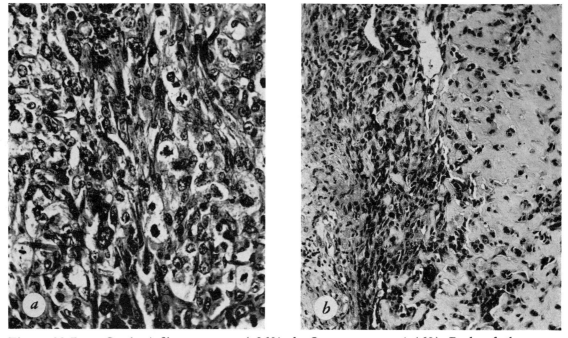

Figure 22-7. *a.* Grade 4 fibrosarcoma. (×260) *b.* Osteosarcoma. (×160) Both of these malignant tumors occurred at sites of benign giant cell tumors that had been treated several years previously by combination of surgery and radiation. (Reproduced with permission from: Williams, R. R., Dahlin, D. C., and Ghormley, R. K.: *Cancer, 7:*764-773, 1954.)

Treatment

When indisputable evidence of malignant change is found in a giant cell tumor or in the zone previously occupied by one, ablative surgical treatment is the procedure of choice. The sarcoma that develops is characteristically radioresistant, being either fibrosarcoma or osteosarcoma. The same principles outlined for the treatment of these sarcomas when they occur primarily should be followed. Radiation, at least as a palliative measure, may be employed for tumors not amenable to ablation.

Prognosis

When frankly malignant transformation has occurred in a benign giant cell tumor, its prognosis is that of the sarcoma present. Approximately 80 percent of those with secondary malignancy have died despite ablative surgery. When mixtures of benign giant cell tumor and frank sarcoma are found, a combination very rare in our experience, ablation is necessary.

Bibliography

1953 Jaffe, H. L.: Giant-cell Tumour (Osteoclastoma) of Bone: Its Pathologic Delimitation and the Inherent Clinical Implications. *Ann R Coll Surg Engl, 13:*343-355.

1956 Murphy, W. R., and Ackerman, L. V.: Benign and Malignant Giant-cell Tumors of Bone, *Cancer, 9:*317-339.

1960 Troup, J. B., Dahlin, D. C., and Coventry, M. B.: The Significance of Giant Cells in Osteogenic Sarcoma: Do They Indicate a Relationship Between Osteogenic Sarcoma and Giant Cell Tumor of Bone? *Proc Staff Meet Mayo Clin, 35:*179-186.

1962 Hutter, R. V. P., Worcester, J. N., Jr., Francis, K. C., Foote, F. W., Jr., and Stewart, F. W.: Benign and Malignant Giant Cell Tumors of Bone. A Clinicopathological Analysis of the Natural History of the Disease. *Cancer, 15:*653-690.

1963 Copeland, M. M., and Geschickter, C. F.: Malignant Bone Tumors: Primary and Metastatic. *CA, 13:*149-155, 187-196, 232-238.

1970 Dahlin, D. C., Cupps, R. E., and Johnson, E. W., Jr.: Giant-Cell Tumor: A Study of 195 Cases. *Cancer, 25:*1061-1070 (May).

Chapter 23

"Adamantinoma" of Long Bones

"A DAMANTINOMA" of long bones is a peculiar neoplasm which on the basis of roentgenographic and pathologic features arises within the osseous substance. The origin of the epitheliumlike islands in this tumor is unknown. Some have postulated traumatic implantation of epithelium because almost all reported "adamantinomas" have occurred in bones that are near the cutaneous surface. Others have considered that congenital rests of epithelium may be the source of these tumors. Still others have stated the view that the so-called adamantinoma of long bones is not epithelial at all but represents rather an unusual manifestation of some sarcoma, especially synovial sarcoma.

Perhaps the most acceptable view, advanced by Changus, Speed, and Stewart in 1957, is that the tumor is angioblastic in origin. Many of the pertinent cases available for my review strongly favor this concept.

Electron microscopic observations have indicated an epithelial quality of these lesions. It is obvious from hematoxylin-eosin preparations that part of at least some of these lesions exhibit squamous differentiation. The malignant cells of these tumors likely are capable of various expressions.

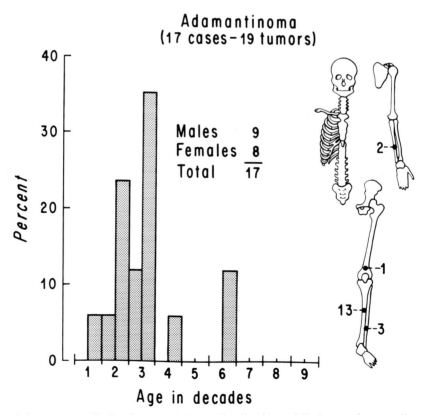

Figure 23-1. Skeletal, age, and sex distribution of "adamantinomas."

Despite this controversial literature, the fact remains that "adamantinoma" of long bones comprises a small group of distinctive tumors that present as primary lesions of bone. It may be that several histogenetically different tumors can produce the features of "adamantinoma." None of the proposed theories of origin explains its peculiar predilection for the tibia.

The name "adamantinoma" was given to these tumors because of their histologic resemblance to the common adamantinoma (ameloblastoma) of the jawbones. These odontogenic tumors of the jaws and the histologically related tumor that arises from Rathke's pouch are obviously not related and are excluded from the discussion that follows.

Incidence

Somewhat more than one hundred examples of adamantinoma of long bones have been recorded in the literature. The seventeen cases in the Mayo Clinic series comprised only about one third of 1 percent of the malignant primary tumors of bone.

Sex

Slightly more than one half of the patients reported have been males.

Age

In collected series, the second, third, fourth, and fifth decades have contributed nearly equal numbers of patients. In 1965, Moon found that two of ninety-one patients were less than eleven years old and the two were more than sixty years of age.

Localization

Of all reported adamantinomas of long bones, 90 percent have involved the tibia, but examples have been found in all of the long tubular bones. Most of these tumors have been in the middle portion of the affected bone.

Symptoms

The prolonged clinical course of many patients with this tumor indicates its general slow growth. Pain is the most common initial symptom, whereas local tumefaction is the first complaint in a few cases. The duration of symptoms prior to diagnosis has varied from a few months to fifty years.

Physical Examination

A mass, which may be painful, is the only physical finding of consequence.

Roentgenologic Features

Seventeen cases from our files provided the following information. The most common or "typical" appearance was that of multiple, sharply circumscribed, lucent defects of different sizes, with sclerotic bone interspersed between the zones and extending above and below the lucent zones. Some of the lucent zones were small, entirely cortical, and similar to such lesions of fibrous dysplasia. Rarely, the rarefied area was elongated and predominantly within the medullary cavity, with a zone of irregular sclerosis at its margins. Typically, one of the lytic areas, usually in the midshaft, was the largest and most destructive-appearing, actually destroying the cortex. When both tibia and fibula were involved, the appearance was consistently as described. The multiple lucent zones may represent multifocal involvement initially, but because the intervening bone is abnormally sclerotic, these zones probably represent one lesion.

Rare lesions of various bones have presented as large, multiloculated cystic areas with a soap-bubble appearance.

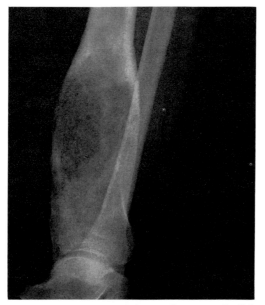 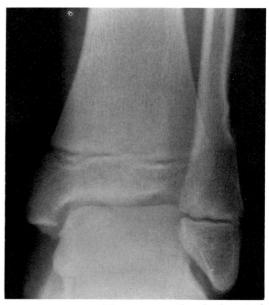

Figure 23-2. *Left.* Adamantinoma of tibia of twenty-seven-year-old woman who had noted swelling for eight years. Lesion, which is illustrated in Figure 23-6, was removed by curettage, but despite initial improvement, amputation became necessary sixteen years later. Nature of lesion at time of amputation was not known. *Right.* Juxtafibular adamantinoma in twelve-year-old boy who had noted swelling for four months. Tumor, which eroded cortex from without, was 3.5 by 2 by 1 cm.

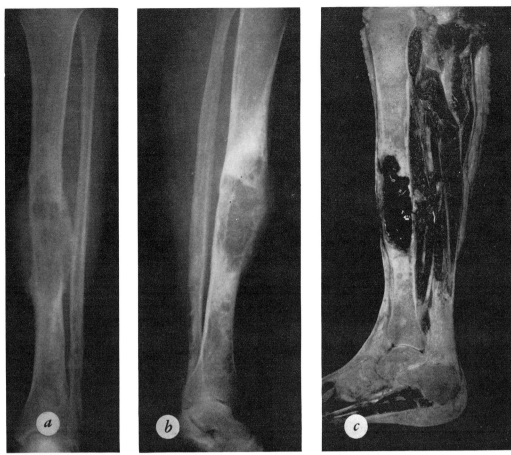

Figure 23-3. *a* and *b*. Anteroposterior and lateral views of adamantinoma of tibia of twenty-four-year-old man. Surgical procedure had been performed elsewhere fifteen months previously. Defects seen in fibula and in lower portion of tibia were composed of fibrous tissue. *c*. Amputated specimen showing defect produced by curettage that had been performed nine days previously. Fourteen months after amputation, patient died of unknown cause, but inguinal nodal metastasis had been verified in interim. (Reproduced with permission from: Dockerty, M. B., and Meyerding, H. W.: *JAMA, 119*:932-937, 1942.)

Gross Pathology

Ordinarily, "adamantinomas" are clearly delimited peripherally as indicated by the roentgenograms. Their contour is often somewhat lobulated. Most of the tumors are gray or white, and they vary in consistency from firm and fibrous to soft and brainlike. They may contain spicules of bone and calcareous material. Cystic cavities, which may contain blood or straw-colored fluid, are sometimes encountered. Some of the tumors burst through the overlying cortex, but this is unusual in patients who have not been subjected to surgical therapy. As previously mentioned, a few "adamantinomas" have been distinctly eccentric, not involving the medulla.

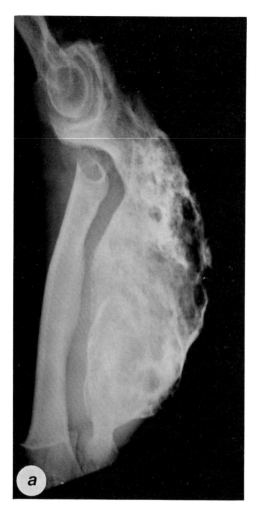 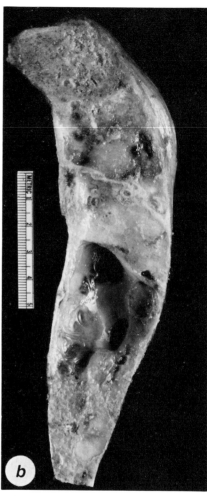

Figure 23-4. *a.* Adamantinoma expanding and distorting most of ulna of fifty-seven-year-old man who had had complaints for fifty years and had cystlike defect known for forty-three years. *b.* Resected specimen was partially cystic but microscopically was characteristic of adamantinoma in solid zones. Lesion is shown histologically in Figure 23-12*a*. (Reproduced with permission from: Unni, K. K., Dahlin, D. C., Beabout, J. W., and Ivins, J. C.: *Cancer, 34:*1796-1805, 1974.)

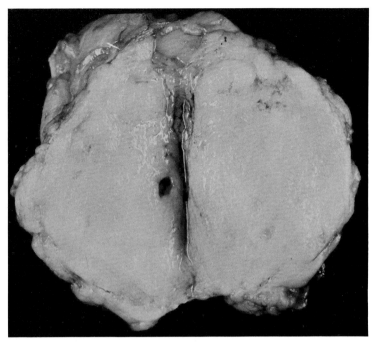

Figure 23-5. Metastatic adamantinoma to groin that developed, along with pulmonary metastasis, fifteen years after amputation for adamantinoma of midshaft of tibia. Lesion is shown histologically in Figure 23-12*b*.

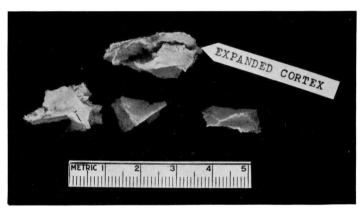

Figure 23-6. Fragments of tumor illustrated in Figure 23-2 *left*. Note that tissue is firm and fibrous, and cortex is expanded, although intact.

Histopathology

Various histologic patterns have been described, but all of them have an epithelial quality. There is variation from tumor to tumor and even within different fields of the same tumor. A common pattern consists of neoplastic islands in which the peripheral cells, often columnar, are arranged in palisaded fashion. In the centers of some of these islands, a stellate reticulumlike appearance is observed. Even cyst formation may occur within these islands, and this basic pattern has prompted use of the term "adamantinoma." A second pattern consists of islands of cells that resemble cutaneous basal cells. As in the preceding type, these cellular aggregates often show peripheral palisading of nuclei, and they are ordinarily disposed in a fibrous stroma. The appearance of this second type is very similar to that of basal cell carcinoma of the skin. Additional variation in the histopathologic appearance is afforded by fields that closely resemble squamous cell carcinoma and by other fields that mimic ordinary adenocarcinoma.

Differentiating adamantinoma from metastatic carcinoma may be difficult, especially if one considers only the histopathologic features.

The vascular origin of "adamantinoma" of long bones was strongly supported in the evidence presented by Changus and coworkers in 1957. They pointed out the histologic similarity of the proliferating cells of these tumors to the angioblasts in the embryologic formation of normal blood vessels. The angioblastic character of the cells was further supported by histochemical studies. The tumors in the present series have features in accord with their views.

The relationship of the fibrous-dysplasia-like lesions, separate from but in the vicinity of these "'adamantinomas," to the neoplasm is still obscure. When present, however, they afford the roentgenologist additional evidence that the principal lesion is an "adamantinoma." They may pose a problem in that the abundant fibroblastic tissue may obscure small islands of adamantinoma.

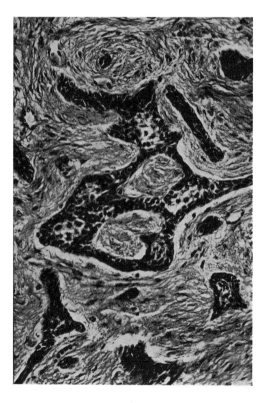

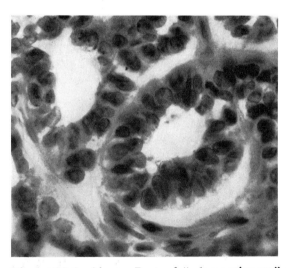

Figure 23-8. Above. Part of "adamantinoma" shown in Figure 23-3 had glandular pattern, as shown above, whereas other zones resembles squamous cell carcinoma. (×600) (Reproduced with permission from: Dockerty, M. B., and Meyerding, H. W.: *JAMA, 119:* 932-937, 1942.)

Figure 23-7. Left. Multiple sections of tumor illustrated in Figures 23-2 *left* and 23-6 showed this pattern. (×200)

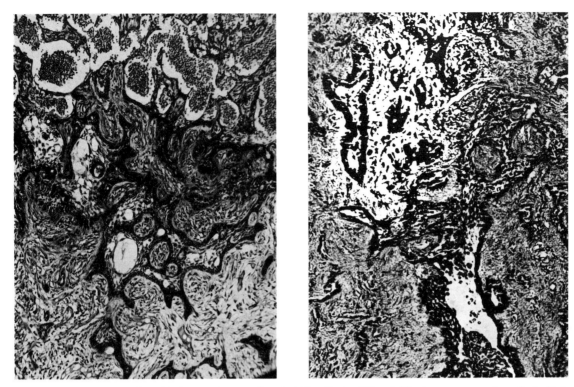

Figure 23-9. Two other "adamantinomas" of tibia. *Left.* Blood-filled spaces and endothelial-type cells above shade into classic "adamantinoma" pattern below. (×125) *Right.* Here, glandular pattern has become prominent. (×175)

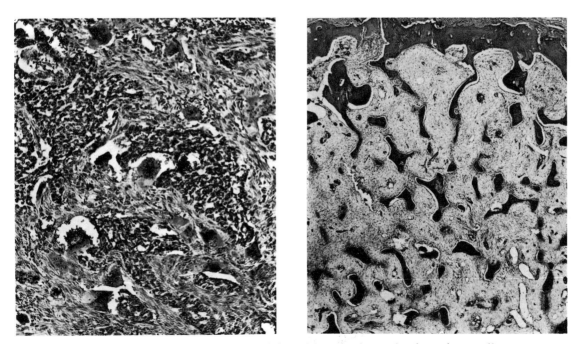

Figure 23-10. *Left.* "Adamantinoma" of tibia with prominent benign giant cell component. This is an unusual finding. (×116) *Right.* One of fibrous zones near tibial "adamantinoma." Some such zones that we have studied have not contained recognizable neoplasm. (×22)

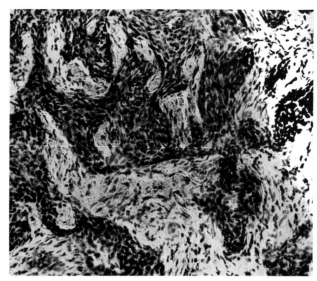

Figure 23-11. Markedly squamous appearance seen in some of these tumors. (×100) Actual squamous "pearl" formation and intercellular bridges are sometimes seen.

Treatment

After carefully reviewing all the recorded cases and amplifying the available information by sending questionnaires to the authors who reported the cases, Baker and his associates concluded that amputation is the treatment of choice. This conclusion was based upon the finding that recurrence followed local excision in two thirds of the cases and recurrence was followed by death in eight instances.

One might be justifiably tempted to employ wide block excision of the involved segment of bone if the lesion is small and well located. This less radical approach for selected lesions has been recommended by a number of authors. Our own experience, based on a study of twenty-nine patients with adamantinoma, of which only three were known to have died of their disease, favors resection of the tumor whenever possible.

Prognosis

Early radical therapy should effect a high proportion of cures. However, temporizing with inadequate attempts at local excision has caused death owing to metastasis. Although the average "adamantinoma" runs an indolent course, some otherwise typical examples metastasize early. Metastasis may be by either the hematogenous or the lymphatic route. The lungs are most often the site, but metastasis may be "widespread," to other bones, abdominal organs, or lymph nodes.

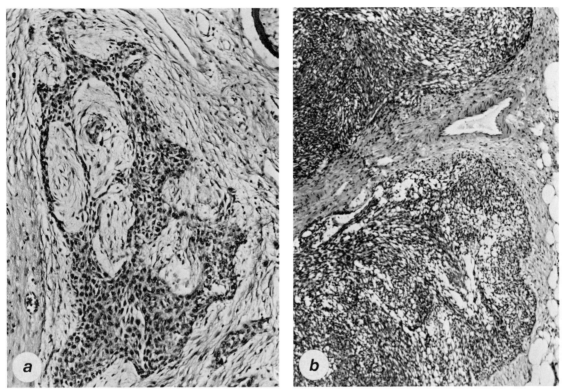

Figure 23-12. *a.* Adamantinoma from ulnar lesion of fifty years' duration shown in Figure 23-4. (×160) *b.* Adamantinoma metastasis to groin shown in Figure 23-5. This lesion is similar histologically to pulmonary mass found at that time and to tibial adamantinoma that led to amputation fifteen years previously. (×100)

Bibliography

1913   Fischer, B.: Über ein Primares Admantinom der Tibia. *Frankfurt Z, Pathol, 12:*422-441.

1930   Richter, C. S.: Ein Fall von Adamantinomartiger Geschwulst des Scheinbeins. *Z Krebsforsch, 32:*273-279.

1940   Hebbel, R.: Adamantinoma of the Tibia. *Surgery, 7:*860-868.

1942   Dockerty, M. B., and Meyerding, H. W.: Adamantinoma of the Tibia: Report of Two New Cases. *JAMA, 119:*932-937.

1954   Baker, P. L., Dockerty, M. B., and Coventry, M. B.: Adamantinoma (So-called) of the Long Bones: Review of the Literature and a Report of Three New Cases. *J Bone Joint Surg, 36A:*704-720.

1954   Lederer, H., and Sinclair, A. J.: Malignant Synovioma Simulating "Adamantinoma of the Tibia." *J Pathol Bacteriol, 67:*163-168.

1954   Hicks, J. D.: Synovial Sarcoma of the Tibia. *J Pathol Bacteriol, 67:*115-161.

1957   Changus, G. W., Speed, J. S., and Stewart, F. W.: Malignant Angioblastoma of Bone. A Reappraisal of Adamantinoma of Long Bone. *Cancer, 10:*540-559.

1960   D'Aubigne, R. M.: Adamantinome Du Tibia. *Rev Chir Orthop, 46:*92-96.

1962   Cohen, D. M., Dahlin, D. C., and Pugh, D. G.: Fibrous Dysplasia Associated With Adamantinoma of the Long Bones. *Cancer, 15:*515-521.

1962   Elliott, G. B.: Malignant Angioblastoma of Long Bones, So-called "Tibial Adamantinoma." *J Bone Joint Surg, 44B:*25-33.

1963   Gloor, F.: Das Sogenannte Adamantinom der Langen Röhrenknochen. *Virchows Arch [Pathol Anat], 336:*489-502.

1965   Moon, N. F.: Adamantinoma of the Appendicular Skeleton: A Statistical Review of
       Reported Cases and Inclusion of 10 New Cases. *Clin Orthop, 43:*189-213 (No-
       vember-December).

1969   Rosai, J.: Adamantinoma of the Tibia: Electron Microscopic Evidence of Its Epi-
       thelial Origin. *Am J Clin Pathol, 51:*786-792 (June).

1974   Unni, K. K., Dahlin, D. C., Beabout, J. W., and Ivins, J. C.: Admantinomas of Long
       Bones. *Cancer, 34:*1796-1805 (November).

1975   Huvos, A. G., and Marcove, R. C.: Adamantinoma of Long Bones: A Clinicopatho-
       logical Study of Fourteen Cases With Vascular Origin Suggested. *J Bone Joint Surg,
       57A:*148-154 (March).

Chapter 24

Malignant (Fibrous) Histiocytoma

NUMEROUS REPORTS of this type of tumor of bone have appeared in recent years. A typical neoplasm is one that shows fibrogenic differentiation, often in a "storiform" pattern, and other areas of cells with nuclei that are similar but appear to be histiocytic. The nuclei are often indented, cytoplasm is usually abundant and may be slightly foamy, nucleoli are often large, and multinucleated malignant giant cells are usually a prominent feature.

Many osteosarcoma, fibrosarcomas, and dedifferentiated chondrosarcomas contain areas that resemble what we regard as malignant (fibrous) histiocytoma. It seems appropriate to place the word "fibrous" in parentheses because a few neoplasms that are in the spectrum show no fibrogenesis. When sections of all parts of a malignant tumor fit the histologic pattern, the designation of malignant (fibrous) histiocytoma seems appropriate.

Because they appeared to be properly designated as malignant (fibrous) histio-

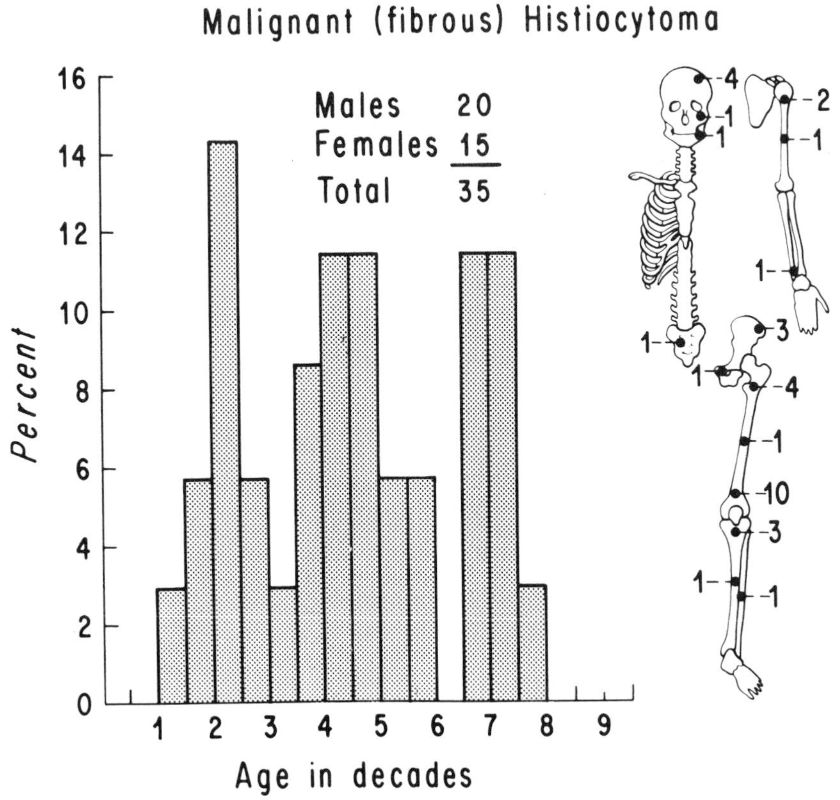

Figure 24-1. Skeletal, age, and sex distribution of malignant (fibrous) histiocytomas. (Reproduced with permission from: Dahlin, D. C., Unni, K. K., and Matsuno, T.: *Cancer, 39*:1508-1516, 1977.)

cytoma, 35 tumors were segregated from 158 fibrosarcomas and 962 osteosarcomas in this series. There were seventeen fibrosarcomas and eighteen osteosarcomas. No tumors that fulfilled the histologic criteria were found among our other bone tumors. Details of the thirty-five cases are given in this chapter. Even electron microscopic studies have not clarified the veracity of this new diagnosis.

It seems that when cells become malignant they have the capability of differentiating into the pattern that we call malignant (fibrous) histiocytoma.

Incidence

Only 35 examples of malignant (fibrous) histiocytoma were culled from a total of 4,774 malignant primary bone tumors.

Sex

Twenty of the thirty-five patients were males. This slight preponderance of lesions in males is in accord with the literature.

Age

Nearly any age may be affected. One patient was only six years old.

Localization

Many different bones were affected, but long bones were the site in twenty-four cases.

Symptoms

As with other varieties of bone tumors, pain (twenty-three cases) and swelling (eighteen cases) were most frequent. One patient had had symptoms for only one week; nearly half of the lesions had produced symptoms for six months to two years. Three of the tumors complicated Paget's disease of bone, and four developed in bone that had been affected by prior radiation therapy. In no case was nodal metastasis proved or even strongly suggested clinically.

Physical Findings

Pain or swelling or both as a consequence of the local lesion were noted.

Roentgenologic Features

As detailed by Feldman and Norman, these features nearly always indicated that the suspect area harbored a malignant tumor. Metastatic carcinoma or malignant lymphoma of bone might produce a similar pattern. In one case, margination of the lesion suggested that it was benign.

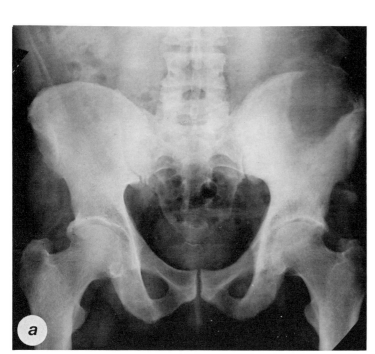
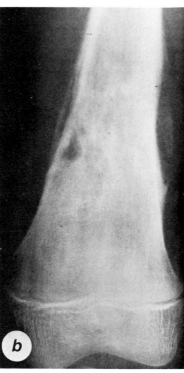

Figure 24-2. *a.* Malignant (fibrous) histiocytoma complicating Paget's disease in sixty-four-year-old man. This lesion was deemed to be inoperable, but patient survived seventeen years after radiation therapy. *b.* Malignant (fibrous) histiocytoma in ten-year-old girl. Features, although indicating malignancy, do not specifically suggest histologic diagnosis. (Figure 24-2*a* reproduced with permission from: Dahlin, D. C., and Coventry, M. B.: *J Bone Joint Surg, 49A:*101-110, 1967.)

Gross Pathology

The tumors varied from fibrous to soft. A few lesions were yellowish owing to lipid content or were brown or tan. A few contained necrotic zones. Benign heterotopic ossification occurred within one lesion, which is illustrated in Figure 24-3 *right*. This was the only periosteally located tumor; the remainder were prominently intraosseous. Only one tumor had produced pathologic fracture. Three of the tumors arose in Paget's disease.

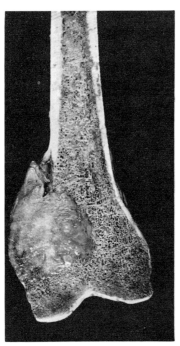 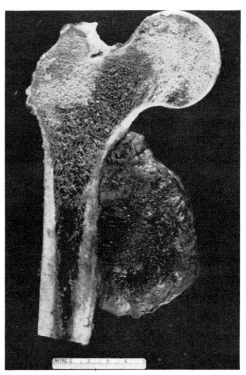

Figure 24-3. *Left.* Malignant (fibrous) histiocytoma in twenty-six-year-old man, originally coded as fibroblastic osteosarcoma. Location of this lesion is typical of osteosarcoma, but osteoid in it is of questionable veracity. Generalized metastasis developed sixty-two months after amputation for this sarcoma, and death occurred at seventy-three months. *Right.* Similar tumor centered in periosteal location in forty-two-year-old man. He died with metastasis eleven months after hindquarter amputation for this tumor.

Histopathology

Microscopic quality determined inclusion of tumors in this series. The features observed represent what dominated the fields studied; marked variation existed within these tumors. Multinucleated tumor cells (malignant giant cells) with nuclei usually possessing a histiocytic appearance were found in every tumor, but these varied from numerous to few. The histiocytic appearance was provided by grooving or indentation of nuclei, nucleoli that were often acidophilic and large, and a frequently prominent, well-defined cytoplasmic mass. A few tumors contained prominent foci of histiocytic mononuclear cells, which were suggestive of reticulum cell sarcoma of bone. Fibrosis varied from slight to prominent throughout many fields, and it was recognized to some degree in twenty-eight of the thirty-five tumors. The fibrogenic areas frequently exhibited a storiform or "cartwheel" pattern, with the fascicles appearing to radiate irregularly from focal zones. Osteoid, "debatable" or relatively definite, was present in small foci in nearly half of these lesions. Such "osteoid" is debatable because subjective interpretation of pink homogeneous material is involved. Chronic inflammatory cells, usually lymphocytes, were found in twenty-four tumors. These inflammatory cells occurred in small clusters, or were scattered diffusely through the tumors, or were most prominent at the periphery of neoplasms. A few tumors had what appeared to be immaturity of these cells, and the cells resembled lymphoblasts; these cells possibly were part of the neoplasia. Although myofibrils and cross-striations were not identified, the abundant granular cytoplasm of the cells produced a myogenic aura in sixteen of the thirty-five tumors. The foamy cytoplasm in the cells of eighteen tumors was so prominent that the diagnosis of liposarcoma was considered. Hemosiderin was recognized in a few of these cells. Necrosis was present in sections of ten tumors, and osteoclastlike benign giant cells were seen in eight. The tumors usually had a well-circumscribed pushing border when they extended outside bone, but a few lesions invaded fat or striated muscle.

Most of the tumors were highly malignant with pronounced nuclear anisocytosis and many mitotic figures, which were often atypical. Only two tumors were moderately well differentiated and thus somewhat difficult to be judged malignant.

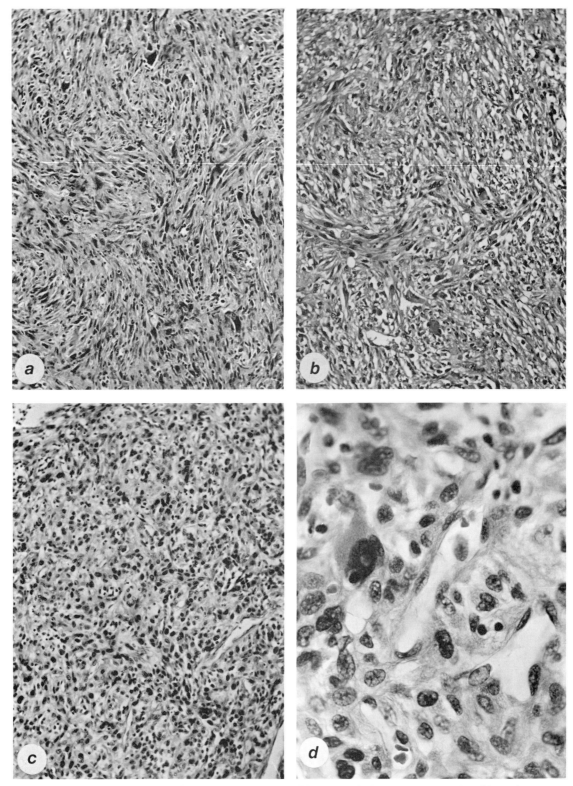

Figure 24-4. Patterns recognized as malignant (fibrous) histiocytoma. *a.* "Storiform" pattern of fibrogenesis and atypical nuclei. (×160) *b.* Similar "storiform" pattern in distal femoral tumor. (×160) *c.* Mandibular tumor with histiocytic nature of neoplastic cells evident and only slight fibrogenesis. (×160) *d.* At higher magnification, histiocytic quality of malignant cells of this mandibular tumor is more evident. (×600) (Reproduced with permission from: Dahlin, D. C., Unni, K. K., and Matsuno, T.: *Cancer, 39:*1508-1516, 1977.)

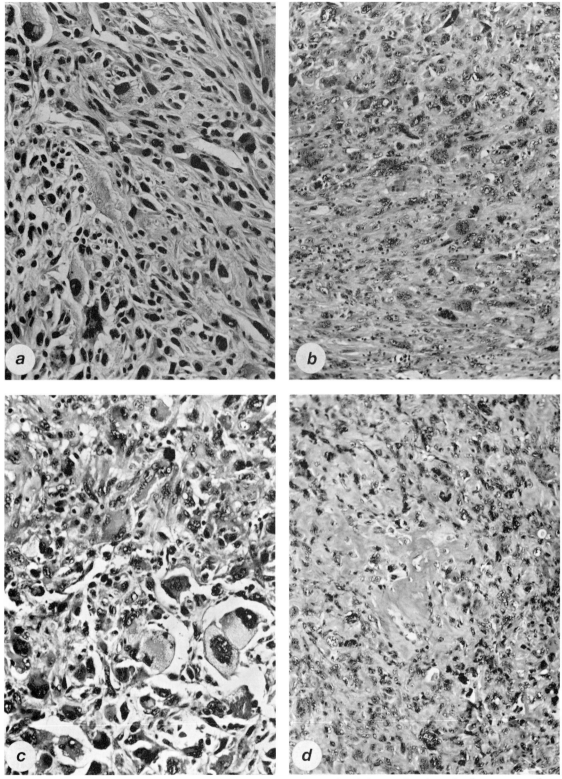

Figure 24-5. *a.* Malignant (fibrous) histiocytoma of parietal bone developed nine years after radiation therapy for brain tumor. (×250) *b.* Similar malignant tumor of distal part of femoral shaft of twenty-four-year-old woman. Benign and malignant multinucleated cells are numerous. (×160) *c.* Another area of tumor shown in *b.* Many of the large malignant cells contain foamy cytoplasm. *d.* Osteoidlike material in same tumor. Problem is whether one can allow malignant (fibrous) histiocytoma to produce such matrix. (×160) (Reproduced with permission from: Dahlin, D. C., Unni, K. K., and Matsuno, T.: *Cancer, 39:*1508-1516, 1977.)

Treatment

Although this series did not provide definitive information, the tumors probably are relatively radioresistant. All nineteen tumors of the tubular long bones in patients treated more than five years previously were managed by amputation. Interestingly, radiation resulted in long-term survival of two patients who had inoperable pelvic tumors. Four of the thirty-five tumors developed, however, in previously radiated bone.

I currently believe that therapeutic principles like those for fibrosarcoma or for fibroblastic osteosarcoma are appropriate. Our series provided no information as to the value of cytotoxic therapy.

Prognosis

Of twenty-eight patients treated more than five years previous to our study, sixteen survived for five years or longer. Four of these died of their tumors six to seven years after resection for or amputation of the primary lesion.

The earlier designation of osteosarcoma in fourteen of the twenty-eight patients eligible for five-year survival was not associated with a significantly worse prognosis than was the original diagnosis of fibrosarcoma for the other fourteen.

For some unexplained reason, the patients documented by Feldman and Norman and by Spanier, Enneking, and Enriquez fared more poorly than ours did.

Bibliography

1972 Kempson, R. L., and Kyriakos, M.: Fibroxanthosarcoma of the Soft Tissues: A Type of Malignant Fibrous Histiocytoma. *Cancer, 29:*961-976 (April).

1972 Soule, E. H., and Enriquez, P.: Atypical Fibrous Histiocytoma, Malignant Fibrous Histiocytoma, Malignant Histiocytoma, and Epithelioid Sarcoma, A Comparative Study of 65 Tumors. *Cancer, 30:*128-143 (July).

1974 Mirra, J. M., Bullough, P. G., Marcove, R. C., Jacobs, B., and Huvos, A. G.: Malignant Fibrous Histiocytoma and Osteosarcoma in Association With Bone Infarcts: Report of Four Cases, Two in Caisson Workers. *J Bone Joint Surg, 56A:* 932-940 (July).

1975 Fu, Y.-S., Gabbiani, G., Kaye, G. I., and Lattes, R.: Malignant Soft Tissue Tumors of Probable Histiocytic Origin (Malignant Fibrous Histiocytomas): General Considerations and Electron Microscopic and Tissue Culture Studies. *Cancer, 35:*176-198 (January).

1975 Newland, R. C., Harrison, M. A., and Wright, R. G.: Fibroxanthosarcoma of Bone. *Pathology, 7:*203-208 (July).

1975 Spanier, S. S., Enneking, W. F., and Enriquez, P.: Primary Malignant Fibrous Histiocytoma of Bone. *Cancer, 36:*2084-2098 (December).

1976 Alquacil-Garcia, A.: Personal Communication.

1976 Huvos, A. G.: Primary Malignant Fibrous Histiocytoma of Bone: Clinicopathologic Study of 18 Patients. *NY State J Med, 76:*552-559 (April).

(See also Chapter 10 Bibliography.)

Chapter 25

Fibrosarcoma and Desmoplastic Fibroma

FIBROSARCOMA occurring in bone is defined as a malignant tumor of spindle-shaped cells that produce no osteoid material in the primary lesion or in secondary deposits. Collagen production varies from abundant to none, tending to be less in the highly anaplastic examples. Fibrosarcoma may be so well differentiated that it is difficult to distinguish from benign conditions such as fibrous dysplasia.

It is somewhat didactic to differentiate fibrosarcoma of bone from its close relative, fibroblastic osteosarcoma. Relatively minor clinical features distinguish these two entities, and both are best treated by ablative surgical means. Occasionally, one finds osteoid substance only after prolonged search through many sections of a tumor that is predominantly fibroblastic, indicating that the separation is an artificial one.

After exclusion of the tumors that merely abutted on bone, on the premise that they were probably of soft-tissue origin, there remained in the Mayo Clinic series no distinct group of tumors that one might logically call "periosteal fibrosarcomas." This manner of selection perhaps excludes some sarcomas of periosteal origin. From the gross pathologic features, it is apparent that most fibrosarcomas of bone arise in the medullary or the cortical regions, although a few undoubtedly begin in the periosteum.

"Secondary" fibrosarcoma accounted for 27 percent of the 158 in this series. Twenty-nine occurred after radiation, four developed in giant cell tumors that had had no prior radiation, five occurred in Paget's disease, and five in other conditions. Several sarcomas complicating infarcts of bone have been described.

Multicentric origin is suggested in some cases of fibrosarcoma of bone. I have seen several examples, especially in material sent in for consultation, in which two or more skeletal foci were present when the patient first sought medical care.

Myxosarcomalike foci may be prominent in fibrosarcoma of bone. Rarely, the entire tumor has an appearance that tempts one to designate it as a myxosarcoma. Transitional types between these and obvious fibrosarcomas make me prefer to include such lesions with the fibrosarcomas.

Desmoplastic Fibroma

This rare tumor was listed among the benign conditions in Tables 1, 2, and 3 in Chapter 1. Its locally infiltrative quality puts it in a "borderline" position with regard to malignancy. Hence, the four examples in this total series of bone tumors are briefly described in this chapter.

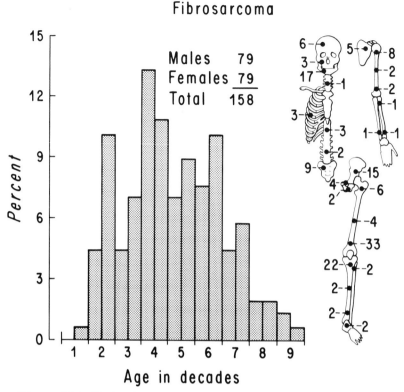

Figure 25-1. Skeletal, age, and sex distribution of fibrosarcomas.

Incidence

The 158 fibrosarcomas in this series comprised 3.3 percent of the total primary malignant bone tumors. Fibrosarcoma was less than one-sixth as common as osteosarcoma.

Sex

Males and females were equally affected.

Age

The fibrosarcomas were rather evenly distributed among the second through the sixth decades of life. The tendency of fibrosarcoma to occur among older people as commonly as among the younger is the major clinical difference between it and osteosarcoma; forty-three tumors occurred as late complications of preexisting conditions.

Localization

The sites involved by fibrosarcoma do not differ remarkably from those involved by osteosarcoma. The long bones, where the tumor is usually found in the metaphyseal region, contributed more than 50 percent of cases. Several tumors that affected the maxillary antrum, including its bony walls, were excluded for lack of evidence of osseous origin. One patient in this series presented with multifocal skeletal disease.

Symptoms

Fibrosarcoma produces the ordinary symptoms of malignant tumor in bone, namely pain and swelling. Generally, these are of short duration. Patients whose fibrosarcomas arise secondarily give an appropriate history of the original condition and often have had radiation therapy many years before the malignant tumor appears.

Physical Examination

Painful swelling in the region of the tumor is usually found, unless the tumor is covered by a thick layer of uninvolved tissue. Spindle cell sarcoma and even carcinomas with spindle-shaped cells may metastasize to the skeleton and mimic primary fibrosarcoma, so evidence for such hidden lesions should be sought. Only one patient had Recklinghausen's neurofibromatosis, but her tibial fibrosarcoma contained no stigmata that could make it definitely neurogenic.

The symptoms and physical examination are sometimes altered in fibrosarcoma secondary to the other conditions listed in Table 7. Fibrosarcomas that result from dedifferentiation of chondrosarcomas as described in Chapter 17 are not included in these data.

TABLE 7

PREDISPOSING CONDITIONS IN "SECONDARY" FIBROSARCOMA
IN 158 FIBROSARCOMAS OF BONE

Condition		*Number of Cases*
Paget's disease		5
Giant cell tumor		16
Prior radiation therapy	12*	
Prior surgical therapy	2	
No prior therapy	2	
Ameloblastic fibroma		2
Desmoplastic fibroma		1
Radiated miscellaneous benign bone lesions		10*
Radiation for nonosseous disease		7*
Benign osseous lesions		2
Total		43

* A total of 29 arose in previously radiated bone.

Roentgenologic Features

As Pugh (1954) has so aptly stated, there are no roentgenologic features that distinguish fibrosarcoma of bone from osteolytic osteosarcoma. The essential destructive characteristics of the latter tumor have been described previously. Periosteal, reactive new bone formation may be seen. There are no pathognomonic features of fibrosarcoma of bone, but generally, the diagnosis of malignant tumor can be made with reasonable assurance. The neoplastic tissue often permeates the affected bone well beyond the lytic zone seen in the roentgenogram.

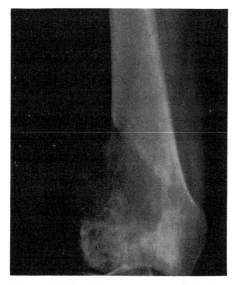

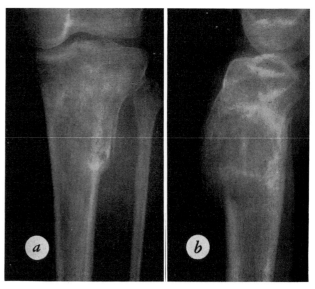

Figure 25-2. Fibrosarcoma producing irregular destruction of lower portion of femur. (Reproduced with permission from: McLeod, J. J., Dahlin, D. C., and Ivins, J. C.: *Am J Surg, 94:*431-437, 1957.)

Figure 25-3. *a* and *b*. Anteroposterior and lateral views of fibrosarcoma of upper metaphyseal portion of tibia. Note cortical destruction, especially anteriorly. (Reproduced with permission from: McLeod, J. J., Dahlin, D. C., and Ivins, J. C.: *Am J Surg, 94:*431-437, 1957.)

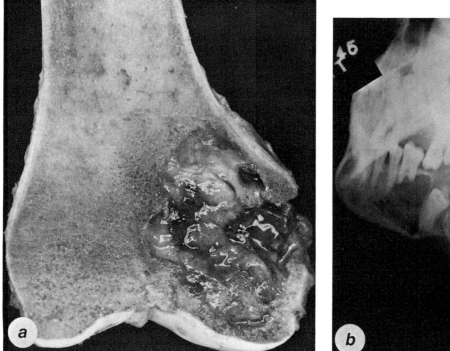

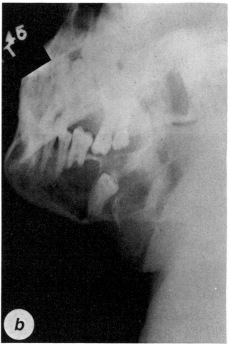

Figure 25-4. *a.* Fibrosarcoma in eighteen-year-old man. Note permeation beyond margins of soft tumor. Patient died with metastasis twenty-two months after amputation. *b.* Grade 2 fibrosarcoma coexisting with benign ameloblastic fibroma in thirty-nine-year-old man.

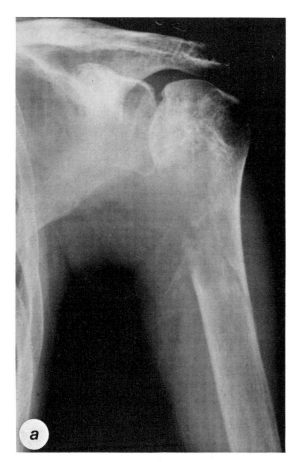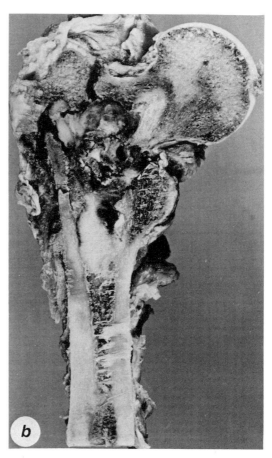

Figure 25-5. *a.* Grade 2 myxoid fibrosarcoma in fifty-six-year-old woman. Lesion developed eighty-one months after radiation for ipsilateral mammary adenocarcinoma. *b.* Fibrosarcoma complicating infarct in sixty-two-year-old woman and associated with pathologic fracture. (Case contributed by Doctor N. Miller of Charleston, South Carolina.)

Gross Pathology

Fibrosarcoma of bone may be composed of a firm, fibrous mass of tissue or of soft, fleshy, friable, and sometimes even myxoid tissue that invades the bone in an irregular fashion. Some tumors of this type, however, are reasonably well circumscribed and can be shelled out of the bone of origin rather readily. Areas of necrosis and hemorrhage may be present. Almost all of the fibrosarcomas of central origin break through the cortex and present with a large or small extraosseous component. Permeation of bone and invasion through the cortex help differentiate these tumors from benign fibrous conditions. The average tumor of this type has its longest axis parallel to and within the bone of origin. Practically any bone and any portion of it can be affected by this neoplasm. In a few instances, the tumor is chiefly outside the bone and thus is likely to be of periosteal origin.

Fibrosarcoma, like osteosarcoma, metastasizes primarily by the hematogenous route, producing secondary deposits in the lung most commonly, but also in various sites including other bones.

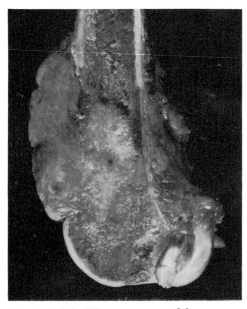

Figure 25-6. Fibrosarcoma of lower portion of femur. This is specimen from case represented in Figure 25-2. (Reproduced with permission from: McLeod, J. J., Dahlin, D. C., and Ivins, J. C.: *Am J Surg, 94*:431-437, 1957.)

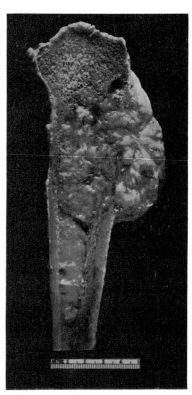

Figure 25-7. Specimen from case illustrated in Figure 25-3. (Reproduced with permission from: McLeod, J. J., Dahlin, D. C., and Ivins, J. C.: *Am J Surg, 94*:431-437, 1957.)

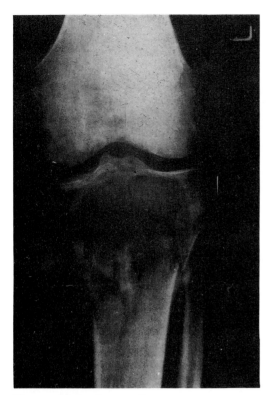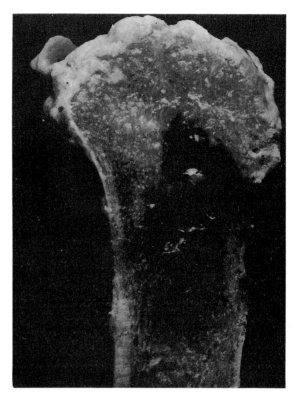

Figure 25-8. *Left.* Fibrosarcoma of tibia. This lytic tumor was markedly myxoid. *Right.* Similar myxoid type of fibrosarcoma. Although not grossly obvious, tumor completely permeated upper end of tibia.

Histopathology

Fibrosarcoma in bone has the same histologic features as its soft-tissue counterpart. However, sections may reveal that it is invading and destroying bone, especially near the periphery of the tumor. There is wide variation in the degree of differentiation of the component fibroblasts and in the amount of collagen produced. The shapes of the nuclei vary from long and slender to oval. Nuclear irregularities and the number of mitotic figures are increased in the more anaplastic (higher-grade) tumors. The collagen is arranged in rather orderly bands and whorls in the lower-grade lesions. Some highly anaplastic spindle cell tumors produce no recognizable collagen, but such tumors are logically included among the fibrosarcomas because of their histologic kinship.

Benign multinucleated cells are sometimes found in fibrosarcomas, but they are more commonly seen among the malignant cells of osteosarcomas.

A few fibrosarcomas are so low grade that the problem of differentiation from benign lesions arises. The benign conditions that may enter into the problem of differentiation include cellular lesions of fibrous dysplasia and nonosteogenic fibroma of bone. I have seen a number of cases in which the original specimen from a fibrosarcoma had been underdiagnosed as some benign condition. Attention to signs of aggressiveness as may be indicated in the roentgenogram or by permeation of tumor among preexisting trabeculae or destruction of the overlying bony cortex helps one avoid this error.

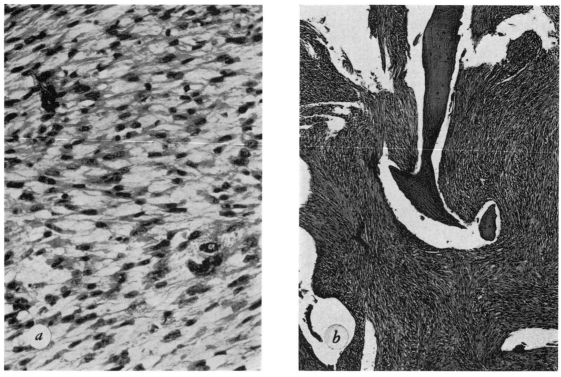

Figure 25-9. *a.* Grade 2 fibrosarcoma. (×200) This section, which shows only slight collagen production, came from tumor illustrated in Figures 25-3 and 25-7. *b.* Periphery of fairly well differentiated fibrosarcoma shown invading bone. (×75) (Reproduced with permission from: McLeod, J. J., Dahlin, D. C., and Ivins, J. C.: *Am J Surg, 94:*431-437, 1957.)

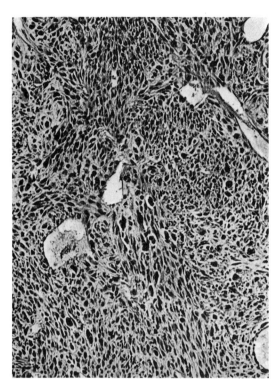 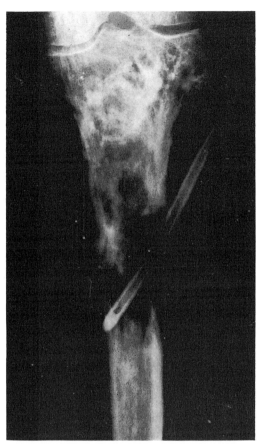

Figure 25-10. *Left.* Relatively anaplastic fibrosarcoma with bizarre and irregular nuclei, but with considerable collagen production. (×100) *Right.* Infected fibrosarcoma destroying junction of upper and middle thirds of tibia. Lesion developed twenty-eight years after radiation of aneurysmal bone cyst in this area.

Fibrosarcoma, as defined here, includes tumors with spindle-shaped cells, usually with distinctly larger nuclei than those of Ewing's sarcoma, but sometimes not definitely collagenous. Metastatic spindle cell sarcoma can mimic the pattern of primary fibrosarcoma of bone. This includes a few that are obviously myogenic, having arisen in the uterus or the gastrointestinal tract. A problem sometimes not resolvable from histologic study is that metastatic carcinoma in bone can show prominent "spindling" of the malignant cells. Sometimes careful physical examination, including special roentgenographic studies and significant historical details, are required in the assessment of a problem case.

The whorled or storiform pattern in some fibrosarcomas of bone has made many of them confused with the rather nebulous "entity" called malignant (fibrous) histiocytoma. Indeed, seventeen of the tumors in this group have such a close resemblance to that group that I have included them and data pertaining to them in the analysis of thirty-five cases in Chapter 24. Because I am not certain of the designation of malignant (fibrous) histiocytoma, data concerning them is also given in this chapter. The problem is illustrated in Figure 25-11.

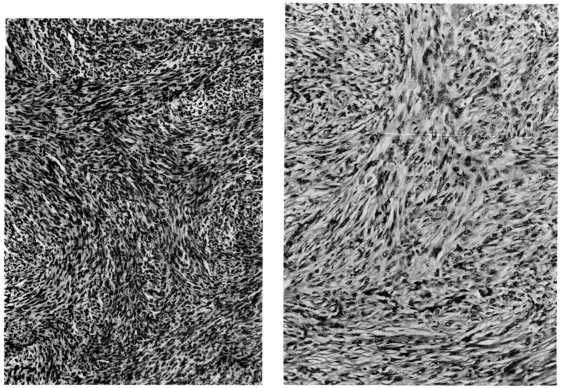

Figure 25-11. *Left.* Fibrosarcoma with moderate differentiation and whorls of cells. (×100) *Right.* Higher magnification to accentuate same quality. (×160) Pattern such as exhibited in these areas of two different tumors makes one consider diagnosis of malignant (fibrous) histiocytoma.

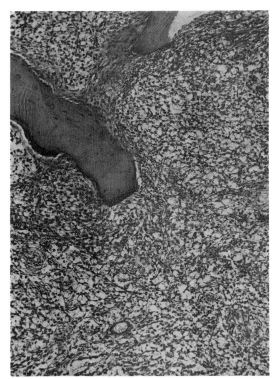 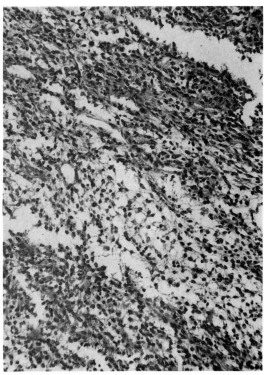

Figure 25-12. *Left.* Section from tumor shown in Figure 25-8 *right*. Parts of this fibrosarcoma, which is permeating bone, resemble myxoid liposarcoma, but stains for fat were negative. (×100) *Right.* Another fibrosarcoma containing foci of loosely arranged myxoid-appearing cells. (×125)

Treatment

Ablative surgical treatment of the type used for osteosarcoma is usually indicated for fibrosarcoma of bone. Details regarding management of tumors of various sites are given in Chapter 19. Fibrosarcoma is relatively radioresistant.

Some have made a convincing plea for conservative block-excisional therapy for some of the well-localized fibrosarcomas of long bones on the premise that they are relatively benign. Experience at the Mayo Clinic indicates, however, that fibrosarcoma is practically as lethal as osteosarcoma and demands prompt, adequate therapy.

Prognosis

Although 26.8 percent of the patients in our earlier series (McLeod and coworkers, 1957) survived five years, more than one fourth of these survivors subsequently died of the effects of their tumors. Most authorities believe that the well-differentiated fibrosarcomas have a prognosis distinctly better than that of osteosarcoma.

Desmoplastic Fibroma

Only about thirty cases of this tumor have been documented. This lesion has affected patients of a wide variety of ages. Long tubular bones have been the sites of predilection, but this lesion also has been found in various sites such as the ilium, os calcis, scapula, mandible, and vertebra. Roentgenologically, the rarefying defect is generally central and reasonably well demarcated, often having an irregular border that produces a "trabeculated" appearance. Grossly, there is a dense, tough, rubbery, whorled mass of fibrous tissue that bears a remarkable similarity to desmoids of soft-tissue origin. Histologically, there are hypocellular bundles of collagenous tissue with sparse, small, slender, spindle-shaped nuclei. Mitotic activity is absent or practically so. The lack of giant cells and hypocellularity contrast with the findings in nonosteogenic fibroma. There is no osseous metaplasia as in fibrous dysplasia or low-grade central (intramedullary) osteosarcoma. Lack of nuclear anaplasia and of mitotic activity allows differentiation from fibrosarcoma. Complete resection is apparently the best therapy; sometimes this may entail segmental resection of the affected part of a bone.

The four desmoplastic fibromas in this series of 6,221 bone tumors attest to their rarity. One was in the os calcis of a twenty-one-year-old woman, one in the radius of a sixteen-year-old boy, one in the mandible of a twenty-five-year-old man, and one in the humerus of a sixteen-year-old boy.

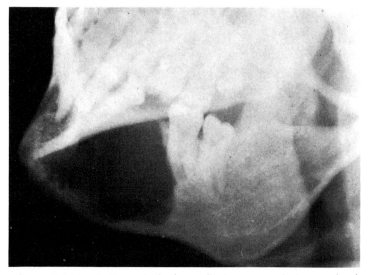
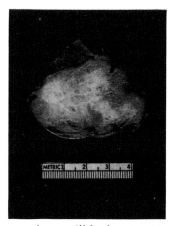

Figure 25-13. *Left.* Relatively well demarcated desmoplastic fibroma of mandible in twenty-five-year-old man who had noted swelling in region for four months. *Right.* Dense, whorled, fibrous mass that was removed by resection of involved segment of mandible. This case illustrates hazard of diagnosing desmoplastic fibroma. Although this tumor was considered typical of that disease, recurrent tumor in same area was grade 2 fibrosarcoma, and despite hemimandibulectomy, patient died thirty-five months later with metastasis.

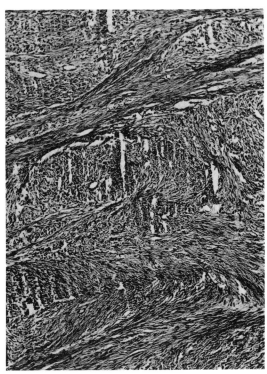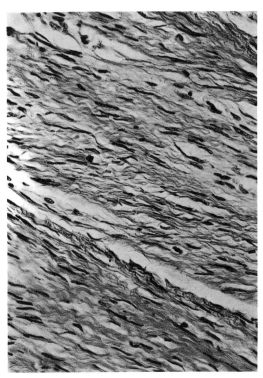

Figure 25-14. *Left*. Fascicles of dense collagenous tissue from desmoplastic fibroma illustrated in Figure 25-13. (×65) Note marked similarity to desmoid tumors of soft-tissue origin. *Right*. Higher magnification to show nuclear details. (×250) Slightly more cellular zones were found retrospectively.

Bibliography

1944 Steiner, P. E.: Multiple Diffuse Fibrosarcoma of Bone. *Am J Pathol, 20:*877-893.

1948 Stout, A. P.: Fibrosarcoma: The Malignant Tumor of Fibroblasts. *Cancer, 1:*30-63.

1954 Pugh, D. G.: *Roentgenologic Diagnosis of Diseases of Bones.* Baltimore, Williams & Wilkins, p. 559AW.

1957 McLeod, J. J., Dahlin, D. C., and Ivins, J. C.: Fibrosarcoma of Bone. *Am J Surg, 94:*431-437.

1958 Goidanich, I. F., and Venturi, R.: I Fibrosarcomi Primitivi Dello Scheletro. *Chir Organi Mov, 46:*1-90.

1958 Jaffe, H. L.: *Tumors and Tumorous Conditions of the Bones and Joints.* Philadelphia, Lea & Febiger, pp. 298-313.

1958 Gilmer, W. S., Jr., and MacEwen, G. D.: Central (Medullary) Fibrosarcoma of Bone. *J Bone Joint Surg, 40A:*121-141.

1960 Furey, J. G., Ferrer-Torells, M., and Reagan, J. W.: Fibrosarcoma Arising at the Site of Bone Infarcts. A Report of 2 Cases. *J Bone Joint Surg, 42A:*802-810.

1960 Whitesides, T. E., Jr., and Ackerman, L. V.: Desmoplastic Fibroma. A Report of Three Cases. *J Bone Joint Surg, 42A:*1143-1150.

1961 Christensen, E., Hojgaard, K., and Winkel Smith, C. C.: Congenital Malignant Mesenchymal Tumors in a Two Month Old Child. *Acta Pathol Microbiol Scand, 53:*237-242.

1962 Nielsen, A. R., and Poulsen, H.: Multiple Diffuse Fibrosarcomata of the Bones. *Acta Pathol Microbiol Scand, 55:*265-272.

1964 Dahlin, D. C., and Hoover, N. W.: Demoplastic Fibroma of Bone. Report of Two Cases. *J A M A, 188:*685-687.

1965 Lichtenstein, L.: *Bone Tumors,* ed. 3. St. Louis, Mosby, pp. 229-240.

1966 Dorfman, H. D., Norman, A., and Wolff, H.: Fibrosarcoma Complicating Bone Infarction in a Caisson Worker: A Case Report. *J Bone Joint Surg, 48A:*528-532 (April).

1969 Dahlin, D. C., and Ivins, J. C.: Fibrosarcoma of Bone: A Study of 114 Cases. *Cancer, 23:*35-41 (January).

1969 Eyre-Brook, A. L., and Price, C. H. G.: Fibrosarcoma of Bone: Review of Fifty Consecutive Cases From the Bristol Bone Tumour Registry. *J Bone Joint Surg, 51B:*20-37 (February).

1974 Mirra, J. M., and Marcove, R. C.: Fibrosarcomatous Dedifferentiation of Primary and Secondary Chondrosarcoma: Review of Five Cases. *J Bone Joint Surg, 56A:* 285-296 (March).

1974 Nilsonne, U., and Mazabraud, A.: Les Fibrosarcomes de L'os. *Rev Chir Orthop, 60:*109-122 (March).

1975 Cunningham, C. D., Smith, R. O., Enriquez, P., and Singleton, G. T.: Desmoplastic Fibroma of the Mandible: A Case Report. *Ann Otol Rhinol Laryngol, 84:*125-129 (January-February).

1976 Hernandez, F. J., and Fernandez, B. B.: Multiple Diffuse Fibrosarcoma of Bone. *Cancer, 37:*939-945 (February).

Chapter 26

Chordoma

CHORDOMA is a neoplasm that develops from remnants of the primitive notochord. It apparently can arise from normal products of the notochord, the nuclei pulposi, or from abnormal "rests" of notochordal tissue. It ordinarily grows slowly and is malignant because of local invasion, but metastasis is relatively uncommon.

Chordoma has a distinct predilection for the ends of the spinal column. Thus, the sacrococcygeal region and the base of the skull near the spheno-occipital synchondrosis account for the great majority of cases. Small, non-neoplastic masses of vestigial notochordal tissue are not uncommonly found in the region of the spheno-occipital junction in the midline.

This tumor is relatively uncommon in the dorsal and lumbar portions of the vertebral column, which is strange because the largest masses of notochordal products, in the form of the nuclei pulposi, occur in these regions.

One might question whether chordoma is correctly classed among the neoplasms of bone. The intimate relationship of the notochord to the skeleton and the clinical and roentgenologic features of these tumors make the inclusion a logical one.

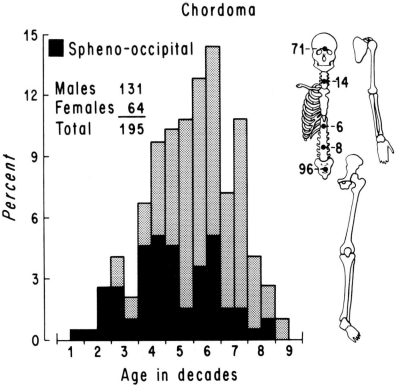

Figure 26-1. Skeletal, age, and sex distribution of chordomas.

329

Incidence

Chordoma is usually referred to as a very rare neoplasm, but it accounted for more than 4 percent of the malignant tumors in this series. Possibly a selection factor operates in a series such as this which includes many referred patients.

Sex

Chordoma affects males approximately twice as frequently as females. Of the sacrococcygeal tumors, 74 percent were in males, whereas only 58 percent of the spheno-occipital lesions were in males.

Age

As indicated in the illustration above, chordoma is distinctly uncommon in patients less than thirty years of age. There was one patient in the first decade, six in the second decade, and twelve in the third decade of life. Spheno-occipital chordomas are recognized clinically approximately a decade earlier in life than those in the sacrococcygeal region.

Localization

Chordoma is so strictly localized to the midline regions of the body that this affords important diagnostic evidence. Nearly half of the tumors occurred in the sacrococcygeal region, and 35 percent occurred at the base of the brain. Most of the remainder involved the cervical vertebrae. The dorsal and lumbar vertebral regions are rarely affected.

Symptoms

The duration of symptoms prior to the time the patient seeks medical care varies from months to several years. Pain is a practically constant feature of sacrococcygeal chordoma, and characteristically it occurs at the tip of the spinal column. Constipation because of the presence of the tumor and complaints resulting from pressure on or destruction of nerves emerging from the distal portion of the spinal cord may develop. In rare instances, a sacrococcygeal chordoma produces a post-sacral mass.

Spheno-occipital chordoma may cause symptoms referable to any of the cranial nerves, but those resulting from involvement of the nerves to the eye are by far the most common. This tumor may destroy the pituitary gland and produce evidence of its dysfunction, protrude laterally and give signs suggestive of a tumor of the cerebellopontine angle, or even erode inferiorly and obstruct the nasal passages. Large intracranial extension may evoke the general features of intracranial neoplasm.

Chordomas arising along the remainder of the spinal column frequently produce symptoms from compression of nerve roots or the spinal cord, or they produce a mass.

Physical Findings

Almost every sacrococcygeal chordoma has a presacral extension that may be detected on careful rectal examination. The mass is, of course, firm and fixed to the sacrum. Digital and proctoscopic examination discloses that it is extrarectal. Evidences of nerve dysfunction, such as "cord" bladder, anesthesias, and paraesthesias, are relatively unusual and late features.

Those chordomas that arise at the base of the brain may, as already indicated, produce signs referable to any of the cranial nerves or to involvement of the pituitary. Examination of the visual fields may disclose defects that suggest the correct diagnosis. Only rarely does a patient complain of nasal obstruction.

Since chordoma of the cervical, thoracic, and lumbar portions of the vertebral column may present posteriorly, laterally, or anteriorly, a great variety of symptoms may be produced. For example, one in the cervical region of the spinal column may give clinical features that are suggestive of chronic retropharyngeal abscess. Physical examination often discloses evidence of encroachment on the nerves or spinal cord.

Roentgenologic Features

Roentgenographic study reveals evidence of osseous involvement or a soft-tissue mass in more than 90 percent of cases. An irregular zone of destruction that begins in the midline of the sacrum characterizes 75 percent of sacrococcygeal examples. Residual osseous trabeculae and amorphous masses of calcification may be seen in the lesion. The sacrum is often expanded owing to the slow growth of the neoplasm. A soft-tissue mass, almost always anterior, is usually visible.

Cranial chordoma nearly always produces roentgenographic changes and may contain radiopaque masses. Destruction of bone in the spheno-occipital or hypophyseal region is usually evident. Some portion of the sella turcica is affected in most cases. Invasion and destruction of the sphenoid and petrous bones occasionally are seen. Ventriculography and cerebral angiography may aid in localizing the lesion.

The chordomas that involve the cervical, thoracic, and lumbar segments of the spinal column usually produce significant roentgenographic changes. Zones of bone destruction, sometimes containing sclerotic foci, are seen involving one or more vertebrae. Some of these tumors, especially if they displace the pharynx or trachea, produce a significant soft-tissue mass.

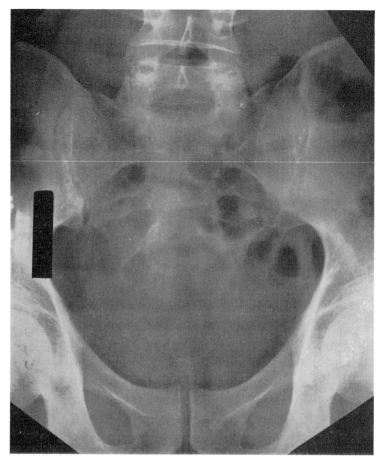

Figure 26-2. Destruction of sacrum and coccyx by chordoma that has also produced large soft-tissue mass in pelvis. (Reproduced with permission from: Utne, J. R., and Pugh, D. G.: *Am J Roentgenol, 74:*593-608, 1955.)

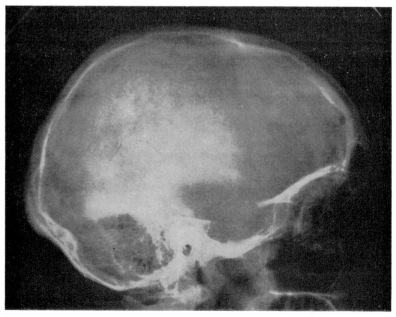

Figure 26-3. Marked involvement in region of sella by chordoma of spheno-occipital zone. (Reproduced with permission from: Dahlin, D. C., and MacCarty, C. S.: *Cancer, 5:*1170-1178, 1952.)

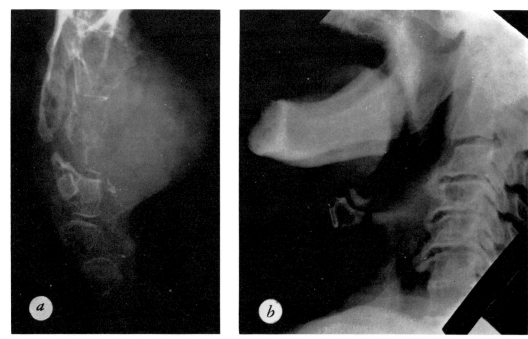

Figure 26-4. *a.* Lateral view of surgically excised chordoma. There is expansion of sacral cortex by antesacral soft-tissue mass. *b.* Lateral view of cervical segment of spinal column demonstrating soft-tissue shadow of cervical chordoma anterior to third, fourth, and fifth cervical vertebrae. (Reproduced with permission from: Utne, J. R., and Pugh, D. G.: *Am J Roentgenol, 74:*593-608, 1955.)

Gross Pathology

A chordoma is a soft, lobulated, grayish tumor that is semitranslucent and resembles chondrosarcoma or even mucous adenocarcinoma. It is usually well encapsulated except in the region of bone invasion, where no distinct edge of the tumor may be delineated. Sacral chordoma practically always has a presacral extension that is usually covered by the elevated periosteum. It may extend into the spinal canal. A spheno-occipital chordoma almost always bulges into the cranial cavity and distorts or destroys structures at the base of the brain.

Sometimes chordoma at the base of the brain penetrates and fills the sphenoid sinus or even the nasal or nasopharyngeal cavities.

An occasional chordoma contains focal calcification or ossification, but such foci are rarely prominent. Like chondrosarcomas, some chordomas are relatively firm and others are extremely myxoid and semiliquid.

Perhaps 10 percent of chordomas metastasize, usually by the hematogenous route. Deposits may develop in unusual locations, including the skin. Recurrence often produces multiple nodules in the region of previous surgical excision.

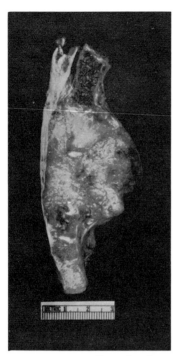

Figure 26-5. Sacral chordoma with anterior extension. This is smallest surgically excised tumor of this region in present series. (Reproduced with permission from: Dahlin, D. C., and MacCarty, C. S.: *Cancer, 5:* 1170-1178, 1952.)

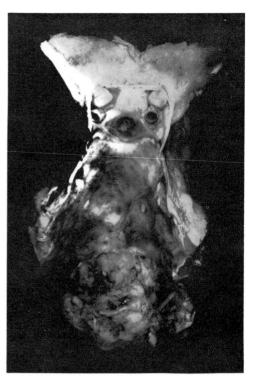

Figure 26-6. Spheno-occipital chordoma removed at autopsy. Note mass posterior to region of optic nerves, carotid vessels, and pituitary body.

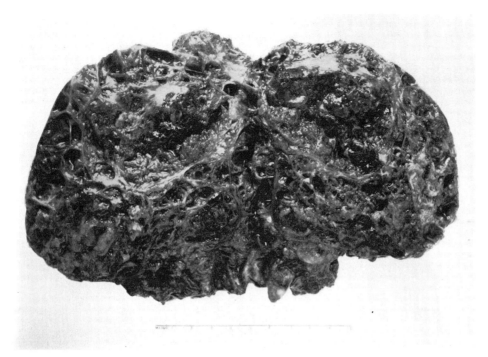

Figure 26-7. Sacral chordoma more than 10 cm in diameter. Specimen shows lobular feature of chordoma especially well.

Histopathology

Chordoma cells are characteristically disposed in lobules. Physaliferous cells that are vacuolated because of intracytoplasmic, mucous droplets are usually described as characteristic of chordoma, and they can be found in most of these tumors. Sometimes, however, they are present in only small numbers and constitute an insignificant portion of the histologic pattern. The intracellular vacuoles, when they are present, vary in size from those that are barely visible to those that are several times the diameter of the cell's nucleus. Syncytial strands of cells lying in a mass of mucus that has been formed by the cells are almost as characteristic as are the physaliferous cells. Cell boundaries in these syncytial strands are indistinct.

Considerable variation of nuclear size and chromatin is seen in some of these tumors, and rarely, mitotic figures also may be present. Such evidence of cellular activity did not alter the clinical course of the sacrococcygeal chordomas in the present series.

Chordoma cells often give a positive reaction to glycogen stains, but a similar type of reaction is observed in chondrosarcoma. Mucous stains are likewise of little value because the other differential diagnostic problem, mucous adenocarcinoma, as well as chordoma, produces mucicarmine-positive material.

Chordoma that arises in the spheno-occipital region is sometimes histologically very similar to chondrosarcoma. Such an association of chordoma with areas that are similar to chondrosarcoma is distinctly unusual for chordomas at other sites, including the sacrococcygeal region.

The diagnosis of chordoma nearly always must be verified histologically because other lesions may simulate it. In the sacral region, other primary bone neoplasms such as giant cell tumor, metastatic carcinoma, and even ependymomas or meningoceles may be found. Unusual zones in a chordoma, in rare instances, have the histologic appearance of fibrosarcoma, chondrosarcoma, or even osteosarcoma.

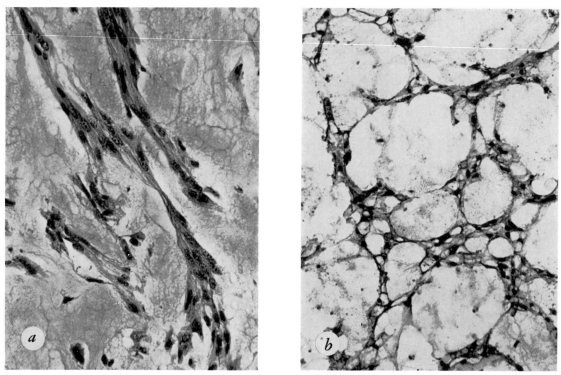

Figure 26-8. *a*. Cells with scanty eosinophilic cytoplasm and indistinct cell boundaries lying in mass of mucus. (×325) This is common finding in chordoma. *b*. Physaliferous cells arranged in strands separated by mucus. (×205) This is another of the patterns produced in chordoma.

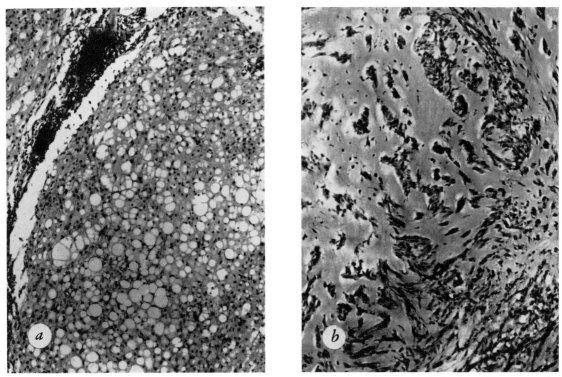

Figure 26-9. *a*. Mucous vacuoles in cytoplasm of chordoma cells, so-called physaliferous cells. (×100) *b*. Syncytial strands of cells in sea of mucus, a very common pattern in chordoma. (×100) (Reproduced with permission from: Dahlin, D. C., and MacCarty, C. S.: *Cancer, 5:* 1170-1178, 1952.)

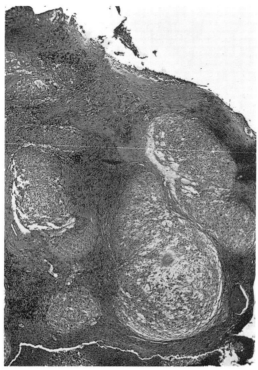

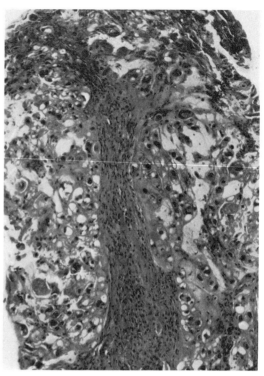

Figure 26-10. Periphery of chordoma to show characteristic lobular pattern seen in these tumors. (×30) (Reproduced with permission from: Dahlin, D. C., and MacCarty, C. S.: *Cancer, 5:*1170-1178, 1952.)

Figure 26-11. Nuclear abnormalities and even fairly abundant mitotic figures are seen in a minority of chordomas. (×100) (Reproduced with permission from: Dahlin, D. C., and MacCarty, C. S.: *Cancer, 5:* 1170-1178, 1952.)

Figure 26-12. Surgically excised sacrococcygeal chordoma showing tumor in sacrum and prominent presacral extension. Its histologic features are shown in Figure 26-13. This was one of three sacrococcygeal chordomas that contained foci indistinguishable from chondrosarcoma. Patient has survived more than five years after operation was performed.

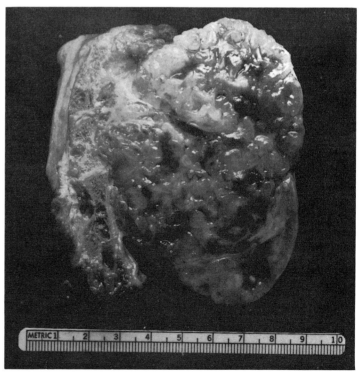

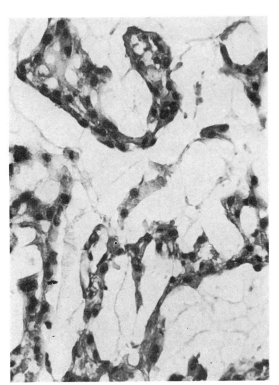
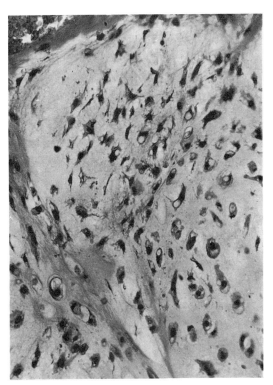

Figure 26-13. *Left.* Chordoma illustrated in Figure 26-12. Typical cords of cells and intercellular mucus. (×400) *Right.* Lobules of classic chondrosarcoma, as depicted here, were present in same tumor and were indistinguishable grossly from main mass of chordoma. (×225)

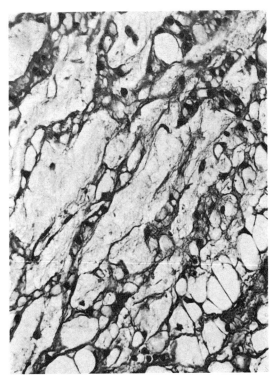
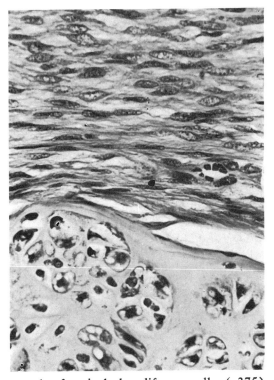

Figure 26-14. *Left.* Another sacral chordoma with strands of typical physaliferous cells. (×375) *Right.* Chondrosarcoma and fibrosarcoma in same tumor as shown at *left.* Foci of osteosarcoma also were present, and metastasis developed promptly. (×445)

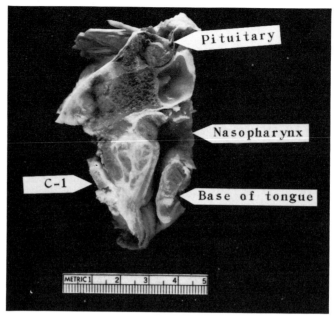

Figure 26-15. Spheno-occipital chordoma removed at autopsy. Infiltration of bone with extension up behind pituitary gland and down into tissues behind naso-pharynx indicates surgical inaccessibility of chordomas in this location. (Case contributed by Doctor P. T. Sloss of Grand Island, Nebraska.)

Treatment

Until recently, the treatment of chordoma was unsatisfactory. The tumor was only partially removed, and the patient was afforded palliative benefit at best. The only hopeful aspects were that, owing to the slow growth of the tumor, a few patients obtained several years of freedom of symptoms after subtotal removal and that some chordomas proved to be radiosensitive.

It has now been established that radical, complete removal of some sacrococcygeal tumors is feasible and should be attempted. The plane of excision must be well beyond the edge of the tumor to avoid recurrence due to implantation. For tumors not amenable to complete removal and for inoperable recurrent lesions after surgical therapy, radiation should be employed.

As illustrated in Figure 26-15, spheno-occipital chordomas are so located as to preclude complete surgical removal. If radiation therapy fails and a chordoma in this location produces increased intracranial pressure, surgical intervention may be necessary.

Transnasal biopsy of the sphenoid sinus region may provide tissue for verification of the diagnosis of chordoma prior to institution of radiation therapy, since many spheno-occipital chordomas extend into this sinus.

Prognosis

Prior to adoption of the more radical surgical technique, even the patient with sacrococcygeal chordoma was doomed to eventual, though perhaps delayed, death from local extension of the tumor. The sacrococcygeal neoplasm often extended to block the genitourinary or gastrointestinal tract, and the spheno-occipital tumor produced lethal intracranial complications. Subtotal surgical removal sometimes produces gratifying remissions. A number of reports have lauded radiation therapy of chordomas, but it is impossible to predict which tumors will respond.

Radical surgical techniques have produced prolonged survival and will no doubt afford permanent cure for some patients with less extensive sacrococcygeal chordoma. It must be remembered, however, that this tumor usually grows slowly and that long-term follow-up is necessary in the evaluation of any therapeutic regimen.

Interestingly, nearly all cartilaginous tumors arising from the base of the cranium arise from or near the spheno-occipital synchondrosis. As indicated in Figure 26-18, approximately one third of such tumors are partially or nearly completely chondroid in appearance. Their prognosis is, paradoxically, much better than that suggested by their histologic appearance.

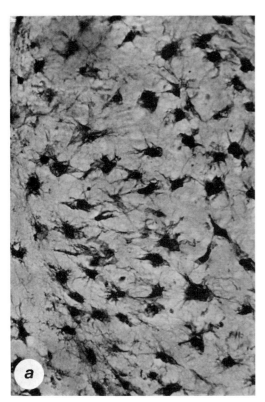 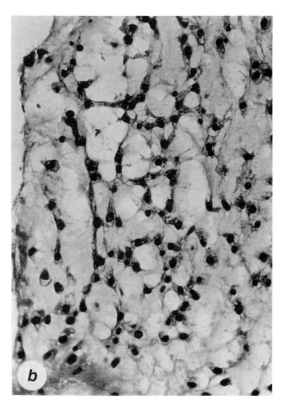

Figure 26-16. *a.* Area resembling grade 1 chondrosarcoma in spheno-occipital chondroid chordoma. (×350) *b.* Area of typical chordoma from same tumor. Cells occur in syncytial anastomosing strands of cytoplasm. (×350)

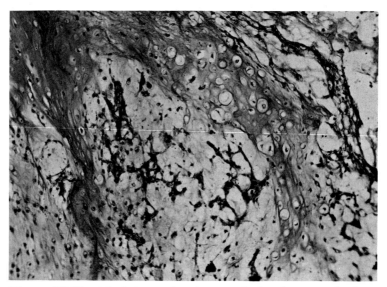

Figure 26-17. Admixture of patterns of chordoma and chondromatous tumor in same field. (×95)

Figure 26-18. There was a pronounced increased likelihood that patients with spheno-occipital chordomas would survive long intervals if their chordomas were nearly completely or even partially chondroid. Histologic appearance of these chondroid areas varied from that of cellular, "active" chondroma to that of grade 1 or grade 2 chondrosarcoma. (Reproduced with permission from: Heffelfinger, M. J., Dahlin, D. C., MacCarty, C. S., and Beabout, J. W.: *Cancer, 32:*410-420, 1973.)

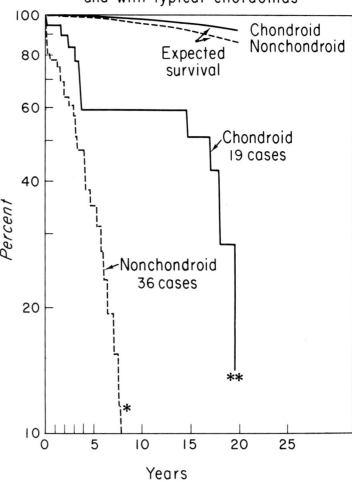

Survival of patients with chondroid and with typical chordomas

Bibliography

1935 Fletcher, E. M., Woltman, H. W., and Adson, A. W.: Sacrococcygeal Chordomas; A Clinical and Pathological Study. *Arch Neurol Psychiatr, 33:*283-299.

1935 Adson, A. W., Kernohan, J. W., and Woltman, A. W.: Cranial and Cervical Chordomas; A Clinical and Histologic Study. *Arch Neurol Psychiatr, 33:*247-261.

1935 Mabrey, R. E.: Chordoma: A Study of 150 Cases. *Am J Cancer, 25:*501-517.

1945 Givner, I.: Ophthalmologic Features of Intracranial Chordoma and Allied Tumors of the Clivus. *Arch Ophthalmol, 33:*397-402.

1952 Dahlin, D. C., and MacCarty, C. S.: Chordoma: A Study of Fifty-nine Cases. *Cancer, 5:*1170-1178.

1952 MacCarty, C. S., Waugh, J. M., Mayo, C. W., and Coventry, M. B.: The Surgical Treatment of Presacral Tumors: A Combined Problem. *Proc Staff Meet Mayo Clin, 27:*73-84.

1955 Utne, J. R., and Pugh, D. G.: The Roentgenologic Aspects of Chordoma. *Am J Roentgenol, 74:*593-608.

1957 Greenwald, C. M., Meaney, T. F., and Hughes, C. R.: Chordoma—Uncommon Destructive Lesion of Cerebrospinal Axis. *J A M A, 163:*1240-1244.

1960 Forti, E., and Venturini, G.: Contributo alla Conoscenza delle Neoplasie Notocordali. *Riv Anat Patol Oncol, 17:*317-396.

1961 MacCarty, C. S., Waugh, J. M., Coventry, M. B., and O'Sullivan, D. C.: Sacrococcygeal Chordomas. *Surg Gynecol Obstet,113:*551-554.

1964 Spjut, H. J., and Luse, S. A.: Chordoma: An Electron Microscopic Study. *Cancer, 17:*643-656.

1964 Kamrin, R. P., Potanos, J. N., and Pool, J. L.: An Evaluation of the Diagnosis and Treatment of Chordoma. *J Neurol Neurosurg Psychiatry, 27:*157-165.

1967 Higinbotham, N. L., Phillips, R. F., Farr, H. W., and Hustu, H. O.: Chordoma: Thirty-Five-Year Study at Memorial Hospital. *Cancer, 20:*1841-1850 (November).

1968 Falconer, M. A., Bailey, I. C., and Duchen, L. W.: Surgical Treatment of Chordoma and Chondroma of the Skull Base. *J Neurosurg, 29:*261-275 (September).

1970 Knechtges, T. C.: Sacrococcygeal Chordoma With Sarcomatous Features (Spindle Cell Metaplasia). *Am J Clin Pathol, 53:*612-616 (May).

1973 Heffelfinger, M. J., Dahlin, D. C., MacCarty, C. S., and Beabout, J. W.: Chordomas and Cartilaginous Tumors at the Skull Base. *Cancer, 32:*410-420 (August).

1975 Kerr, W. A., Allen, K. L., Haynes, D. R., and Sellars, S. L.: Familial Nasopharyngeal Chordoma: Letter to the Editor. *S Afr Med J, 49:*1584 (September).

1975 Richter, H. J., Jr., Batsakis, J. G., and Boles, R.: Chordomas: Nasopharyngeal Presentation and Atypical Long Survival. *Ann Otol Rhinol Laryngol, 84:*327-332 (May-June).

Chapter 27

Hemangioendothelioma (Hemangiosarcoma) and Hemangiopericytoma

MALIGNANT VASOFORMATIVE tumors comprised less than 1 percent of malignant neoplasms in this series. These lesions have varied from such highly anaplastic lesions that their recognition as spindle cell sarcomas with vasoformative capability was difficult and sometimes only manifest in part of the tumor to well-differentiated neoplasms that have been called hemangioendothelioma.

Hemangiosarcoma and hemangioendothelioma are used interchangeably in this discussion because there is no valid method of differentiating one from the other.

Vascular spindle cell sarcomas that are not of provable endothelial origin and metastatic carcinoma are differential diagnostic problems. Metastatic cancer to bone may be very vascular, and its aggregates of plump cells mimic those of some angiosarcomas.

Multifocality, especially in a limited portion of the skeleton (for example, in one extremity), occurs in approximately one third of hemangiosarcomas.

Malignant hemangiopericytoma of bone is exceedingly rare. Only five such cases were recognized in this series.

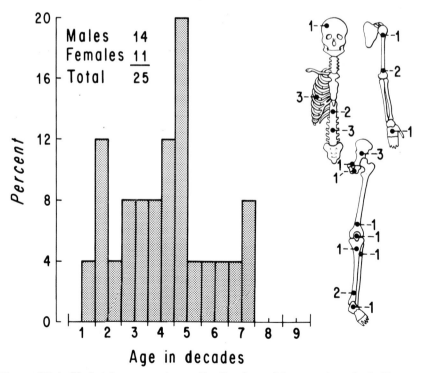

Figure 27-1. Skeletal, age, and sex distribution of hemangioendotheliomas.

Incidence

These twenty-five cases comprised less than 1 percent of malignant tumors of bone in the Mayo Clinic experience. Fifteen of these cases were diagnosed during the last five years.

Sex

Fourteen of the twenty-five patients were males.

Age

Nearly all ages were represented, with no particular predominance for any group.

Localization

More than one third of the tumors were in the long tubular bones, but other skeletal regions were commonly affected.

The five hemangiopericytomas involved a dorsal vertebra, a rib, the ischium, the ilium, and the mandible.

Symptoms

These tumors produced no specific features. Pain was the usual symptom.

Physical Findings

There were no specific features. Sometimes tenderness was elicited locally.

Roentgenologic Features

These neoplasms produced osteolytic zones and rarely any reactive new bone formation. In the more anaplastic, higher-grade (Broders) lesions, the margins were indistinct and irregular, and no trabeculae remained within the tumor. In the low-grade tumors, scattered trabeculae persisted and the margins were more sharply demarcated. It was not definite from the roentgenograms whether some of the low-grade lesions were malignant or benign. Multifocality, when present, suggested the vascular nature of the process.

Gross Pathology

The lesional tissue was typically bloody, suggesting its primary vascular nature. The tumors were usually soft. Occasionally, they showed zones of necrosis, and some had permeated bone beyond the zone of destruction seen on roentgenogram.

Histopathology

At one end of the spectrum, in the highly anaplastic tumors, the vasoformative nature of the spindle-shaped malignant cells may be difficult to determine. Silver staining for reticulum fibers may accentuate the vascular nature of the tumor and thus help in the differentiation from other spindle cell malignant tumors such as fibrosarcoma.

Furthermore, such stain determines whether the proliferating cells are inside the channels, as is true of hemangiosarcoma, or outside them, as is true of hemangiopericytoma. As with hemangiopericytomas arising in soft tissues, tumors often show distortion of vascular contour because of bulgings of masses of cells from outside reticulin-outlined spaces. The pattern of hemangiopericytoma must be found consistently throughout all areas of a tumor because many lesions contain foci that simulate the pattern of hemangiopericytoma.

The plump cells of some hemangiosarcomas are confusingly similar to cells in metastatic carcinoma. The pronounced vascularity of some such carcinomas may complicate the problem. Awareness of the possibility of a lesion being primarily vascular helps in its recognition.

The least anaplastic tumors may be difficult to distinguish from capillary hemangioma. The following criteria for malignancy seem correct when assessing intraosseous endothelial neoplasms. The lining cells of the channels must be plump and usually produce intravascular papillations or tufting. Sometimes moderate distension of vascular channels is produced by solid masses of such proliferating cells. Rare mitotic figures should be found in such cells.

Capillary vascular proliferations may be exuberant in some benign conditions, such as aneurysmal bone cysts, and these must not be mistaken for evidence of a primary neoplasm of blood vessels.

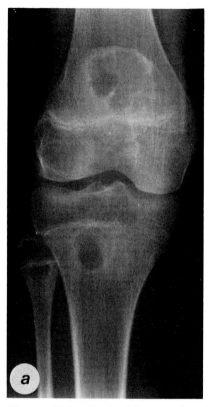

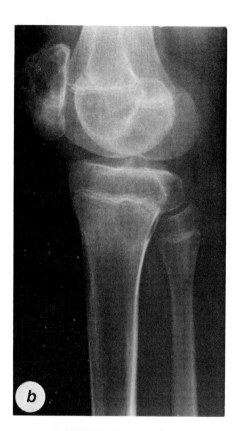

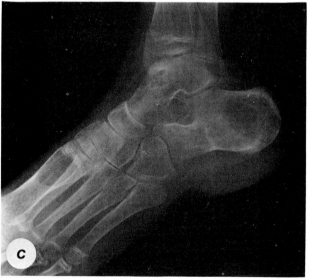

Figure 27-2. Grade 1 hemangioendothelioma shown in Figure 27-3 *bottom left*. *a.* Lytic zones are present in patella, tibia, and fibula. *b.* Lateral view to indicate patellar lesion more clearly. *c.* Similar lesions in first metatarsal, calcaneus, and talus. After patellar removal, patient has responded well for two years, having had systemic chemotherapy and radiation therapy to the lesions.

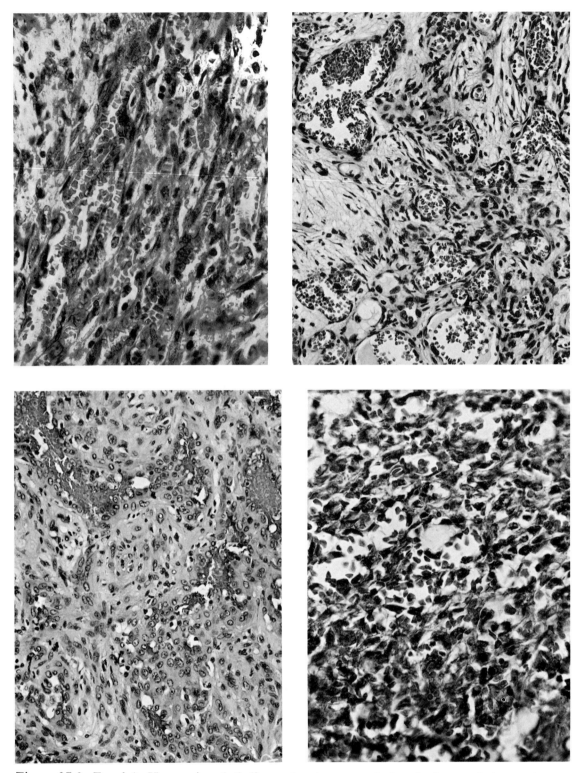

Figure 27-3. *Top left*. Hemangioendothelioma (angiosarcoma) that had caused destruction of second lumbar vertebra of thirty-eight-year-old man. (×360) Note capillary formation, plump cells, and mitotic figure. *Top right*. Grade 1 hemangioendothelioma that had produced questionably malignant destruction of 4 cm of upper part of humeral shaft in fourteen-year-old girl. In some areas, endothelial cells were plump. (×200) *Bottom left*. Grade 1 hemangioendothelioma illustrated in Figure 27-2. Distended channels filled by plump neoplastic cells were found in resected patellar lesion. (×250) *Bottom right*. Highly malignant hemangioendothelioma from fibular lesion shown in Figure 27-4. (×400)

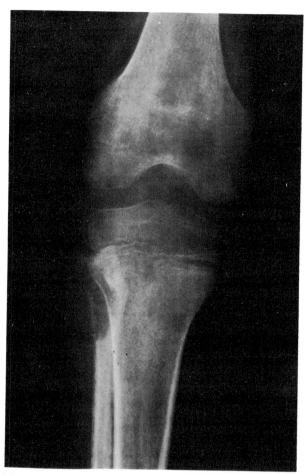

Figure 27-4. Angiosarcoma with malignant destruction of fibula of eight-year-old boy. Other bones about knee and foot were considered unremarkable.

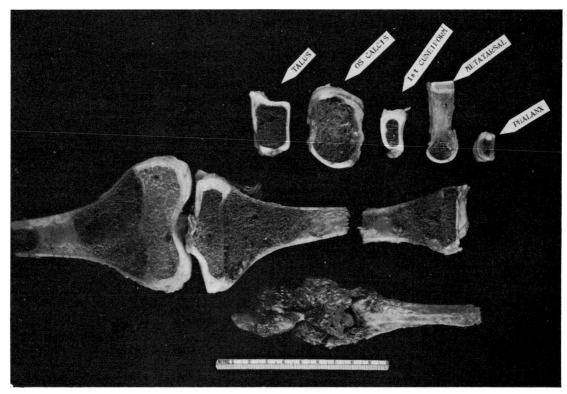

Figure 27-5. Amputated specimen with destruction of fibula (near scale), but also showing multicentric foci of angiosarcoma in femur, tibia, and bones of foot. Malignant tissue had permeated bone in all of dark zones. Patient died of sarcoma within six months.

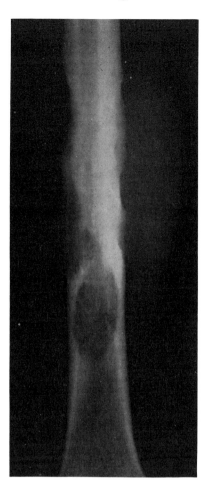

Figure 27-6. Hemangiosarcoma of large portion of femoral shaft, showing multiple zones of central and cortical destruction with tumor extending into adjacent soft tissue.

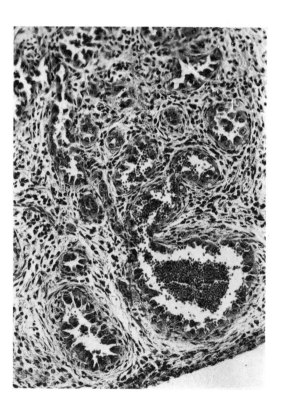

Figure 27-7. Microscopic appearance of part of tumor illustrated in Figure 27-6. Here angiosarcoma is reasonably well differentiated, with plump, malignant endothelial cells producing spaces, some of which contain blood. (×200)

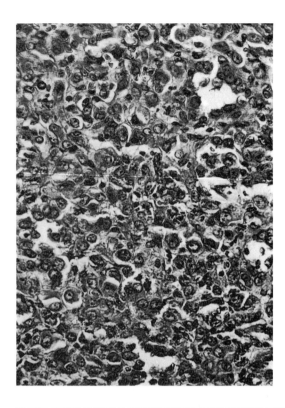

Figure 27-8. In other regions, angiosarcoma of Figure 27-6 was highly anaplastic, as shown here. Transitions from well-differentiated zones were observed. Anaplastic portions taken out of context may have been misinterpreted as some other sarcoma. (×300) (Case contributed by Doctor Manuel Sarmina of Findlay, Ohio, who stated that patient was well twenty-seven months after disarticulation at the hip.)

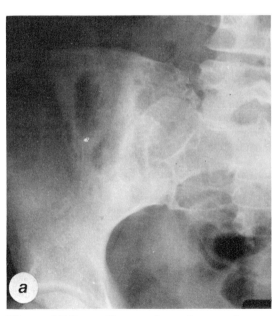

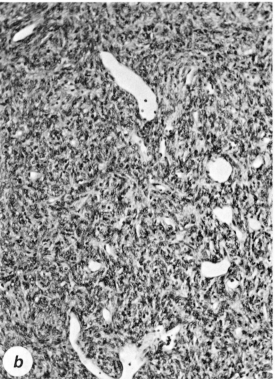

Figure 27-9. *a.* Destruction of posterior part of ilium at sacrum produced by malignant hemangiopericytoma in thirty-seven-year-old woman. *b.* Histologic pattern of this lesion. Fairly abundant mitotic figures were present. (×160) Patient was well forty-seven months after subtotal resection and radiation therapy, but she died with recurrence and metastasis seventeen months later.

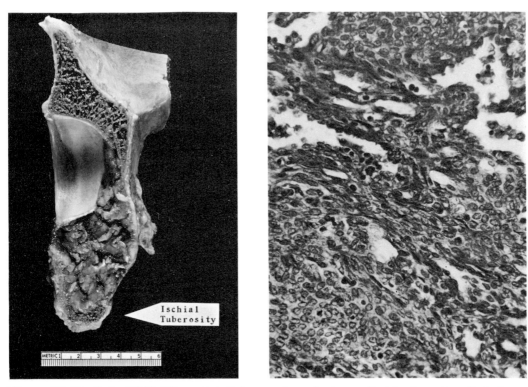

Figure 27-10. *Left.* Well-differentiated hemangiopericytoma that had produced destruction and slight expansion of ischium. The sixty-four-year-old man was well five years after hemipelvectomy. *Right.* Reticulin stain verified that proliferating neoplastic cells were pericytes. (×300)

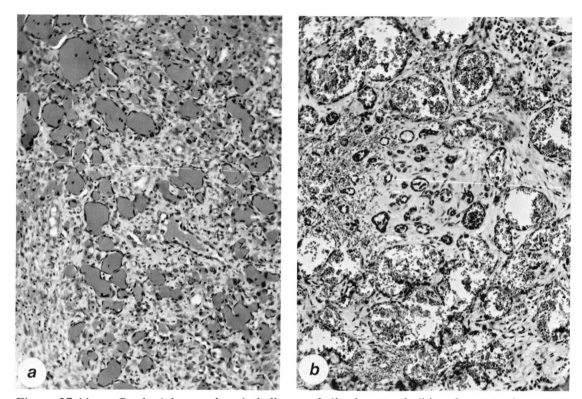

Figure 27-11. *a.* Grade 1 hemangioendothelioma of distal part of tibia of twenty-three-year-old woman. Lesion was considered to be a malignant but well-differentiated tumor because of plump and irregularly shaped neoplastic cells among capillary vascular spaces. Patient was well twenty-six months after excision of lesion and radiation therapy. (×160) *b.* Grade 1 hemangioendothelioma shown in Figure 27-3 *top right.* In zones like this, some of the neoplastic cells produced solid epitheliumlike clusters reminiscent of adamantinoma of long-bone type.

Treatment

Evidence of multicentricity in the skeleton, present in about one third of patients with hemangiosarcomas, must be sought before deciding on therapy for a lesion. Surgical resection plus radiation therapy seems appropriate and is usually effective for the neoplasms that are better differentiated. The value of each of these modalities is not strictly known.

More anaplastic tumors are, apparently, likewise relatively radioresistant and are best treated by surgical ablation. Radiation therapy may produce marked palliation.

Prognosis

Exact information on prognosis is not available partly because so many angiosarcomas are multifocal. Well-differentiated tumors are often associated with long survival. Highly anaplastic angiosarcomas and hemangiopericytomas are associated with poor prognosis. More long-term studies are necessary and, hopefully, will help provide data relative to prognosis.

Bibliography

1956 Carter, J. H., Dickerson, R., and Needy, C.: Angiosarcoma of Bone: A Review of the Literature and Presentation of a Case. *Ann Surg, 144:*107-117 (July).

1962 Hartmann, W. H., and Stewart, F. W.: Hemangioendothelioma of Bone: Unusual Tumor Characterized by Indolent Course. *Cancer, 15:*846-854 (July-August).

1965 Bundens, W. D., Jr., and Brighton, C. T.: Malignant Hemangioendothelioma of Bone: Report of Two Cases and Review of the Literature. *J Bone Joint Surg, 47A:*762-772 (June).

1968 Otis, J., Hutter, R. V. P., Foote, F. W. Jr., Marcove, R. C., and Stewart, F. W.: Hemangioendothelioma of Bone. *Surg Gynecol Obstet, 127:*295-305 (August).

1969 Campanacci, M., Cenni, F., and Giunti, A.: Angiectasie, Amartoma, e Neoplasmi Vascolari dello Scheletro ("Angioma," emangioendotelioma, emangiosarcoma). *La Chirurgia degli Organi di Movimento, 58:*472-498.

1971 Dorfman, H. D., Steiner, G. C., and Jaffe, H. L.: Vascular Tumors of Bone. *Hum Pathol, 2:*349-376.

1971 Unni, K. K., Ivins, J. C., Beabout, J. W., and Dahlin, D. C.: Hemangioma, Hemangiopericytoma, and Hemangioendothelioma. *Cancer, 27:*1403-1414.

1972 Dube, V. E., and Fisher, D. E.: Hemangioendothelioma of the Leg Following Metallic Fixation of the Tibia. *Cancer, 30:*1260-1266 (November).

1972 Garcia-Moral, C. A.: Malignant Hemangioendothelioma of Bone: Review of World Literature and Report of Two Cases. *Clin Orthop, 82:*70-79 (January-February).

1973 Dunlop, J.: Primary Haemangiopericytoma of Bone: Report of Two Cases. *J Bone Joint Surg, 55B:*854-857 (November).

1975 Larsson, S.-E., Lorentzon, R., and Boquist, L.: Malignant Hemangioendothelioma of Bone. *J Bone Joint Surg, 57A:*84-89 (January).

Chapter 28

Conditions That Commonly Simulate Primary Neoplasms of Bone

AᴅᴇQᴜᴀᴛᴇ ᴄᴏɴsɪᴅᴇʀᴀᴛɪᴏɴ of all of the reactive, traumatic, infectious, metabolic, congenital, and other conditions of bone that may simulate benign or malignant neoplasms would require a volume larger than this one. My purpose in this chapter is to indicate the types of problems that are encountered and to document briefly some of those most often seen in material sent to me for consultation from other pathologists. Pseudotumors of bone in hemophiliacs (Ghormley and Clegg, 1948) and hydatid disease of bone that produces a severe problem not seen in the United States (Alldred and Nisbet, 1964) are among the conditions that will not be elaborated.

Amyloid deposits within bone may simulate neoplasms. Such deposits may not be associated with myeloma. Abnormally prominent costal cartilages may be mistaken for neoplasms; microscopic determination that the cartilage is not neoplastic is essential. Improper views or misinterpretation may promote the erroneous assumption clinically and roentgenologically that neoplasm is present; for example, the rhomboid impression near the medial end of the clavicle may pose a problem.

Metastatic Carcinomas

Metastatic deposits from carcinomas are by far the most common malignant tumors affecting the skeleton. Although the correct diagnosis is usually obvious when the clinical history is considered, it is often unsafe to assume that any given skeletal lesion or lesions are necessarily related to a proved carcinoma. The punched-out areas of destruction characteristic of myeloma, for example, may be mistaken for areas of lytic metastatic deposit. Metastatic carcinoma is especially likely to afford a diagnostic problem when only one skeletal lesion is found and no "primary" is known. A destructive process secondary to hypernephroma is particularly likely to simulate a primary lesion of bone, because this cancer has a tendency to produce a clinically solitary metastatic lesion and the primary tumor is in an obscure location. Carcinomas may invade bone by direct extension.

Metastatic carcinoma chiefly affects the older age-groups. It is especially likely to involve the vertebral column, the pelvis, the ribs, the calvarium, and even the large bones of the limbs near the body. Metastasis of carcinoma distal to the levels of the knees and elbows, however, is uncommon.

Physical Findings

The osseous lesions of metastatic carcinoma may closely simulate primary malignant tumor. Pain, with or without swelling, and symptoms resulting from pressure on neighboring structures or from pathologic fracture are the most prominent.

Roentgenologic Features

Metastatic tumors usually produce irregular destruction of bone indicative of their malignant quality. Although most such lesions are osteolytic, many metastatic deposits from carcinoma of the prostate and some of those from other tumors are osteoblastic. Even malignant lymphomas sometimes evoke considerable sclerosis. Occasionally, especially in the pelvic bones, broadening of the osseous outline may result from periosteal elevation by the growing tumor and subperiosteal formation of new bone. The region of actual involvement by metastatic carcinoma is frequently more extensive than is seen roentgenographically.

Gross Pathology

The lesions of metastatic carcinoma in bone do not present gross diagnostic characteristics. Lesions vary from those that are fibrotic owing to scirrhous reaction produced by the tumor to those that are extremely soft and mushy. The osteoblastic metastatic lesions so often seen from prostatic carcinoma are very dense and relatively characteristic. Rarely, the osteoid and bone that may result from reaction to a deposit of metastatic carcinoma is confusingly similar to that produced by osteosarcoma. It may be difficult to determine that the osteoid is not produced by the malignant cells.

Histopathology

The average metastatic carcinoma to bone, with its glandular or squamous elements, is readily diagnosed. Even if these are absent, the characteristic pattern of small islands of epithelial cells interspersed within a fibrous stroma is practically pathognomonic. Some highly anaplastic carcinomas with spindling nuclei closely simulate fibrosarcoma. In such instances, when one encounters a single metastatic lesion from a hidden primary, it may be extremely difficult to decide whether or not one is dealing with a primary malignant tumor. This is especially true of certain hypernephromas.

Treatment

The treatment of patients with skeletal metastasis is becoming increasingly important. Certain carcinomas, especially those from the prostate and breast, are benefited by both medical and surgical hormonal therapy. Carcinoma metastatic from the thyroid may be held in abeyance for protracted periods by the use of radioactive iodine. Orthopedic surgical procedures in combination with radiation or other therapy are often of much value in the management of metastatic carcinoma to the skeleton. Amputation for solitary skeletal metastatic lesions must occasionally be considered. The present series contains a case in which a solitary metastatic deposit developed in the distal part of the femur eight years after removal of a hypernephroma, and amputation was followed by known survival for eleven additional years. Chemotherapeutic agents sometimes provide palliation.

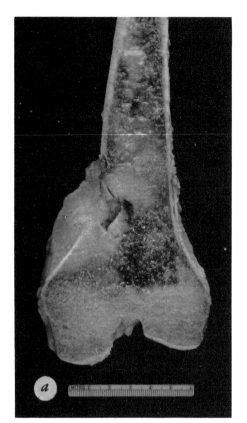 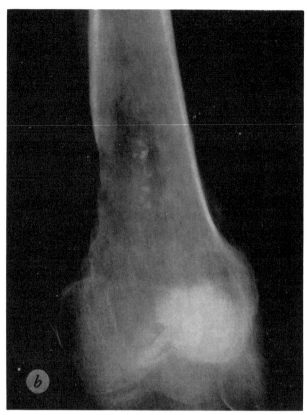

Figure 28-1. *a.* Gross specimen, and *b,* roentgenogram of metastatic squamous cell carcinoma, grade 1. This lesion developed ten years after below-knee amputation for grade 1 squamous cell carcinoma of foot. Popliteal lymph nodes were uninvolved, and route of metastasis is obscure. Interestingly, metastasis was to an area containing benign enchondroma.

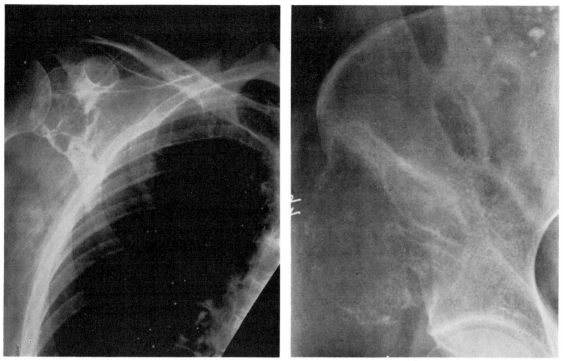

Figure 28-2. *Left.* Slightly expansile metastatic hypernephroma of neck of scapula. Renal tumor had been removed six years previously. Patient had had shoulder pain for eighteen months. *Right.* Metastatic renal cell adenocarcinoma producing destruction and "expansile" lesion of ilium of sixty-five-year-old woman.

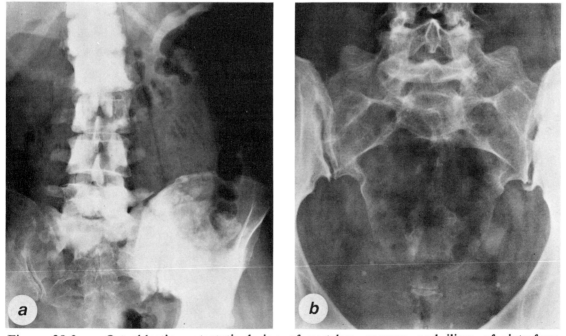

Figure 28-3. *a.* Osteoblastic metastatic lesion of vertebra, sacrum, and ilium of sixty-four-year-old woman. Although such osteoblastic metastases strongly suggest metastatic prostatic carcinoma, primary lesion was pulmonary adenocarcinoma. *b.* Metastatic mammary adenocarcinoma simulating sacral chordoma.

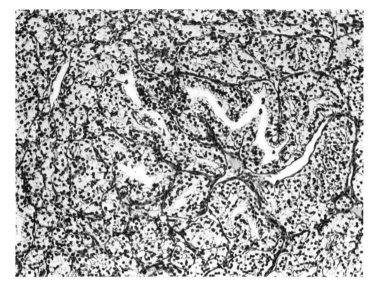

Figure 28-4. Typical metastatic hypernephroma with clear cells in an organoid pattern. (×150)

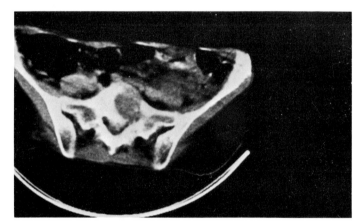

Figure 28-5. Computerized tomography showing metastasis in body of sacrum. Lesion was poorly visualized on conventional roentgenogram.

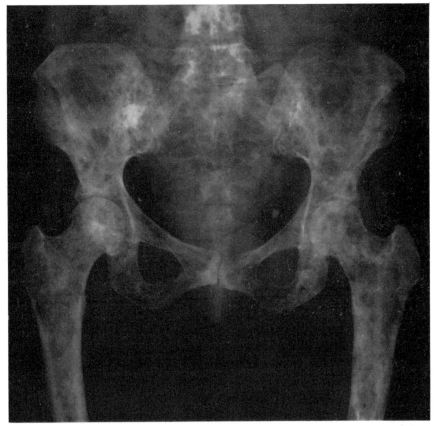

Figure 28-6. Extensive lytic carcinomatous deposits secondary to primary lesion in breast. (Reproduced with permission from: Pugh, D. G.: *Roentgenologic Diagnosis of Diseases of Bones.* Baltimore, Williams & Wilkins, 1954.)

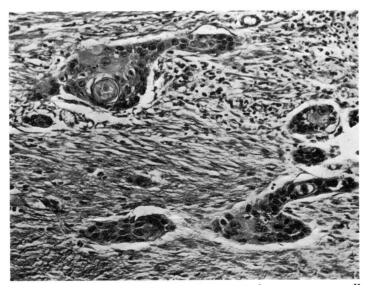

Figure 28-7. Nests of cells of metastatic squamous cell carcinoma in skeleton. Note extensive fibrogenic reaction and clusters of lymphocytes. (×150)

Fibrous Dysplasias

Fibrous dysplasia is probably the result of an anomaly in the development of bone. It is characterized by the occurrence of one, a few, or numerous discrete skeletal defects. Yellow or brown patches of cutaneous pigmentation may accompany the bone lesions, especially in patients with a severe disseminated form of the disease. When, in addition to cutaneous pigmentation, such polyostotic disease is accompanied by signs of endocrine abnormality, especially precocious puberty in girls, the condition is commonly called "Albright's syndrome."

"Fibro-osseous dysplasia" is a term that is gaining acceptance for many of the defects of this type that involve the base of the skull and the jawbones. Dysplastic lesions at these sites often contain such an abundance of osseous trabeculae intermingled with the fibrous tissue that they are distinctly hard and may cast a dense shadow in the roentgenogram. Many, if not all, of the so-called osteofibromas and fibro-osteomas in these locations are actually examples of fibro-osseous dysplasia.

Polyostotic fibrous dysplasia usually manifests itself early in life, as does also the monostotic form. The latter disease is relatively common, Pritchard being able to review 256 cases from the literature in 1951. Almost any bone in the body may be affected, and those lesions in the jawbones or at the base of the brain are especially likely to come to clinical and surgical attention.

Physical Findings

Many of the lesions of fibrous dysplasia are completely asymptomatic and never discovered, as evidenced by the finding of occasional "silent" lesions in roentgenologic examination of the thorax. The dysplasia may produce defective growth and deformity and pain in any bone. The upper part of the femur is especially predilected. Those lesions that involve the bones of the face and skull usually produce signs and symptoms because of their size, such as focal swelling and exophthalmos. Deformity due to the mass is the usual problem presented by patients with lesions in the jaws. The lesions may become quiescent after puberty but this is by no means always the case. A lesion of fibrous dysplasia may produce its first symptoms in adulthood.

Mazabraud discussed the rare disease in which multiple myxomas of soft somatic tissue coexist in patients who have fibrous dysplasia with or without Albright's syndrome. The files of the Mayo Clinic contain three cases with these associated diseases of soft tissue and bone.

Roentgenologic Features

The defects of fibrous dysplasia are usually well-defined zones of rarefaction. The rarefied zone is often surrounded by a narrow rim of relatively sclerotic bone. Expansion with thinning of the cortex is especially likely to occur in narrow bones such as the ribs. Those lesions with a large osseous component such as are commonly seen around the base of the skull and the maxilla are likely to be relatively radiopaque. This characteristic is accentuated if the lesion bulges into an air-containing sinus.

Gross Pathology

Examination reveals considerable variation in the lesions of fibrous dysplasia, but the average one is well defined and composed of dense fibrous tissue. Embedded in this fibrous tissue are usually enough small osteoid trabeculae to impart a distinctly gritty quality. Slight to extensive cyst formation may be present, whereas those with marked ossification may resemble osteoma. Those lesions that arose from thin bones such as the maxilla may bulge into adjacent cavities or soft-tissue zones in a polypoid fashion.

Histopathology

The major feature is a proliferation of fibroblasts that produce dense collagenous matrix. The fibroblastic cells may exhibit, in areas, a storiform or cartwheel arrangement like that of so-called fibrous histiocytoma. The fibrous element typically contains trabeculae of osteoid and bone. These may show reversal lines mimicking those of Paget's disease. The trabeculae have a completely meaningless arrangement concerning function. Metaplastic chondroid substance is sometimes present, and on rare occasions, it is so prominent that the question of a neoplasm of hyaline cartilage arises. Areas of degeneration may contain only relatively acellular fibrous or myxoid tissue. These tend to be central, and the rim only may show the metaplastic osteoid of the basic process. Some lesions of fibro-osseous dysplasia are composed predominantly of osteoid and bone, with only sparse fibroblastic elements separating the trabeculae. Sometimes, especially in lesions of the jaws and at the base of the brain, the osseous component is in the form of little spherical masses, which are surrounded by the proliferating spindle cells in such a fashion that psammomatous meningioma is simulated. Mitotic figures may be found in the actively proliferating lesions of fibrous dysplasia. Benign giant cells and masses of lipophages are commonly associated with degenerative foci.

Treatment

Treatment should be conservative. The lesions commonly stop growing at puberty. Therapy should be directed at restoring the normal configuration when the skull or jawbones are affected. In large bones, deformity secondary to the disease may require correction. Radiation therapy is probably of no value and introduces the hazard of sarcomatous change. Fibrous dysplasia has little tendency to undergo spontaneous malignant change.

Prognosis

The prognosis in fibrous dysplasia is generally good. The deforming lesions of the jawbones or skull may sometimes recur, but ordinarily they respond favorably to additional conservative surgical therapy. Some of the large lesions in weight-bearing bones require curettage and bone grafting for the maintenance of function. Occasionally, recurrence is a problem, but the long-term prognosis is usually good.

The vast majority of cases of fibrous dysplasia we have encountered that later exhibited sarcoma had had radiation for the benign disease. We had seven postradiation sarcomas in our files, another one in which chondrosarcoma developed in a femur with atypical fibrous dysplasia, a second had chondrosarcoma and fibrous dysplasia intermixed in a lesion of the innominate bone, and a third had osteosarcoma of the ischium and fibrous dysplasia nearby in the innominate bone.

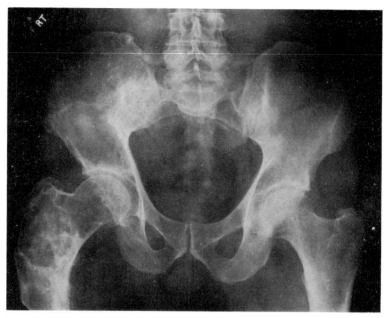

Figure 28-8. Fibrous dysplasia involving right side of pelvis and upper part of femur. Roentgen therapy had been given twenty years previously. Although roentgenogram does not suggest it, sarcoma shown in Figure 28-14 has now complicated femoral lesion. Increasing pain had been noted for four months. Patient died with metastasis twenty-three months after hemipelvectomy.

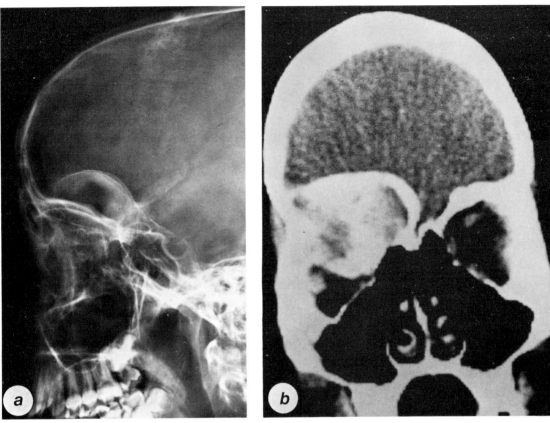

Figure 28-9. *a.* Fibrous dysplasia of orbital bone area of right side in fourteen-year-old girl. She had noticed increasing proptosis for nine years. Skull, including its base, is commonly site of fibrous dysplasia. *b.* Computerized tomography aided in delimiting zone of involvement.

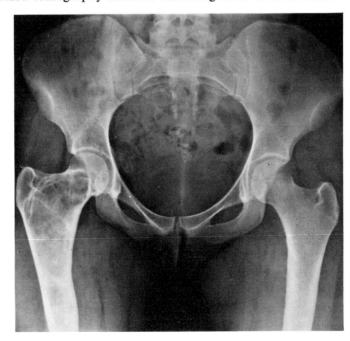

Figure 28-10. Typical fibrous dysplasia affecting neck and shaft of right femur of twenty-one-year-old woman. Lesion had produced pain for five years.

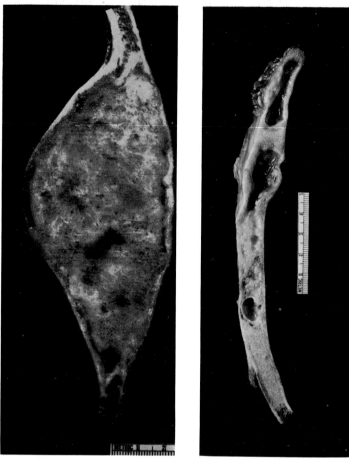

Figure 28-11. *Left.* Longitudinal section of rib expanded by fibrous dysplasia. *Right.* Fibrous dysplasia of rib showing multicystic degenerative change. Such alteration is not uncommon in fibrous dysplasia. (Figure 28-11 *left* reproduced with permission from: Zimmer, J. F., Dahlin, D. C., and Clagett, O. T.: *J Thorac Surg, 31:*488-496, 1956.)

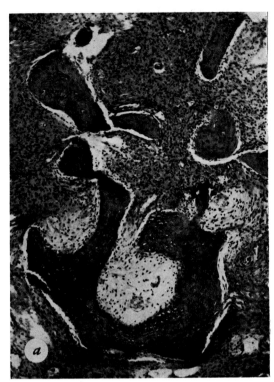
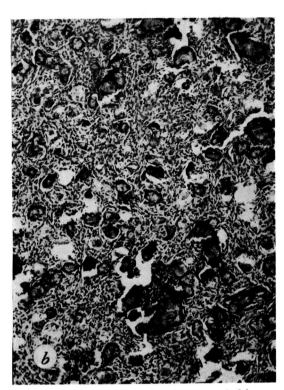

Figure 28-12. *a.* Classic fibrous dysplasia with proliferating fibroblastic tissue and bizarre masses and trabeculae of osteoid tissue and bone. (×75) *b.* Fibro-osseous dysplasia, in this instance producing spherical masses of osseous tissue. This pattern is often seen in lesions at base of skull and has been mistaken for meningioma. (×100)

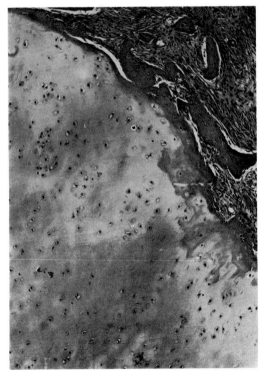
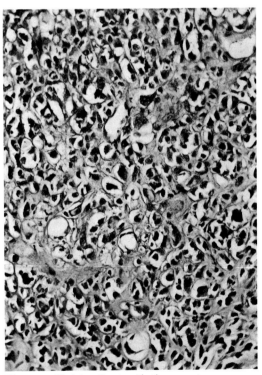

Figure 28-13. Chondroid zones such as this may occur in fibrous dysplasia, and in rare instances, they dominate the histologic pattern.

Figure 28-14. Postradiation osteosarcoma complicating femoral lesion of fibrous dysplasia shown in Figure 28-8.

Osteofibrous Dysplasias (Ossifying Fibroma of Long Bones)

This is characteristically a tibial lesion that is seen in patients who are less than ten years of age. Long-term prognosis is good from Campanacci's personal study of twenty-two cases. Histopathologic study indicates that this is a variant of fibrous dysplasia, but it is primarily a cortical lesion. Kempson has called these lesions "ossifying fibroma." Osteoblasts mantling the trabeculae are prominent, in contrast to their inconspicuousness in the typical areas of ordinary fibrous dysplasia.

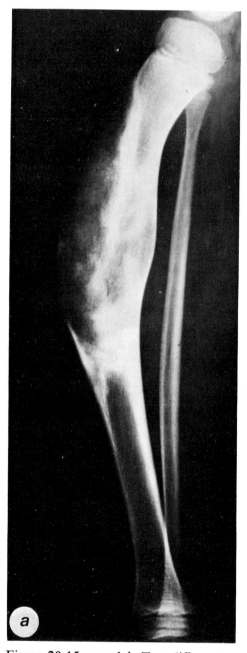
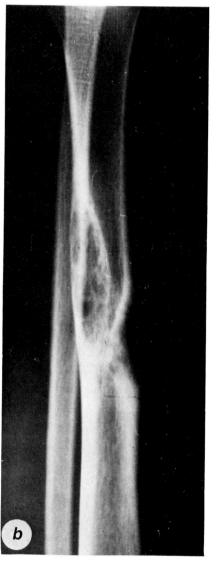

Figure 28-15. *a* and *b*. Two different cases of osteofibrous dysplasia of tibia. *c*. Zone in lesion showing somewhat endematous fibrous tissue and osteoid trabeculae similar to those of ordinary fibrous dysplasia. *d*. More abundant and more mature trabeculae near periphery of lesion. (Cases contributed by Doctor M. Campanacci of Bologna, Italy.)

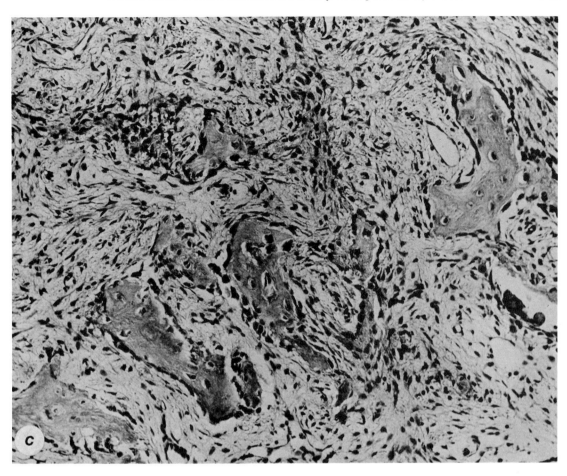

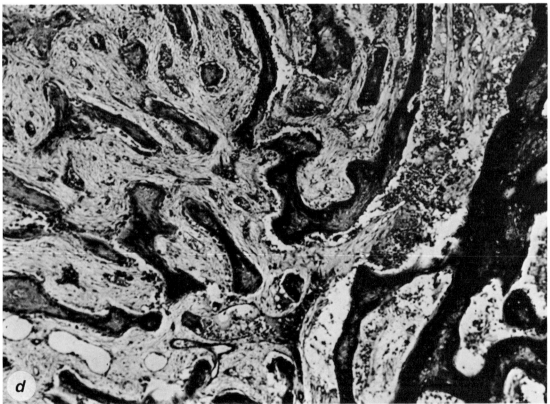

Aneurysmal Bone Cysts

Aneurysmal bone cyst is one of the "variants" that has been justifiably excluded from the bona fide giant cell tumors. Features that make it logical to exclude this lesion from the neoplastic category include the observation that examples of it have regressed following incomplete removal. The cause of this strange process in bone is unknown. It is similar to and probably related to other reactive non-neoplastic processes, including giant cell "reparative" granuloma of jaws, traumatic reactions observed in periosteum and bone, and even florid heterotopic ossification.

Aneurysmal bone cysts may arise *de novo* in bone, in which case no definite pre-existing lesion can be demonstrated in the tissue. The data shown here relate to such cases. Aneurysmal-bone-cyst-like areas are found in various benign conditions, including giant cell tumor, chondroblastoma, chondromyxoid fibroma, and fibrous dysplasia. Even malignant tumors of bone may contain such benign aneurysmal-bone-cyst-like areas. Obviously, it is necessary for one to be assured that he has recognized any underlying causative process, because it will dictate the clinical capability of the process.

In the present series, aneurysmal bone cyst has been only half as common as giant cell tumor. Males accounted for 43 percent of the 134 cases. In striking contrast to the age distribution of giant cell tumors, 85 percent of which occurred in

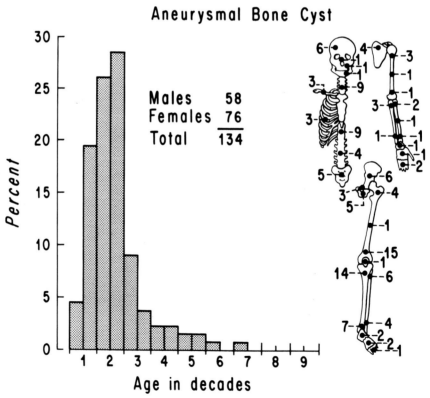

Figure 28-16. Skeletal, age, and sex distribution of aneurysmal bone cysts.

patients who were twenty years old or older, 78 percent of the patients with aneurysmal bone cyst were less than twenty years old.

The roentgenographic shadow is sometimes confusingly like the lysis produced by a malignant tumor.

Physical Findings

Pain and swelling are the important features and they vary in duration from weeks to a few years. The lesion tends to increase in size until therapy is instituted. Vertebrae are relatively commonly involved (Cohen and co-workers, 1964), with the production of signs and symptoms owing to compression of the spinal cord and emerging nerves.

Roentgenologic Features

The lesion often has a characteristic appearance. A zone of rarefaction, which is usually well circumscribed and eccentric, is associated with an obvious soft-tissue extension of the process. In the classic case, this soft-tissue extension is produced by bulging of the periosteum and a resultant layer of roentgenologically visible new bone that delimits the periphery of the tumor. The lesional area tends to show trabeculation. Fusiform expansion may be produced when small bones such as a rib or a fibula are affected.

Gross Pathology

An aneurysmal bone cyst contains anastomosing cavernomatous spaces that ordinarily comprise the bulk of the lesion. The spaces are usually filled with unclotted blood, in which event blood may well up into, but does not spurt from, the tumor when it is unroofed. The eggshell-thick layer of subperiosteal new bone which delimits the lesion is ordinarily readily discernible. Some of these lesions contain solid fleshy and friable or fibrous and granular zones that may comprise half of their bulk.

Histopathology

The essential feature is the presence of cavernomatous spaces, the walls of which lack the normal features of blood vessels. Thin strands of bone are often present in the fibrous tissue of these walls. Sometimes the mineralizing formed elements have a chondroid aura that is unusual in any other lesion of bone. An endothelial lining is unusual. Reconstruction of these cavernomatous spaces from curetted fragments may be extremely difficult. The solid portions of an aneurysmal bone cyst may be fibrous, but they ordinarily contain a lacework of osteoid trabeculae similar to that observed in benign osteoblastoma. Benign giant cells are often present in large numbers, thus accounting for the confusion of this lesion with genuine giant cell tumor. These solid zones with giant cells may resemble giant cell reparative granuloma of jawbones, which is likely a related lesion. The histopathology of aneurysmal bone cyst overlaps that of simple bone cyst, making differentiation difficult or impossible in some cases.

The most important histological problem is to recognize that this lesion is benign. Although mitotic figures may be numerous in the spindle cell areas, the nuclei lack anaplasia, as manifested by hyperchromatism and irregular shape. The osteoid that shades from the dominantly spindle cell regions is disposed in regular trabeculae. Telangiectatic osteosarcoma often simulates aneurysmal bone cyst when viewed at low magnification.

Treatment

The most successful treatment has been surgical removal of the entire lesion or as much of it as possible. Occasionally, bone grafting of the resultant defect may be necessary. Recurrence sometimes develops. It may be difficult to determine when roentgenographic evidence of recurrence is sufficient to warrant additional treatment. Although radiation has been advocated, especially for vertebral examples with compression of the spinal cord, three late postradiation sarcomas have made us cautious about its use. These sarcomas developed at the sites of aneurysmal bone cysts of the tibia, the femur, and a vertebra.

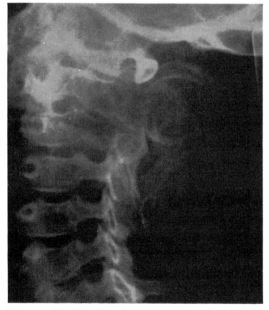

Figure 28-17. Classic aneurysmal bone cyst of second cervical vertebra. (Reproduced with permission from: Dahlin, D. C., Besse, B. E., Jr., Pugh, D. G., and Ghormley, R. K.: *Radiology, 64:*56-65, 1955.)

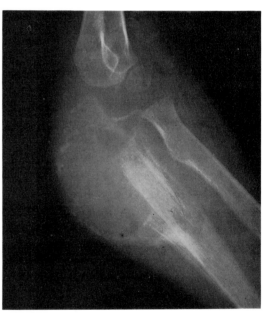

Figure 28-18. Another typical example, here affecting ulna. (Reproduced with permission from: Besse, B. E., Jr., Dahlin, D. C., Pugh, D. G., and Ghormley, R. K.: *Clin Orthop, 7:*93-102, 1956.)

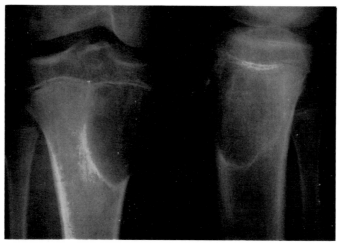

Figure 28-19. This aneurysmal bone cyst of the tibia had not yet produced much expansion.

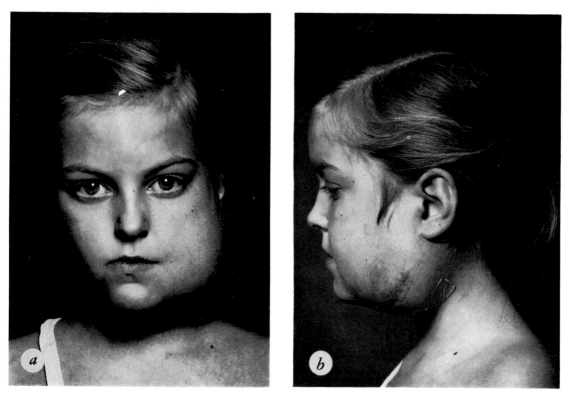

Figure 28-20. *a* and *b*. Aneurysmal bone cyst of mandible. Lesion had produced swelling for three months and had recurred after incomplete removal. Wide excision with preservation of mandible resulted in cure.

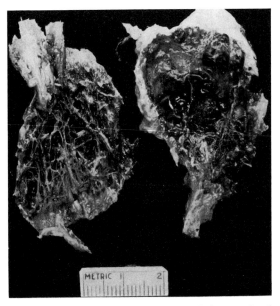

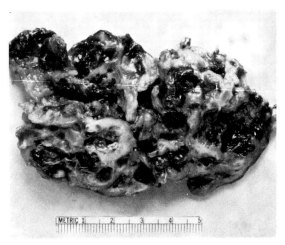

Figure 28-21. Surfaces produced by sagittal section of aneurysmal bone cyst of upper portion of fibula. (Reproduced with permission from: Dahlin, D. C., Besse, B. E., Jr., Pugh, D. G., and Ghormley, R. K.: *Radiology, 64:*56-65, 1955.)

Figure 28-22. Specimen from mandible of patient illustrated in Figure 28-20. Portions of this aneurysmal bone cyst exhibited features of giant cell reparative granuloma.

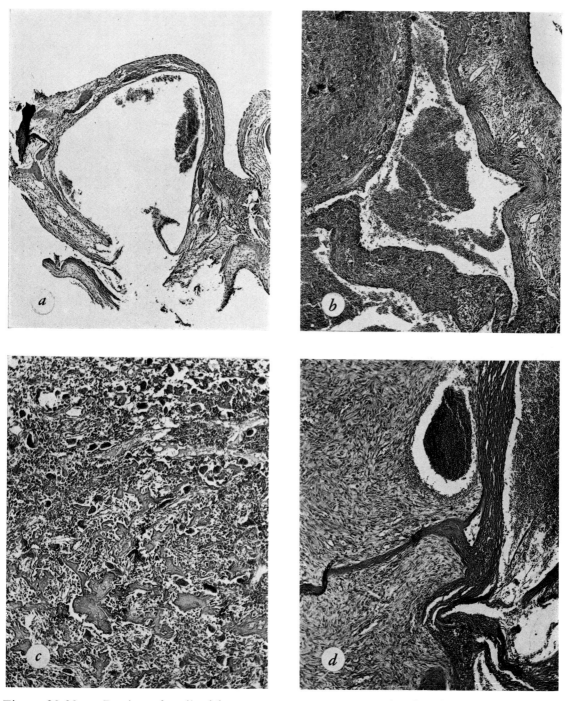

Figure 28-23. *a*. Portion of wall of large cavernomatous space, showing that a smaller blood space is present in wall. (×40) *b*. Thicker and more cellular walls of blood spaces, here containing a few giant cells. (×55) *c*. Solid portion of aneurysmal bone cyst, here containing osteoid trabeculae and numerous benign giant cells. (×80) *d*. Solid fibrous area with cavernous space on right. (×65) (Figures 28-23*b, c,* and *d* reproduced with permission from: Dahlin, D. C., Besse, B. E., Jr., Pugh, D. G., and Ghormley, R. K.: *Radiology, 64*:56-65, 1955.)

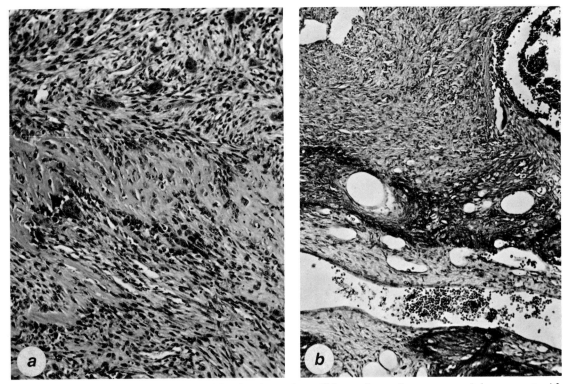

Figure 28-24. *a*. Proliferating fibroblastic tissue in solid portion of aneurysmal bone cyst. Although mitotic figures may be relatively numerous, no significant nuclear anaplasia exists and relatively orderly osteoid trabeculae, as across the center of the picture, are produced. (×160) *b*. Peculiar chondroidlike zones of calcification in solid portions of septa of aneurysmal bone cyst. Such islands are commonly found and are relatively specific. (×150)

Heterotopic Ossification

Heterotopic ossification, often erroneously called myositis ossificans, may occur in muscle or other soft tissues. In its early or "florid" phase, it may present such pronounced cellular activity that it may be mistaken for sarcoma. The lesions of this troublesome disease are rarely explored surgically in their "florid" stage, so they are not commonly encountered. The relative rarity of this disease, however, has delayed understanding of the peculiar tissue reaction associated with it.

Physical Findings

The patient may or may not have experienced significant recent trauma. Sometimes there is a history of unusual muscular exertion. A mass is present in most patients treated surgically. The mass commonly develops in as short a time as a week or two, and rarely, it recurs just as rapidly after surgical removal. This rate of development affords a diagnostic clue, since sarcomas rarely grow so fast.

Roentgenologic Features

In the earliest stages, it may show no evidence of calcific substance. Usually, however, there is a rather well circumscribed, partially osseous tumor, which may give the false appearance of being attached to bone when viewed with only one projection. Some of the deeper-lying tumors may abut on the cortex of a bone and may even be associated with some periosteal reaction. Ordinarily, however, special studies reveal that the bone's cortex is not involved, a feature that aids materially in the differentiation from osteosarcoma. With progression of the lesion, increased ossification develops until finally it is obvious roentgenologically that the process is benign. The mineralized material is typically in the form of trabeculae of bone and begins peripherally in the mass.

Gross Pathology

The tumor is well circumscribed except in the very early phases. It may be completely contained in the belly of a muscle, although an entirely similar process sometimes develops with no apparent relationship to a muscle. It is usually obvious that the lesion did not arise in bone, but a similar reactive change may be related to periosteum and even deeper osseous structures. Ossification is characteristically most pronounced at the periphery of the mass. The central portion may contain small cysts.

Histopathology

Active fibroblastic proliferation is the dominant feature and mitotic figures may be numerous. In all but the earliest lesions of this type, evidence that the fibroblasts are undergoing metaplasia to osteoblasts is present. These osteoblasts produce strands of new osteoid tissue that rapidly become well-formed osseous trabeculae. These are disposed in a somewhat parallel fashion that simulates the appearance of a callus. This "functional" arrangement of the osteoid and osseous trabecula, combined with the lack of true anaplasia in the proliferating cells, affords the histopathologist with the necessary diagnostic clues for the exclusion of sarcoma. Sometimes a chondroid phase is interposed between that of the proliferating fibroblasts and that of the osseous trabecula.

Treatment

Treatment is usually unnecessary if one knows the correct diagnosis.

Prognosis

The prognosis is good whether the lesion is excised or amputation is performed because of an erroneous diagnosis. As indicated, rarely the tumor recurs rather rapidly after excision, but such recurrences are, likewise, benign. One must be certain that he is not merely studying reaction to a more ominous process.

A few instances of malignant transformation of "myositis ossificans" have been recorded, but it is difficult to assess the authenticity of such cases. I believe that most of them represent erroneous interpretation of other processes. None were encountered in the Mayo Clinic material.

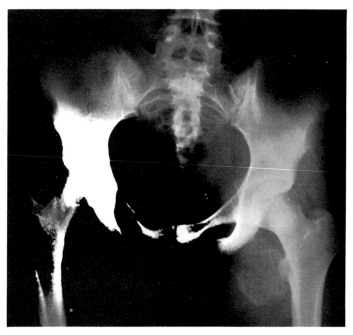

Figure 28-25. Florid heterotopic ossification. Patient had had local pain for one month that began after strenuous gymnastics.

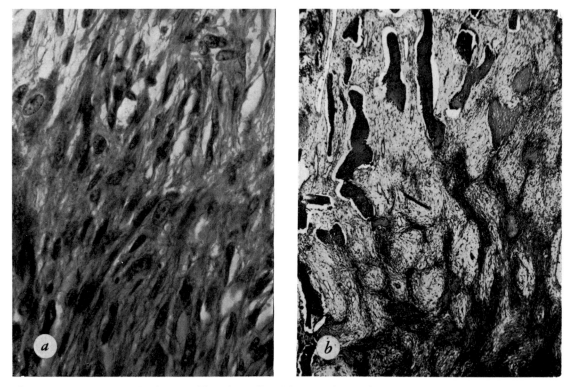

Figure 28-26. *a.* Actively proliferating fibroblasts with mitotic figure in early lesion of heterotopic ossification. Note that nuclei do not appear anaplastic. (×520) *b.* Here fibroblasts have undergone metaplasia and are producing parallel strands of bone. (×45)

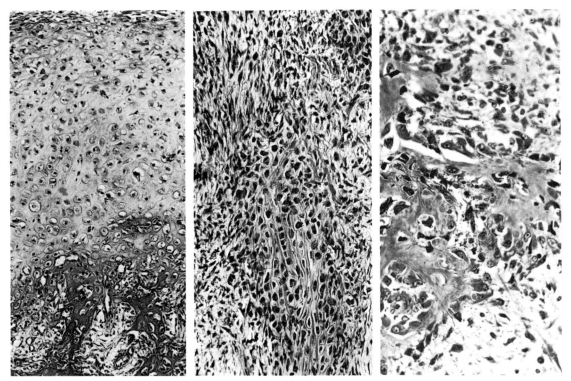

Figure 28-27. "Florid" heterotopic ossification. *Left.* Chondroid foci may stimulate chondrosarcoma. Maturation to bony trabeculae at bottom affords important evidence of their benign nature. (×75) *Middle.* Actively proliferating fibroblasts with focus of osteoid tissue near center. (×125) *Right.* More mature bony trabeculae. Relatively large amount of cytoplasm favors benign nature of osteoblasts. (×300)

Exuberant Callus

A healing fracture, in its early phases, exhibits marked cellular activity with abundant mitotic figures. At this stage, osteoid and chondroid material may not show the obvious functional arrangement of the reparative process, and the histologic appearance is ominous when studied out of context. Later, maturation of these substances resolves the problem. Baker, in 1946, emphasized that healing fractures are especially likely to simulate sarcoma in patients with fragilitas ossium. If the callus is the result of fatigue (march) fracture, which most commonly affects a metatarsal or the tibia, the underlying fracture may be roentgenographically obscure. A somewhat unusual site of stress fracture is in the pubic ramus after "total hip" surgery; in this location especially, the roentgenographic changes have been mistaken for those of neoplasm. Traumatic avulsion of the periosteum can evoke the same type of healing reaction.

As in heterotopic ossification, nuclear evidences of malignancy are lacking. Again, the tendency for maturation of the proliferating elements into regularly arranged trabeculae is an important clue. In this type of reaction, the earliest signs of ossification appear adjacent to the bone, and the periphery of the lesion tends to be most cellular.

I am illustrating this problem because it is one commonly seen in material sent in for consultation from other pathologists. Even the proliferative subperiosteal new bone in Caffey's infantile cortical hyperostosis can pose a problem of this type to the histopathologist.

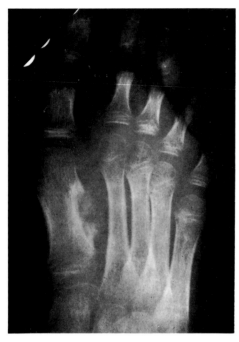

Figure 28-28. Subperiosteal ossification as it appeared one month after injury. Histologic appearance is illustrated in Figure 28-30.

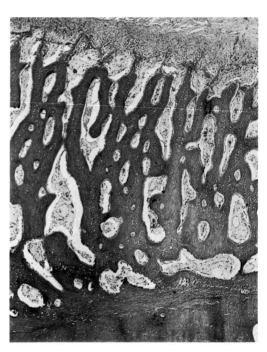

Figure 28-29. Even at this late stage of subperiosteal new bone formation, there is cellular activity just beneath periosteum. (×40)

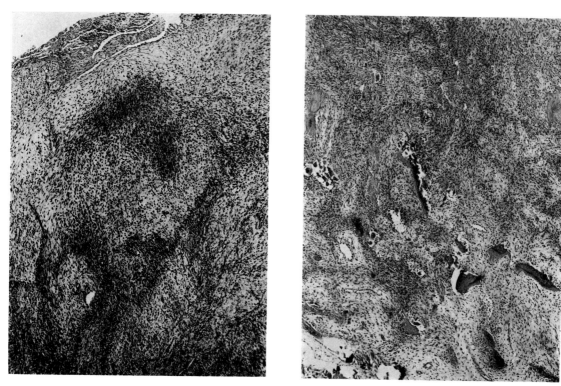

Figure 28-30. Early callus that was mistaken for osteosarcoma. These photomicrographs are from tissue taken from lesion shown in Figure 28-28. Patient had injured his foot a month previously. *Left.* Periphery of reactive process. Maturation to bone is not evident, and mitotic figures are numerous. (×35) *Right.* Near metatarsal, an orderly arrangement of bony trabeculae is beginning to form. (×40)

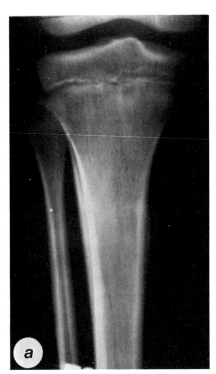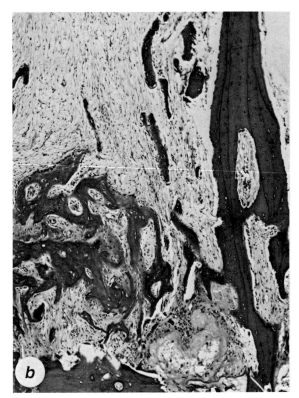

Figure 28-31. *a.* "Stress" fracture in common location. Fracture line may be obscure; attention focused on reactive proliferative cartilage and bone removed for biopsy from callus. *b.* Reactive new bone at site of stress fracture. It is disposed generally at right angles to long trabeculae of preexisting bone, which here shows layer of new bone on its surface. (×64)

Giant Cell Reparative Granulomas

This lesion is peculiar to the jawbones. It has been commonly confused with genuine benign giant cell tumor of bone. The concept that it is not a neoplasm but rather some peculiar reactive lesion is gaining acceptance. The lesion consists of proliferating fibroblasts and often zones in which metaplasia is resulting in the formation of orderly osseous trabeculae. A variable amount of vascularity and microcyst formation may be seen. The basically fibrogenic quality of the lesional tissue is the main feature that differentiates giant cell reparative granuloma from true giant cell tumor. Actually, true giant cell tumors are found so rarely, if ever, in the jawbones that one can practically exclude the possibility. The differentiation of these two lesions is important. Complete removal of giant cell reparative granuloma almost always effects cure, whereas true giant cell tumors recur in 50 percent of cases and 10 percent of them become malignant. Giant cell reparative granuloma commonly occurs in persons in the first decade or two of life as well as in older people.

There appears to be little difference between the lesions within bone that present the histologic characteristics of giant cell reparative granuloma and those that are bascially soft-tissue tumors of the gums with little or no osseous involvement.

A lesion histologically indistinguishable from giant cell reparative granuloma sometimes affects the jaw of a patient with hyperparathyroidism and is, no doubt, evoked by the endocrine disease.

As previously suggested and implied, these lesions probably result from some reactive process, a likelihood suggested by their histologic similarity to aneurysmal bone cyst. Lesions of this type present with involvement of bones well superior to the jaws, and similar lesions, including so-called giant cell reaction of the small bones of the hands and feet, are seen in other parts of the skeleton.

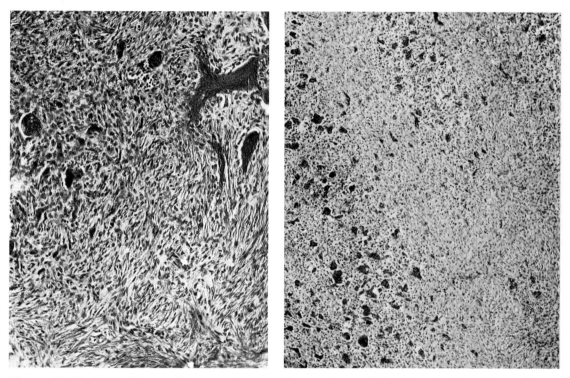

Figure 28-32. *Left.* Giant cell reparative granuloma of mandible. Few benign giant cells are present, but histologic pattern is dominated by fibroblastic cells. Osseous metaplasia, which is almost always present, is seen at upper right. (×100) *Right.* There is greater similarity to giant cell tumor in this field, but fibrogenesis is obvious. (×64)

Giant Cell Reaction or "Lesion"

This lesion was illustrated in the Armed Forces Institute of Pathology fascicle on *Tumors of Bone and Cartilage* by Ackerman and Spjut. Although lesions containing benign giant cells in the small bones of the hands and feet are unusual, a few have the characteristics of genuine giant cell tumor, of chondroblastoma, or of aneurysmal bone cyst. There is also a group, apparently non-neoplastic, in which the stroma shows rather prominent fibrogenesis and new bone formation. These are basically solid but small tumefactions. The nuclei are benign. Their major importance is that they may be mistaken for a more ominous process. These lesions are benign and recurrence is unusual.

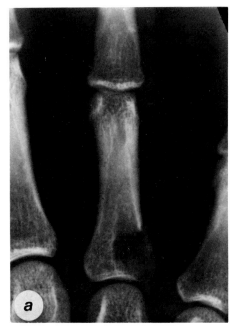
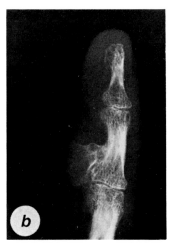

Figure 28-33. *a.* Giant cell "reaction" producing lytic defect at base of proximal phalanx of fourth finger of sixteen-year-old boy. (Case contributed by Doctor M. M. Alvarado, of Dayton, Ohio.) *b.* Similar lesion, which in this instance is exophytic, on middle phalanx of fifth finger of fifty-one-year-old woman. (Case contributed by Doctor A. C. Hoheb and Albany Plastic Surgeons Associated of Albany, New York.)

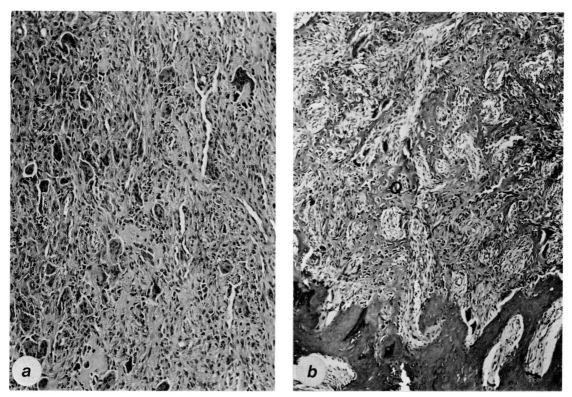

Figure 28-34. *a.* Giant cell "reaction." Lesion differs from true giant cell tumor in that stroma is distinctly fibrogenic, and lesion shows differentiation with production of trabeculae of osteoid. (×160) *b.* In this area, pronounced osteogenesis with production of trabeculae much like that of callus is evident. (×100)

Simple Cysts

Simple or "unicameral" cyst of bone is of unknown cause but apparently results from a disturbance of growth at the epiphyseal line. It is relatively common and usually becomes manifest during the first two decades of life. Generally, the lesion occurs in the upper part of the diaphysis of the humerus, the diaphysis of the femur, or the proximal part of the diaphysis of the tibia, in that order of frequency.

Physical Findings

The patient with a simple cyst of bone may have local pain, but in most cases, the cyst comes to attention only after pathologic fracture has occurred. Occasionally, there is swelling in the region.

Roentgenologic Features

There is often fusiform widening of the bone due to slight expansion in the cystic zone. The cortex is ordinarily eroded and thinned, but it is intact unless pathologic fracture has occurred. Fine trabeculation through the lesion is sometimes seen, and a healed fracture may be evident as a partition through it. A simple cyst usually reaches maximum size before the patient has matured. Frequently, serial roentgenograms reveal that the epiphysis grows away from the region of the cyst so that it lies near the center of the shaft. A cyst not abutting on the epiphysis is referred to as latent.

Gross Pathology

The cystic cavity may contain nothing, but it is usually filled with a clear or yellowish green fluid of low viscosity. The inner surface of the cyst wall frequently displays ridges separating depressed zones, and sometimes it is covered by a layer of fleshy tissue 1 cm or more in thickness. Occasionally, partial or complete septa are seen, the latter type making the cyst multicameral. Recent or old fractures produce modifications of this pattern.

Histopathology

The lining of the cyst may be merely a very thin layer of fibrous tissue. Thicker areas, when present, are composed of fibrogenic connective tissue, which often contains numerous benign giant cells, hemosiderin pigment, a few chronic inflammatory cells, and lipophages. Because of their giant cell component, some of these lesions have been erroneously classed with giant cell tumors. Individual septa, when present, closely resemble those seen in typical aneurysmal bone cyst. The histologic as well as the gross features may have been modified by fracture. Proliferating fibroblastic tissue and callus may be prominent outside and within the cyst. Fibrinous deposits often occur, and these may become mineralized in focal masses resembling those seen in some odontogenic tumors. The lesion has been mistaken for a cementoma.

Treatment

Treatment, when necessary, consists of curettage of the walls of the cyst with complete evacuation of its contents. Bone chips are ordinarily used to fill the defect. It is difficult to determine the optimal time for treatment. Garceau and Gregory (1954) and others have noted a high recurrence rate if patients are less than ten years of age, when the cyst is usually juxtaepiphyseal in location. The chance for permanent cure is good in patients who are more than ten years of age, when the cyst ordinarily has been left behind by the growing epiphyseal line. Johnson and coworkers (1962) described four examples of the extremely rare sarcomatous change in simple cysts. One fibrosarcoma of the femur in our series possibly began in a cyst.

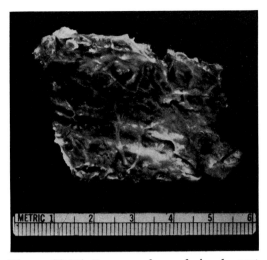

Figure 28-35. Inner surface of simple cyst of upper end of fibula. Note ridges separating depressed areas.

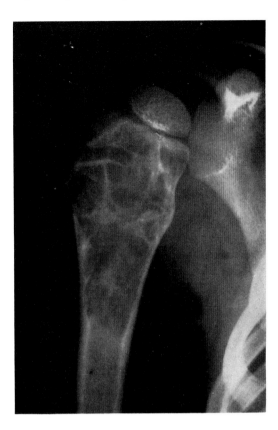

Figure 28-36. Classic appearance of simple cyst of upper portion of shaft of humerus. Fracture had occurred.

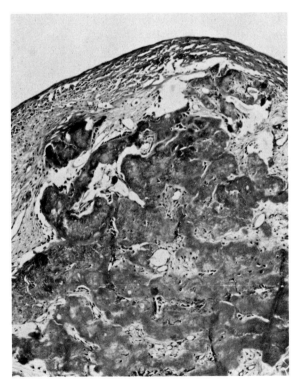

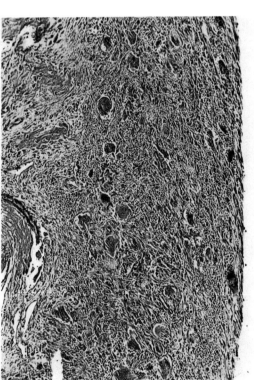

Figure 28-37. *Left.* Wall of simple cyst, in this case, seen as thick and overlying aggregates of degenerating fibrin, probably from prior hemorrhage. Some of these are partially mineralized. (×100) *Right.* Lining of simple cyst. There is thick layer of fibrous tissue, along with fairly numerous benign giant cells. (×100)

Ganglion Cysts

Occasional cysts in bone appear at or near its end and are filled with mucoid, glairy fluid. Typically, they have a thick fibrous wall similar to that of a "ganglion" of tendon sheath, are associated with no significant degenerative changes in the nearby joint, and seem appropriately considered to be collections in synovial spaces in unusual locations.

Epidermoid Cysts

Islands of squamous epithelium sometimes become embedded in bone, and with continued slow growth, a markedly expansile lesion may be produced. The majority of such cysts occur in the bones of the skull, Roth having collected more than 150 cases from the literature to 1964. In addition to causing expansion of the affected bone, the cyst may protrude and displace adjacent soft tissue, including parts of the brain. Accordingly, some of them, especially if they are in roentgenologically obscure locations, may mimic the features of tumors arising in the brain. Sometimes an epidermoid cyst is dumbbell shaped and protrudes beyond both the inner and outer table of the skull.

Roth found records of more than fifty-five cysts of phalanges in the literature. Nearly all of these were in the hand. Except for squamous epithelium-lined cysts in the jaws, where they are common, and in the temporal bone, where they result from middle ear infection, epidermoid cysts are found in practically no bones other than the skull and distal phalanges. The evidence suggests that those in the skull are on a developmental basis and those in the phalanges are probably on the basis of traumatic implantation of epidermis.

Numerous epidermoid cysts of the skull and only three of distal phalanges of the hand were encountered in my study of material from the files of the Mayo Clinic.

Roentgenologic Features

The rarefied defect in bone produced by an epidermoid cyst is typically very sharply defined and surrounded by a thin layer of sclerotic bone.

Pathology

Epidermoid cysts are usually filled with a pearly white mass of inspissated, keratinized squamous epithelium. The microscopic diagnosis depends upon demonstration of a squamous epithelial lining in at least some portion of the cyst wall.

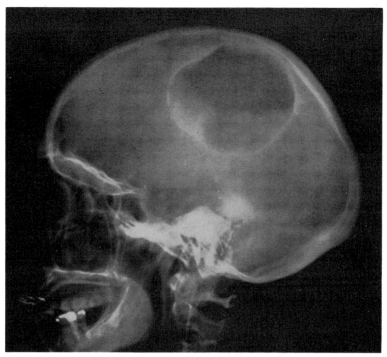

Figure 28-38. Large epidermoid cyst of skull produced mass that bulged into cranial cavity and outwardly as well.

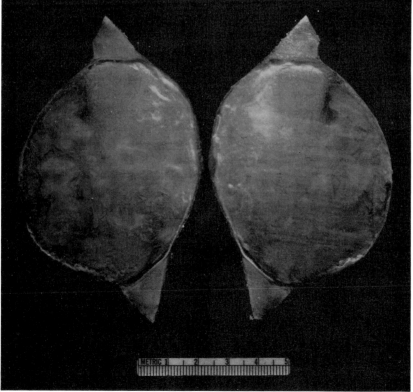

Figure 28-39. Epidermoid cyst shown in Figure 28-38 was excised in its entirety. Since contents were very soft, mass was frozen before it was cut for photography. It bulges internally more than externally.

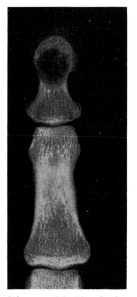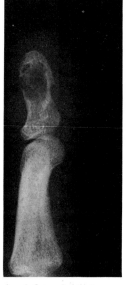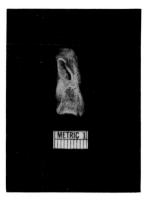

Figure 28-40. *Left* and *right*. Anteroposterior and lateral views of epidermoid cyst of finger. (Case contributed by Doctor J. W. Reagan of Cleveland, Ohio.)

Figure 28-41. Epidermoid cyst destroying part of terminal phalanx of finger.

"Cysts" Associated With Diseases of Joints

One must be suspicious that an osseous defect near a joint may be related to some primary synovial disease.

Severe degenerative joint disease is often accompanied by "cysts" in the juxtaarticular bone. The pathogenesis of these somewhat spherical zones of rarefaction is not clear. They are filled by a degenerative fibromyxoid material. They may be so extensive as to interfere with orthopedic surgical procedures designed to palliate the malfunction of the affected joint. When extensive, they may produce the roentgenographic suggestion that neoplasm of bone is present.

Pigmented villonodular synovitis, especially when it affects the hip joint, sometimes results in similar "degenerative" cysts. Some of the cystlike juxta-articular lesions in pigmented villonodular synovitis result from erosion of the proliferating masses of synovial tissue into the bone. Again, the process may be mistaken for primary disease of bone.

The inflammatory tissue of rheumatoid synovitis often produces rarefactive lesions of bone at the joints in the hands. Less commonly, significant defects adjacent to major joints or in the vertebrae are caused by invading granulomatous masses in rheumatoid disease.

Occasionally, specific infectious processes such as tuberculosis and brucellosis in joints invade and destroy juxta-articular bone.

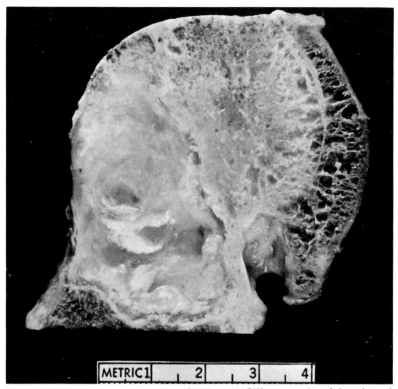

Figure 28-42. Huge "degenerative" cyst filling much of head and neck of femur. Cyst characteristically contains myxoid material and hypocellular fibrous tissue. Note large osteophytic mass overlying femoral head on the right.

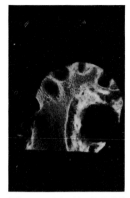

Figure 28-43. Multiple "degenerative" cysts in femoral head of patient with pigmented villonodular synovitis. Cystlike areas were filled with myxoid connective tissue. These cysts were just like those of degenerative arthritis.

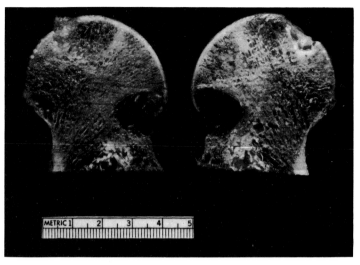

Figure 28-44. Defect in femoral head from patient with rheumatoid synovitis. Defect was filled with granulomatous inflammatory tissue. (Reproduced with permission from: Hunder, G. G., Ward, L. E., and Ivins, J. C.: *Mayo Clin Proc, 40*:766-770, 1965.)

Osteomyelitis

The alterations of bone that result from acute or chronic infection may produce roentgenographic changes that simulate those of bone tumors. Antimicrobial therapy sometimes attenuates the infection to such a degree that normal roentgenographic progression is distorted, thus increasing the likelihood of mistaking an infection of bone for a neoplasm.

Physical Findings

The febrile and septic course of acute osteomyelitis is sometimes obscured by therapy. Furthermore, some of the neoplasms, notably Ewing's sarcoma, produce fever and leukocytosis.

Roentgenologic Features

The earliest sign of osteomyelitis is irregular rarefaction, usually near the end of the shaft of a long bone. Periosteal elevation commonly occurs, and one or more layers of subperiosteal new bone may be produced. Islands of dead bone, which develop later, are relatively radiopaque, owing to the osteoporosis that occurs in the surrounding living bone. On occasion, the roentgeonographic shadow may simulate exactly that produced by a malignant bone tumor. Sometimes, specific chronic infections such as tuberculosis and brucellosis produce a discretely demarcated zone of bone destruction resembling that produced by a slowly growing benign tumor of bone. At other times, a large zone of sclerosis results from an indolent focus of infection in bone, and such a lesion can mimic the appearance of an osteoid osteoma.

Gross Pathology

The granulation tissue present at the site of osteomyelitis may not be identifiable as non-neoplastic.

Histopathology

The differentiation from neoplasm is usually readily apparent. The granulation tissue characteristically contains numerous newly formed capillaries and an admixture of polymorphonuclear leukocytes, plasma cells, and lymphocytes in varied proportions. On some occasions, when an almost pure plasma cell reaction is evoked, the histologic pattern resembles that of multiple myeloma and has resulted in an erroneous diagnosis of neoplasm. Ordinarily, however, the network of proliferating capillaries produces the unmistakable pattern one associates with reaction to infection.

Treatment

The treatment of osteomyelitis varies with the organism responsible for the infection. Management of the condition is sometimes greatly facilitated by examination of fresh-frozen sections at the time of operation. In certain specific mycotic infections, for instance, the diagnosis can be made or strongly suspected from the histologic appearance. Whenever the histologic pattern is that of a granulomatous type of inflammation, bacteriologic investigation can be appropriately directed. A wide variety of bacterial and mycotic infections can produce lesions in bone.

The possibility of malignant change in long-standing chronic osteomyelitis must be considered. The usual malignant tumor is squamous cell carcinoma, which develops from the regenerating skin at the edge of the cutaneous ulceration and invades the underlying already diseased bone. An exacerbation of chronic symptoms or a flare-up in the quiescent stage of osteomyelitis should arouse suspicion of this complication. The carcinoma is usually well differentiated, but successful management depends on amputation. We have encountered twenty-three squamous cell carcinomas in bones affected by chronic osteomyelitis typically of very long duration.

More exotic tumors rarely complicate osteomyelitis, as noted by Morris and Lucas (1964). Our total series includes one osteosarcoma, one malignant lymphoma, and one rapidly lethal myeloma.

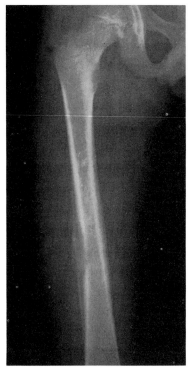

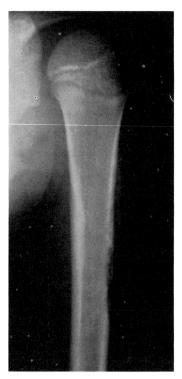

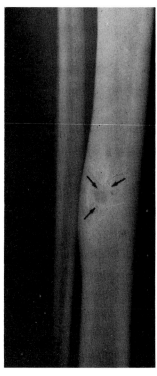

Figure 28-45. Osteomyelitic lesion that roentgenologically simulates sarcoma. This, like one shown in Figure 28-46, was caused by *M. pyogenes* and had destroyed bone and caused periosteal formation of new bone.

Figure 28-46. Osteomyelitis of humerus simulating sarcoma occurred in nine-year-old boy who had noted local pain for one month. Cultures from lesion revealed *M. pyogenes.*

Figure 28-47. Chronic osteomyelitis simulating osteoid osteoma. Lytic lesion is surrounded by sclerotic bone.

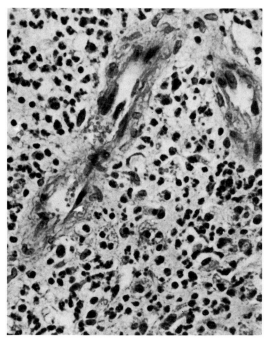

Figure 28-48. Staphylococcal osteomyelitis with neutrophils, plasma cells, and capillary proliferation. (×175)

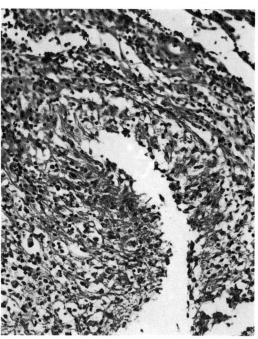

Figure 28-49. Brucellar osteomyelitis. Specific character of infection is suggested by clusters of epithelioid cells. (×170)

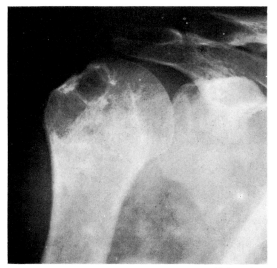

Figure 28-50. Brucellar osteomyelitis simulating chondroblastoma of humerus.

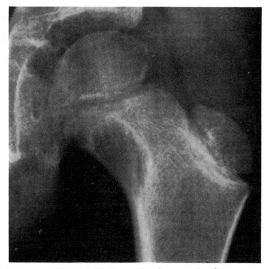

Figure 28-51. Tuberculosis producing neoplasmlike rarefaction of femoral neck.

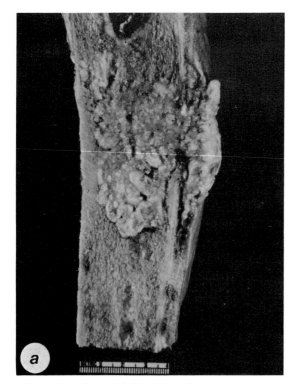 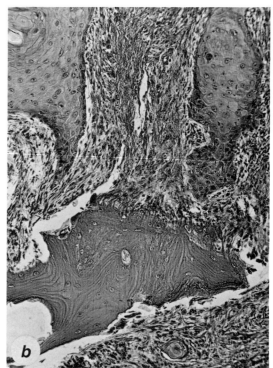

Figure 28-52. *a.* Lighter conglomerate masses of grade 1 squamous cell carcinoma on surface and involving much of medulla of tibia of seventy-seven-year-old man who had had intermittent symptoms of chronic osteomyelitis since fracture through the zone sixty-nine years previously. *b.* Well-differentiated (grade 1, Broders) squamous cell carcinoma deep in focus of chronic osteomyelitis. Such tissue has been mistaken for "benign penetrating epithelium." (×100)

Histiocytosis X (Reticuloendotheliosis)

This category includes conditions that range from the usually solitary and curable eosinophilic granuloma, through the disseminated process that produces the Schüller-Christian syndrome, to the fulminating, rapidly fatal variety known as Letterer-Siwe disease. Osseous lesions ordinarily dominate the pathologic pattern of histiocytosis X, it being basically a disease of the reticuloendothelial system.

Diffuse malignant lymphomas have been mistaken for Letterer-Siwe disease. Letterer-Siwe disease usually affects very young children, whereas the Schüller-Christian syndrome and eosinophilic granuloma are seen most often in children and young adults. Practically any bone of the body may be affected, but there is a predilection for the skull.

Physical Findings

A great variety of symptoms is produced. Ordinarily, patients with eosinophilic granuloma have a solitary painful focus and often a palpable or visible mass. The triad of the Schüller-Christian syndrome classically includes exophthalmos (often unilateral), diabetes insipidus, and rarefied defects of bones of the skull. A partial triad, however, has the same significance if other evidences of dissemination such as anemia, splenomegaly, fatigability, loss of weight, and lymphadenopathy are present. Patients with histiocytosis X may complain of discharge from the ears owning to involvement of the temporal bones, loosening or falling out of the teeth secondary to lesions of the jaw, and any of the symptoms that might be produced by focal destruction of bone. Any bone may be the site of a painful and sometimes expansile lesion. Vertebral involvement may result in collapse of a vertebral body with resultant neurologic symptoms. Cutaneous manifestations, lymphadenopathy, and splenomegaly are most common in the progressing, diffuse form of the disease. Pulmonary infiltration may become clinically important, and on rare occasions, it is the most significant evidence of the disease. Diffuse pulmonary lesions of histiocytosis X, on the other hand, may occur in the absence of osseous lesions; such patients are usually adults who are not seriously ill, may have episodes of spontaneous pneumothorax, and have an unpredictable clinical course.

Roentgenologic Features

The defects in bone are usually discretely defined. Periosteal reaction may be present when the cortex becomes eroded or when pathologic fracture has occurred. If the lesion is solitary, such reaction combined with a poorly defined zone of rarefaction may produce a shadow similar to that of a malignant bone tumor. Multiple adjacent defects often become confluent. Lesions in the mandible are usually concentrated along the alveolar process. The teeth, in consequence, may appear to have no bony support, which indeed is true. Moseley described the roentgenographic features in detail in 1962.

Gross Pathology

The lesional tissue is soft and may be gray, pink, or yellow.

Histopathology

The microscopic appearance is what links these three general conditions together. The salient and pathognomonic feature consists of foci of proliferating histiocytic cells. These histiocytes frequently have ill-defined cytoplasmic boundaries and characteristically contain an oval or indented nucleus. Multinucleated histiocytes may be seen. Although chromatin clumping and nucleoli are inconspicuous, mitotic figures may be common; they contribute to the confusion of histiocytosis X with malignant tumors, especially reticulum cell sarcoma on some occasions. Zones of necrosis are present in many of the lesions. The histiocytes may be swollen owing to cholesterol in their cytoplasm. Varied numbers of eosinophils, lymphocytes, and neutrophils are nearly always present.

Treatment

The treatment of lesions seen in eosinophilic granuloma and of the major ones in Schüller-Christian syndrome is roentgen therapy in moderate dosage. Steroids and other chemotherapeutic agents have been used successfully in the severe, disseminated forms of histiocytosis X.

Prognosis

Complete evaluation of patients who present with a defect characteristic of histiocytosis X is important in estimating prognosis. Those patients who have only one or a few lesions are usually cured by local radiation. Patients with the Schüller-Christian type of disease have a poor long-term outlook, but prolonged palliation can be expected if therapy is administered judiciously. Enriquez, in a study of 116 patients with histiocytosis X at the Mayo Clinic (1966), found that those less than three years of age, those with more than eight bones involved, those with hemorrhagic manifestations, and those with splenomegaly all had an ominous prognosis. Those who survived more than three years after the onset of symptoms had a good prognosis.

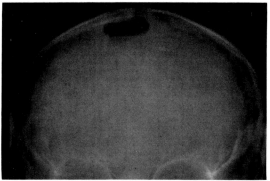

Figure 28-53. Skull defect produced by histiocytosis X. Skull is one of most common sites for lesions in this disease.

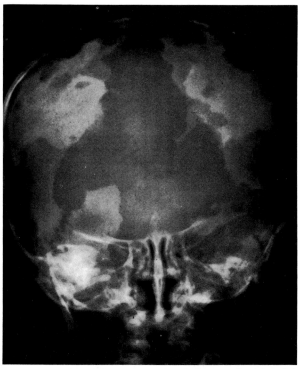

Figure 28-54. Disseminated histiocytosis X with severe involvement of skull. Patient was three-year-old boy who died the following year.

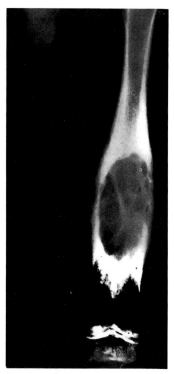

Figure 28-55. Huge solitary lesion of histiocytosis X. Note pronounced sclerosis of adjacent bone.

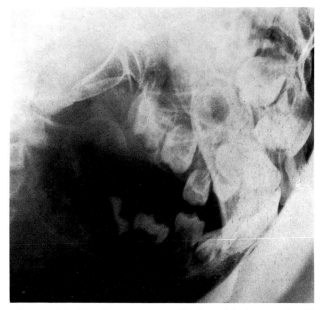

Figure 28-56. Severe mandibular histiocytosis X with teeth about to exfoliate, which is a common complication.

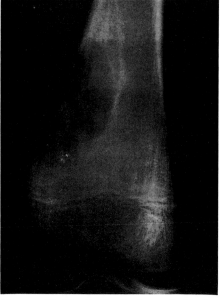

Figure 28-57. Lytic lesion of histiocytosis X showing features suggestive of malignant tumor.

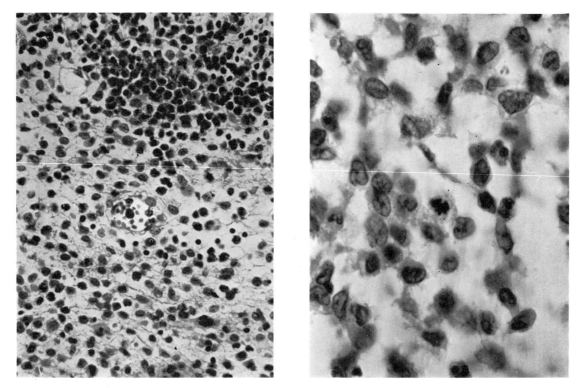

Figure 28-58. *Left*. Lesion of histiocytosis X showing essential pale-staining histiocytes and darker eosinophils that commonly accompany basic cells of lesion. (×385) *Right*. Higher magnification to illustrate details of histiocytes. Note mitotic figure near center of field. (×1000)

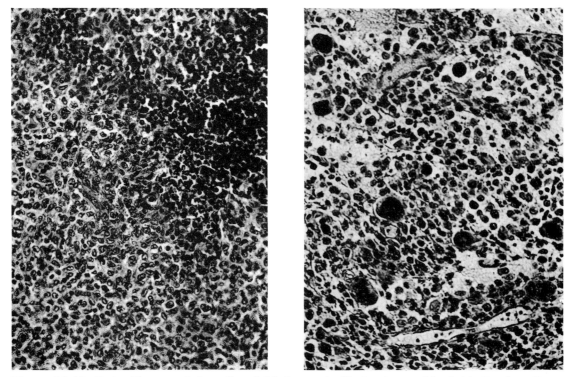

Figure 28-59. *Left*. Characteristic cells of histiocytosis X dominate this field. Dark cells at upper right are eosinophils. (×245) *Right*. Multinucleated histiocytes such as those shown here are found in minority of lesions. (×200)

Paget's Disease

Paget's disease is of unknown cause. It occurs in middle and old age. The pelvis, femur, skull, tibia, and vertebrae are common sites of involvement, although any bone may be affected. In early stages, resorption of bone is prominent. Later there is a mixture of destruction and repair of bone, and in the final stage, the reparative process is predominant and radiopacity is marked. A focal lesion of Paget's disease may simulate primary tumor of bone roentgenologically. With more diffuse involvement of the skeleton, differentiation of it from osteoblastic deposits of metastatic carcinoma may be a problem. Widening of the affected bone is helpful evidence that the sclerosing lesion is a manifestation of Paget's disease.

Histologically, the lesion of Paget's disease may be difficult to identify without roentgenologic bias. Irregular broad trabeculae, reversal or "cement" lines, osteoclastic activity, and fibrous vascular tissue between the trabeculae are characteristic. There may be lesser degrees of these typical alterations. Other diseases such as metastatic carcinoma, malignant lymphoma, callus (from whatever cause), or even mastocytosis can evoke similar roentgenologic changes.

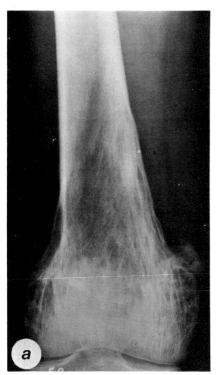 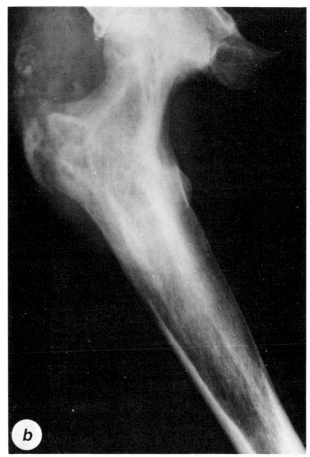

Figure 28-60. *a.* Paget's disease that had produced pain for six months in forty-four-year-old man. Histologically, lesion was benign, although tumefaction was noted at medial condyle. *b.* Paget's disease of upper half of femur. Osteosarcoma had developed at greater trochanter.

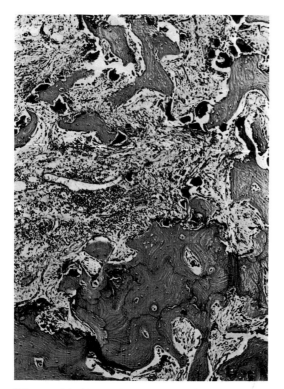 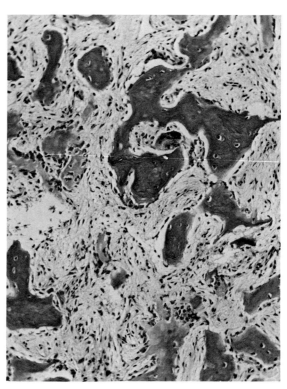

Figure 28-61. *Left.* Paget's disease with characteristic mosaic pattern in irregular osseous trabeculae. Osteoclasts are numerous, and marrow is replaced by vascular fibrous tissue. (×50) *Right.* Earlier Paget's disease with less obvious features. This zone could be mistaken for nondiagnostic fibro-osseous lesion. (×160)

Sarcoma occasionally arises in Paget's disease to complicate the problem of roentgenologic diagnosis. The extensive alteration of bone produced by Paget's disease sometimes obscures early signs of a superimposed malignant process. There were thirty osteosarcomas and five fibrosarcomas complicating Paget's disease of bone in this series.

Hyperparathyroidism

Hyperparathyroidism results from neoplasms or diffuse hyperplasia of the parathyroid glands. Ordinarily, diffuse demineralization of the skeleton occurs, but marked focal absorption sometimes produces a cystlike appearance on the roentgenogram that can simulate the appearance of a primary neoplasm of bone. In some instances, the fibroblastic tissue filling the defect is so exuberant that the contour of the bone bulges, thereby suggesting even more strongly that a neoplasm is present.

Because of the widespread knowledge of the syndrome of hyperparathyroidism, the osseous lesions it produces are rarely subjected to biopsy. The diagnosis is best established by determinations of the serum levels of calcium and phosphorus and by the finding of an increased amount of urinary calcium. Suspicion is aroused when a lesion suggests the diagnosis of giant cell tumor but its histologic appearance or its skeletal location is incorrect for giant cell tumor. Sometimes parathyroid osteopathy produces a lesion similar to aneurysmal bone cyst.

The lesion does not present pathognomonic histologic features. Where the osseous trabeculae are being resorbed, there is proliferating fibroblastic connective tissue usually so richly sprinkled with benign osteoclastlike giant cells that the diagnosis of giant cell tumor may be entertained. The basic fibrogenic quality of the lesion should, however, preclude the diagnosis of giant cell tumor because the latter lesion is not fibrogenic in its proliferating, diagnostic fields. Multifocal giant-cell-rich fibroblastic islands partially separated by fairly well formed trabeculae and the lack of typical features of other giant cell "variants" may alert the histopathologist to the possibility that the lesion may be the result of hyperparathyroidism.

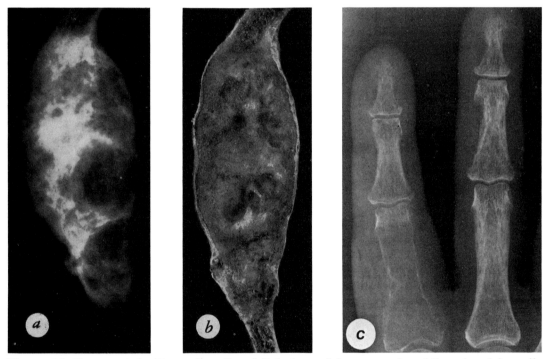

Figure 28-62. *a* and *b*. Expanding "cystic" lesion of hyperparathyroidism involving rib. Note that tumor is composed of fibrous tissue containing prominent foci with trabeculae of bone. *c*. Typical changes of hyperparathyroidism of second and third digits of hand. Tumor of parathyroid osteopathy involves most of first phalanx of second finger.

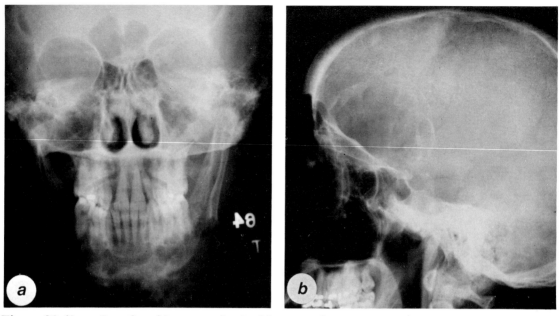

Figure 28-63. *a*. Parathyroid osteopathy in fifty-year-old woman. Left mandibular lesion simulated malignancy. Lesion resolved after removal of parathyroid tumor. On biopsy, lesion had
been called "fibrous dysplasia." *b*. Parathyroid osteopathy producing markedly "expansile"
lesion of orbital plate of frontal bone in twenty-seven-year-old woman. Parathyroid adenoma
of 2,100 g was later removed from mediastinum.

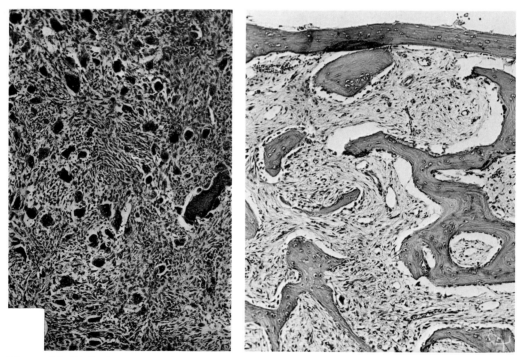

Figure 28-64. *Left*. Osseous lesion of hyperparathyroidism resembling giant cell tumor,
but background "stroma" is somewhat fibrogenic as opposed to that of typical areas
in giant cell tumor. Benign giant cells tend to occur in aggregates separated by fibrogenic tissue in which there may be trabeculae of osteoid or bone. (×100) *Right*. Hyperparathyroidism, probably an older lesion, in which no benign giant cells are seen.
Fibro-osseous tissue fills defect seen by roentgenogram. (×100)

Synovial Chondromatosis and Para-articular Chondromas

Cartilaginous metaplasia of synovium can give rise to one or innumerable cartilaginous bodies, which may undergo partial calcification and ossification. In major joints, this condition is monarticular and most often affects the knee. Numerous loose bodies or a conglomerate mass of osteocartilaginous tissue may develop. The diffuse process, with numerous cartilaginous nodules, may occur in bursae or tendon sheaths and be far from a major articulation.

Of particular interest is that tumors with lobules of characteristic hyaline cartilage occurring in the hands and feet and not of osseous derivation are essentially always benign. Their histologic pattern suggests that nearly all of them are of synovial derivation.

Para-articular chondromas occur in relation to any joint, apparently arising in the capsule. These also are characteristically benign in their clinical evolution, although recurrence is not unusual. They often contain prominent calcific deposits or show extensive ossification.

Histopathology

The histologic appearance of these proliferating cartilaginous tumors is what makes them important to the pathologist. In many instances, the nuclear abnormalities and numbers of multinucleated cells are so great that in the right context, as in the medulla of a major tubular bone, the diagnosis of chondrosarcoma would be strongly supported. Paradoxically, however, these cartilaginous masses are practically never malignant nor even premalignant. Reference to the roentgenogram usually affords convincing evidence that the lesion is extraskeletal. Even parosteal (juxtacortical) osteosarcoma may be suggested by the histologic features.

Prognosis

The prognosis is good, although the diffuse synovial lesions may recur because it is so difficult to remove every vestige of them. The solitary chondromas rarely recur after excision.

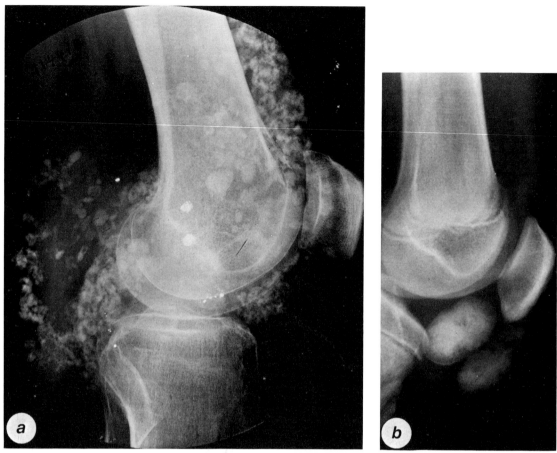

Figure 28-65. *a.* Synovial chondromatosis in forty-nine-year-old man. Note numerous and typically small mineralized aggregates producing prominent enlargement of synovial-lined space. *b.* Para-articular chondromas in twelve-year-old girl. Tumors had been removed from this area two years previously. Note smooth contour of larger extraosseous mineralized mass. Microscopic appearance of lesion is shown in Figure 28-68*b*. (Case contributed by Doctor L. W. Price of Lawrence, Kansas.)

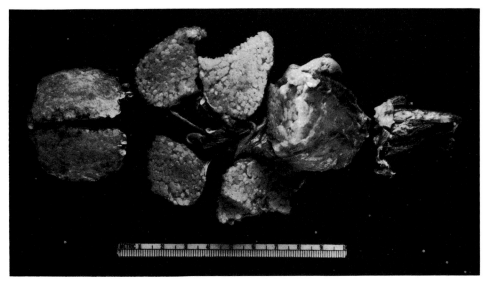

Figure 28-66. Conglomerate mass of cartilage resulting from synovial chondromatosis of iliopectineal bursa. This produced a significant intrapelvic mass. Although cytologically active, diagnosis was established by finding metaplastic cartilage in encapsulating synovium. Excision of mass has given good clinical result more than six years later. This is an extremely unusual location for this disease.

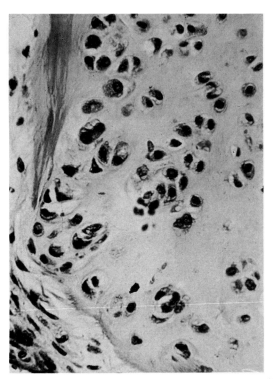 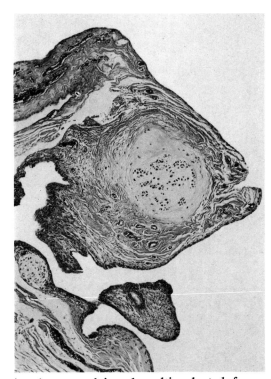

Figure 28-67. *Left.* Synovial chondromatosis showing large nuclei and multinucleated forms that in the proper setting would constitute evidence suggesting malignancy. (×400) *Right.* Demonstration of origin from synovium such as shown here establishes correct benign diagnosis. (×50)

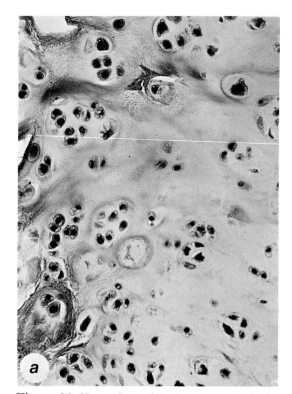 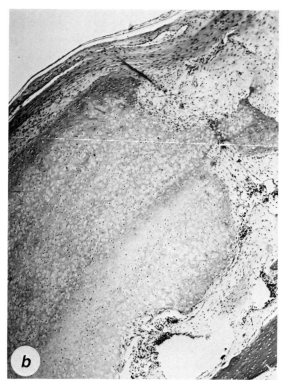

Figure 28-68. *a.* Synovial chondromatosis in extra-articular location near shoulder. Cytologic alterations suggest malignancy, which is essentially precluded when lesion is of synovial origin. (×250) *b.* Chondroid island lacks cytologic atypia and is undergoing maturation to benign osseous trabeculae. (×64)

Bone Infarcts

Infarction of bone is common after decompression sickness, as in caisson workers, and in patients with sickle cell anemia. It is also being reported increasingly often as affecting part of the femoral head in the form of so-called idiopathic aseptic necrosis. Not so well known is that single or multiple osseous infarcts of unknown cause, although rarely seen, can occur in various bones. These may be associated with local pain. In the early stages, according to Bullough and coworkers (1965), there may be no roentgenographic findings. Later, the lesion presents as an irregular area of density, sometimes with a cystlike center. The density is the result of an ingrowth of new bone and impregnation of the necrotic zone with calcium salts. These infarcts may be mistaken for calcifying cartilaginous neoplasms, cysts, and even osteoid osteoma with a surrounding halo of sclerotic bone. Infarcts differ histologically from the relatively common, asymptomatic "bone islands" seen roentgenographically. These latter lesions consist of a focus of bone that is merely too dense for the region in question.

Furey and coworkers, in 1960, described two cases of the extremely rare complication of fibrosarcoma at the sites of bone infarcts. Several other similar examples have been reported since then. One of the osteosarcomas in this series arose in conjunction with an old infarct. Presumably the reparative process associated with a zone of old infarction of bone can result in neoplasia.

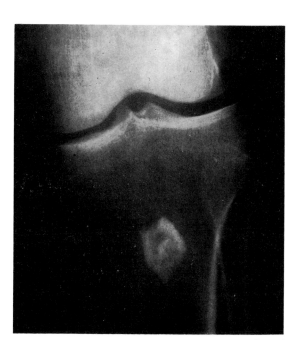
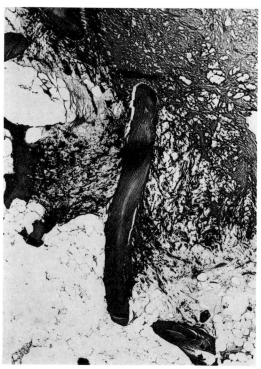

Figure 28-69. *Left.* Bone infarct showing irregular radiodensity. *Right.* Necrotic osseous trabeculae with amorphous mineralization of intervening degenerated marrow. Pattern is characteristic of old infarct of bone. (×30)

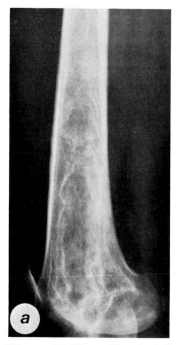
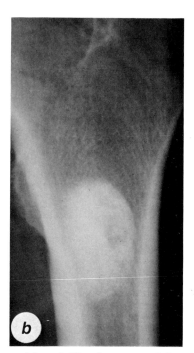
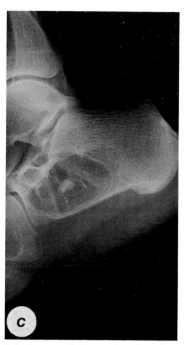

Figure 28-70. *a.* Classic infarct with calcification at periphery of lesion and irregular border, nearly filling distal one third of femoral shaft and condyles. Lesion was found in fifty-four-year-old woman. *b.* Heavily calcified infarct of upper shaft of femur of sixty-three-year-old man. *c.* Infarct with cystic change in os calcis of forty-six-year-old man.

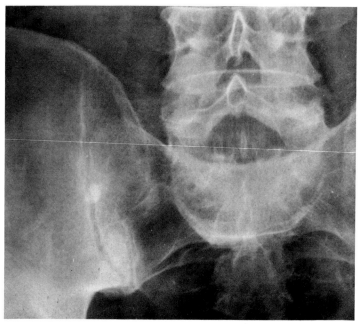

Figure 28-71. Bone "island" in twenty-three-year-old man. Such lesions are ordinarily asymptomatic and are composed of dense "compact" bone. Confusion with neoplasms may be produced, especially by larger lesions of this type.

Bone Islands

These osteosclerotic foci are not uncommonly seen in roentgenograms. When they alter their size, especially becoming larger, they pose the possibility of representing a significant lesion such as osteoblastic metastasis or osteoid osteoma. They seldom exceed 1 cm in size and characteristically do not alter the bone's contour.

Mastocytosis

Mast cell infiltrates can occur in viscera and cause its enlargement. Such infiltrates also can occur in bone. Their important consequence is patchy areas of opacity that are commonly mistaken for those of metastatic carcinoma. By contrast, the course of affected persons, who sometimes have no history of urticaria pigmentosa, is minimally progressive. The clinical findings are important in recognition of the disease.

Specimens from the bone show mast cell infiltrates that may not provide diagnostic cytoplasmic staining quality. These cells are typically small, tend to show spindling and a granulomalike quality, and sometimes occur in relatively small aggregates within normal or slightly fibrotic marrow. The mast cells themselves contain very faintly granular cytoplasm. Eosinophils may be prominent in parts of the infiltrate. Sclerosis with increased size and irregularity of the osseous trabeculae assures the pathologist that he is viewing tissue from the suspected area. Special stains such as alcian blue may disclose metachromasia in the cells of the lesion.

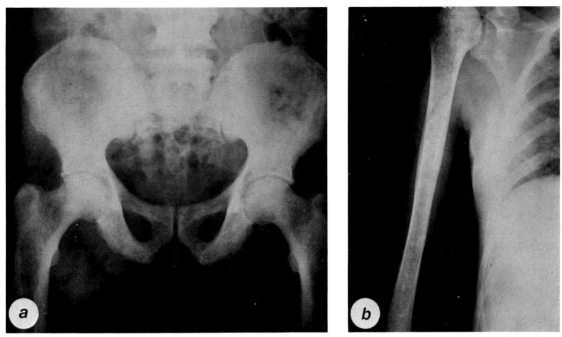

Figure 28-72. *a.* Mastocytosis producing multifocal sclerosing lesions, especially in pelvic bones. These lesions are commonly mistaken for metastatic osteoblastic carcinoma. *b.* Similar sclerosing lesions of humerus in mastocytosis.

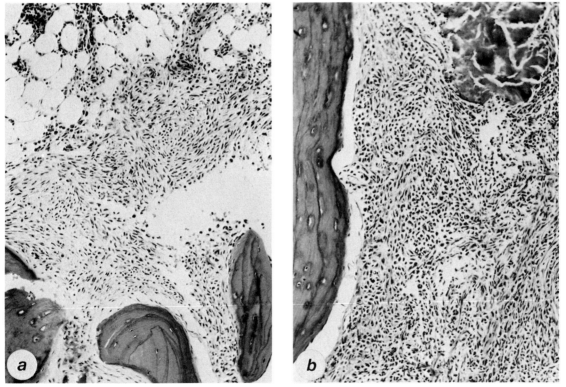

Figure 28-73. *a.* Small "granulomalike" clusters of mast cells are often the only significant histologic finding in the bone. Cells tend to spindle and resemble fibroblasts in areas. Small mast cell nuclei are surrounded by small amount of faintly granular cytoplasm. (×160) *b.* More pronounced infiltrate of similar cells. Note accretion lines on trabecula indicating that this is from an area of osteosclerosis. Amorphous mass at upper right is bone debris forced into this area by processing. (×160)

Mesenchymoma of Chest Wall

This peculiar tumefaction, which seems to have a nearly complete predilection for the chest wall, is important because, though rare, it frequently has been mistaken for sarcoma. The malignant interpretation has been based on the actively proliferating fibroblastic and chondroid elements. A clue that the lesion is benign is the fact that well-formed osseous trabeculae develop from these proliferative tissues. Nuclear evidence of anaplasia is absent. Aneurysmal-bone-cyst-like areas are not uncommon.

This tumor is found in newborns or the very young. The mass involves ribs, either distorting them or arising from them. We have no evidence that any of these lesions has metastasized, but surgical removal may be extremely difficult because of the lesion's size.

No lesion of this type was encountered in the Mayo Clinic series, but we are currently assessing the available information on seven cases sent in for consultation.

Figure 28-74. *a.* Mesenchymoma of left chest wall of one-week-old infant. (Case contributed by Doctor J. Spataro of Phoenix, Arizona.) *b.* Proliferating islands of cartilage from mesenchymoma of chest wall. Note maturation to bony trabeculae at right and sheets of fibroblastic cells. (×100) *c.* Area dominated by proliferating spindling cells separated from cartilaginous island by round cells interspersed with foreign-body giant cells. A few trabeculae are present. (×100) *d.* Cavernomatous spaces like those of aneurysmal bone cyst. Solid tissue in this area is not hypercellular and shows differentiation into obviously benign-appearing trabeculae of bone. (×64).

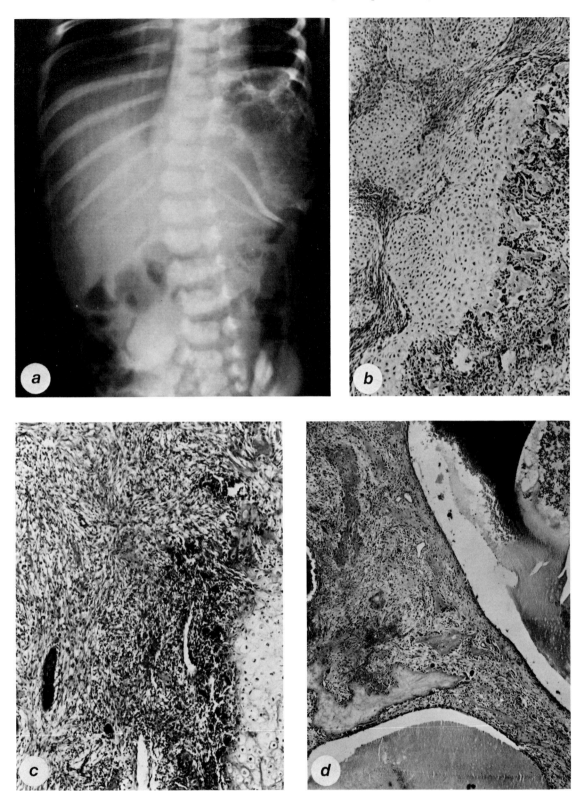

Avulsion Fracture (Ischial Apophyseolysis) and Related Conditions

The tumors formed after avulsion or other trauma at growth centers, including the ischial and tibial tuberosity, may be mistaken for neoplasms. There are hyperplastic masses of cartilage with maturation in areas to bone. Cytologic atypia is absent. Fibrinous and degenerative foci may obscure the histology. Awareness of these conditions and interpretation by a knowledgeable radiologist are necessary in their correct analysis.

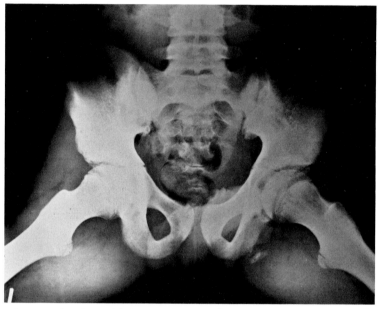

Figure 28-75. Ischial apophyseolysis (avulsion fracture) in twelve-year-old boy whose trouble began with stress. Roentgenologic findings indicate that mass was produced by trauma and was not a neoplasm. (Case contributed by Doctor J. L. Broady of Knoxville, Tennessee.)

Periosteally Located Tumors

A wide variety of tumors involve bone by coaption or erosion from without. Some of these may begin in periosteum, but many obviously arise from periosseous tissues. Desmoid tumors often secondarily involve bone, especially in the region of the forearm. "Giant cell tumors" (fibrous histiocytomas) of tendon-sheath origin occasionally erode, sometimes extensively, into small bones of the hands and feet. Some tumors, for example malignant synovioma, rather frequently invade nearby bone. Some juxtaosseous tumors such as the hemangioma shown in Figure 12-17 *right* and lipomas produce confusingly prominent alteration in nearby bone. A calcifying neoplasm of soft-tissue origin may appear to be a primary bone tumor; this is especially true of synovial chondromatosis or malignant synovioma. Tumoral calcinosis may produce a huge mineralized mass juxtaposed to skeletal structures, especially at the hip and elbow. The lesion is composed of amorphous calcific masses with associated foreign-body giant cell reaction.

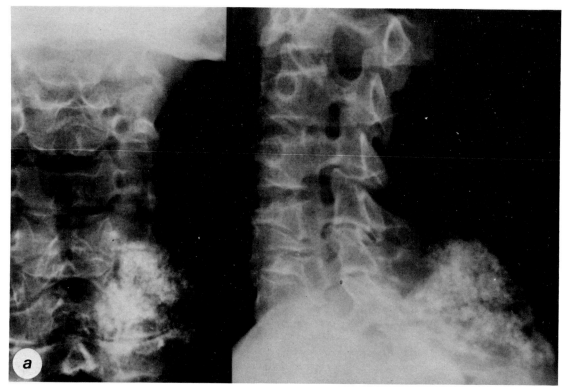

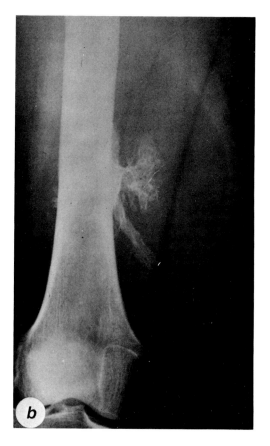

Figure 28-76. *a.* Calcifying malignant synovioma. Tumor presented in posterior left neck region of fifty-eight-year-old man. Preoperatively, mass was considered to be chondrosarcoma. Lesion is intimately associated with and overlies bone structures. (Case contributed by Doctors B. Stener and L. Angervall of Göteborg, Sweden.) *b.* Lipoma characteristically producing large zone of rarefaction and associated with irregular "exostosis" projecting into it from adjacent femur. (Case contributed by Doctor J. Edeiken of Philadelphia, Pennsylvania.)

Misleading Roentgenograms

Although roentgenograms nearly always show the lesion and indicate whether it is benign or malignant, sometimes they are misleading. Infections of bone may simulate neoplasm; benign process may mimic malignant disease; or rarely, roentgenographic findings suggest disease that is not present. Their correct interpretation demands a skilled roentgenologist's analysis.

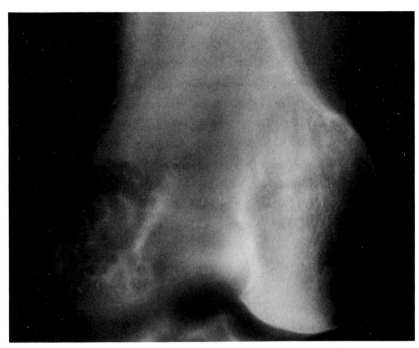

Figure 28-77. Deceptive appearance of lesion provided by roentgenogram. Only cancellous, normal-appearing bone was found on exploration of "zone of rarefaction" in lateral condyle.

Bibliography

1946   Baker, S. L.: Hyperplastic Callus Simulating Sarcoma in Two Cases of Fragilitas Ossium. *J Pathol Bacteriol, 58:*609-623.

1948   Ghormley, R. K., and Clegg, R. S.: Bone and Joint Changes in Hemophilia With Report of Cases of So-Called Hemophilic Pseudotumor. *J Bone Joint Surg, 30A:* 589-600.

1951   Pritchard, J. E.: Fibrous Dysplasia of the Bones. *Am J Med Sci, 222:*313-332.

1953   Jaffe, H. L.: Giant-cell Reparative Granuloma, Traumatic Bone Cyst, and Fibrous (Fibro-osseous) Dysplasia of the Jawbones. *Oral Surg, 6:*159-175.

1954   Garceau, G. J., and Gregory, C. F.: Solitary Unicameral Bone Cyst. *J Bone Joint Surg, 36A:*267-280.

1957   Eversole, S. L., Jr., Holman, G. H., and Robinson, R. A.: Hitherto Undescribed Characteristics of the Pathology of Infantile Cortical Hyperostosis (Caffey's Disease). *Bull Johns Hopkins Hosp, 101:*80-99.

1957   Lichtenstein, L.: Aneurysmal Bone Cyst. Observations on Fifty Cases. *J Bone Joint Surg, 39A:*873-882.

1958   Ackerman, L. V.: Extra-Osseous Localized Non-Neoplastic Bone and Cartilage Formation (So-Called Myositis Ossificans): Clinical and Pathological Confusion With Malignant Neoplasms. *J Bone Joint Surg, 40A:*279-298 (April).

1959 Havard, C. W. H., and Scott, R. B.: Urticaria Pigmentosa With Visceral and Skeletal Lesions. *Q J Med, 24:*459-470.

1960 Furey, J. G., Ferrer-Torells, M., and Reagan, J. W.: Fibrosarcoma Arising at the Site of Bone Infarcts. A Report of 2 Cases. *J Bone Joint Surg, 42A:*802-810.

1960 Wholey, M. H., and Pugh, D. G.: Localized Destructive Lesions in Rheumatoid Spondylitis. *Radiology, 74:*54-56.

1962 Harris, W. H., Dudley, H. R., Jr., and Barry, R. J.: The Natural History of Fibrous Dysplasia: An Orthopaedic, Pathological, and Roentgenographic Study. *J Bone Joint Surg, 44A:*207-233 (March).

1962 Smith, J. H., and Pugh, D. G.: Roentgenographic Aspects of Articular Pigmented Villonodular Synovitis. *Am J Roentgenol, 87:*1146-1156.

1962 Murphy, F. P., Dahlin, D. C., and Sullivan, C. R.: Articular Synovial Chondromatosis. *J Bone Joint Surg, 44A:*77-86.

1962 Linscheid, R. L., and Coventry, M. B.: Unrecognized Fractures of Long Bones Suggesting Primary Bone Tumors. *Proc Staff Meet Mayo Clin, 37:*599-606.

1962 Johnson, L. C., Vetter, H., and Putschar, W. G. J.: Sarcomas Arising in Bone Cysts. *Virchows Arch [Pathol Anat], 335:*428-451.

1962 Moseley, J. E.: Patterns of Bone Change in the Reticuloendothelioses. *J Mt Sinai Hosp, 29:*282-321.

1964 Roth, S. I.: Squamous Cysts Involving the Skull and Distal Phalanges. *J Bone Joint Surg, 46A:*1442-1450.

1964 Lichtenstein, L.: Histiocytosis X (Eosinophilic Granuloma of Bone, Letter-Siwe Disease, and Schüller-Christian Disease). Further Observations of Pathological and Clinical Importance. *J Bone Joint Surg, 46A:*76-90.

1964 Alldred, A. J., and Nisbet, N. W.: Hydatid Disease of Bone in Australasia. *J Bone Joint Surg, 46B:*260-267.

1964 Cohen, D. M., Dahlin, D. C., and MacCarty, C. S.: Vertebral Giant-Cell Tumor and Variants. *Cancer, 17:*461-472.

1964 Morris, J. M., and Lucas, D. B.: Fibrosarcoma Within a Sinus Tract of Chronic Draining Osteomyelitis. Case Report and Review of Literature. *J Bone Joint Surg, 46A:*853-857.

1965 Johnson, L. L., and Kempson, R. L.: Epidermoid Carcinoma in Chronic Osteomyelitis: Diagnostic Problems and Management. *J Bone Joint Surg, 47A:*133-145.

1965 Hunder, G. G., Ward, L. E., and Ivins, J. C.: Rheumatoid Granulomatous Lesion Simulating Malignancy in the Head and Neck of the Femur. *Mayo Clin Proc, 40:*766-770.

1965 Bullough, P. G., Kambolis, C. P., Marcove, R. C., and Jaffe, H. L.: Bone Infarctions Not Associated With Caisson Disease. *J Bone Joint Surg, 47A:*477-491.

1966 Ellis, R., and Greene, A. G.: Ischial Apophyseolysis. *Radiology, 87:*646-648 (October).

1966 Kempson, R. L.: Ossifying Fibroma of the Long Bones. A Light and Electron Microscopic Study. *Arch Pathol, 82:*218-233 (September).

1966 Shauffer, I. A., and Collins, W. V.: The Deep Clavicular Rhomboid Fossa: Clinical Significance and Incidence in 10,000 Routine Chest Photofluorograms. *JAMA, 195:*778-779 (February).

1967 Enriquez, P., Dahlin, D. C., Hayles, A. B., and Henderson, E. D.: Histiocytosis X: A Clinical Study. *Mayo Clin Proc, 42:*88-89 (February).

1967 Harkness, J. W., and Peters, H. J.: Tumoral Calcinosis: A Report of Six Cases. *J Bone Joint Surg, 49A:*721-731 (June).

1967 Mazabraud, A., Semat, P., and Roze, R.: A Propose de L'Association de Fibromyxomes des Tissus Mous à la Dysplasie Fibreuse des Os. *Presse Med, 75:*2223-2228 (October).

1968 Barer, M., Peterson, L. F. A., Dahlin, D. C., Winkelmann, R. K., and Stewart, J. R.: Mastocytosis With Osseous Lesions Resembling Metastatic Malignant Lesions in Bone. *J Bone Joint Surg, 50A:*142-152 (January).

1968 Boseker, E. H., Bickel, W. H., and Dahlin, D. C.: A Clinicopathologic Study of Simple Unicameral Bone Cysts. *Surg Gynecol Obstet, 127:*550-560 (September).

1968 Tillman, B. P., Dahlin, D. C., Lipscomb, P. R., and Stewart, J. R.: Aneurysmal Bone Cyst: An Analysis of Ninety-Five Cases. *Mayo Clin Proc, 43:*478-495 (July).

1970 Campanacci, M., and Leonessa, C.: Displasia Fibrosa dello Scheletro. *Chir Organi Mov, 59:*195-225.

1971 Campanacci, M., and Cervellati, C.: Cisti Aneurismatiche del Bacino a Sviluppo Pseudosarcomatoso. *Chir Organi Mov, 60:*105-112.

1972 Blumenthal, B. I., Capitanio, M. A., Queloz, J. M., and Kirkpatrick, J. A.: Intrathoracic Mesenchymoma: Observations in Two Infants. *Radiology, 104:*107-109 (July).

1973 Feldman, F., and Johnston, A. D.: Ganglia of Bone: Theories, Manifestations, and Presentations. *CRC Crit Rev Clin Radiol Nucl Med, 4:*303-332 (December).

1973 Ireland, D. C. R., Soule, E. H., and Ivins, J. C.: Myxoma of Somatic Soft Tissues: A Report of 58 Patients, 3 With Multiple Tumors and Fibrous Dysplasia of Bone. *Mayo Clin Proc, 48:*401-410 (June).

1973 Smith, J.: Giant Bone Islands. *Radiology, 107:*35-36 (April).

1974 Cabanela, M. E., Sim, F. H., Beabout, J. W., and Dahlin, D. C.: Osteomyelitis Appearing as Neoplasms: A Diagnostic Problem. *Arch Surg, 109:*68-72 (July).

1974 McElfresh, E. C., and Coventry, M. B.: Femoral and Pelvic Fractures After Total Hip Arthroplasty. *J Bone Joint Surg, 56A:*483-492 (April).

1974 Smith, M., McCormack, L. J., Van Ordstrand, H. S., and Mercer, R. D.: "Primary" Pulmonary Histiocytosis X. *Chest, 65:*176-180 (February).

1975 Levy, W. M., Miller, A. S., Bonakdarpour, A., and Aegerter, E.: Aneurysmal Bone Cyst Secondary to Other Osseous Lesions: Report of 57 Cases. *Am J Clin Pathol, 63:*1-8 (January).

1976 Goldman, A. B.: Myositis Ossificans Circumscripta: A Benign Lesion With a Malignant Differential Diagnosis. *Am J Roentgenol, 126:*32-40 (January).

1976 Fitzgerald, R. H. Jr., Brewer, N. S., and Dahlin, D. C.: Squamous-Cell Carcinoma Complicating Chronic Osteomyelitis. *J Bone Joint Surg, 58-A:*1146-1148 (December).

Chapter 29

Odontogenic and Related Tumors

THE JAWBONES provide special tumors that derive from their dental structures. These lesions simulate neoplasms of osseous derivation. The following tabulation of these special tumors, short and somewhat simplified, should be useful to the general pathologist. This short list includes most of these special lesions that the general pathologist is likely to encounter.

Ameloblastoma
Calcifying epithelial odontogenic tumor (Pindborg tumor)
Ameloblastic fibroma
Ameloblastic odontoma
Complex odontoma
Compound odontoma
Myxoma (fibromyxoma)
Adenomatoid odontogenic tumor (Ameloblastic adenomatoid tumor)

Several years ago, we suggested the term "odontogenic mixed tumor" to include ameloblastic fibroma, ameloblastic odontoma, and complex and compound odontoma. This designation acknowledges the histologic overlap seen among members of this group and suggests that they are hamartomatous malformations of the odontogenic anlage. Peculiarly, the fibrous portion of these tumors may become malignant and produce the rare odontogenic sarcomas, including ameloblastic sarcoma.

Bone tumors generally found in the remainder of the skeleton may occur in the jaws; hence, pathologists interested in bone tumors become involved with lesions of odontogenic origin, and therefore, peculiar to the jawbones.

Some special characteristics of tumors of the jaws must be recognized. Osteo chondromas (cartilage-capped benign exostoses) practically never occur in the jaws. Benign chondroblastomas and chondromyxoid fibromas are pathologic curiosities in these bones, and the few recorded tend to be atypical. Osteoblastomas overlap in histopathology with so-called cementoblastomas (*see* Chapter 8). Giant cell tumors of the type found in other bones occur rarely in ever in the jaws, with the exception of those few that develop in Paget's bone. Chondrogenic neoplasms of the jaws are nearly always malignant; one must be aware, however, of chondroid differentiation in a callus or in heterotopic ossification in this region. Osteosarcoma has been easier to cure when it arises in the jaws than it is in other skeletal sites; in these small bones, the lesion develops in somewhat older persons and shows better and often more chondroid differentiation. Adamantinoma of long bones is, of course, a different tumor than ameloblastoma.

Giant cell (reparative) granuloma is distinctively a tumor of the jaw, but a similar process occasionally affects the supramaxillary region, and even bones at distant sites on rare occasions. Aneurysmal bone cyst is probably closely akin to giant cell "tumor" of the jaw, and a classic example is sometimes found there. Synovial chondromatosis sometimes affects the temporomandibular joint.

Metastatic carcinoma can simulate a primary tumor of the jaw.

Although dentinomas are included in many classifications, they probably are but variants of some of the above hamartomalike tumors such as ameloblastic odontoma. Cementifying fibroma (periapical fibrous dysplasia) derives from the specialized bone around the dental roots and thus is not strictly odontogenic. Bulbous masses of densely ossified material surrounding dental roots are considered to be cementomas.

Cysts of the jaws are usually lined by squamous epithelium. Reference to the history and roentgenograms is necessary in determining whether they are related to unerupted teeth, to residual epithelial islands after dental extraction, or whether they have some other genesis. Keratocyst has become recognized as the correct designation for cysts of the jaws that typically have a thinner epithelial lining, lack significant basal zone irregularity like that of rete pegs, and show keratinization at the surface. These cysts have an annoying capability to recur, are often multicentric, and may be associated with the various abnormalities of the basal cell nevus syndrome. Some refer to them as primordial cysts. Occasionally, degenerative alteration with calcification of epithelium produces what has been called "calcifying odontogenic cyst." These cysts and the "hemorrhagic" or "traumatic" cysts of the jaw, which have no lining, pose little diagnostic problem for the histopathologist.

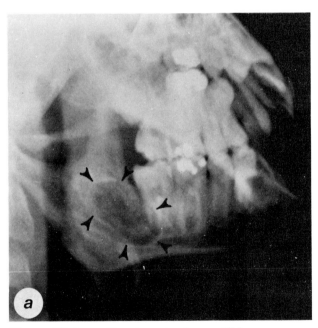
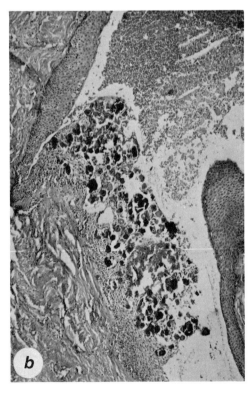

Figure 29-1. *a.* Keratocyst of mandible. *b.* Keratocyst showing in this area zone of degeneration of epithelial cells, some of which have become mineralized. (×64).

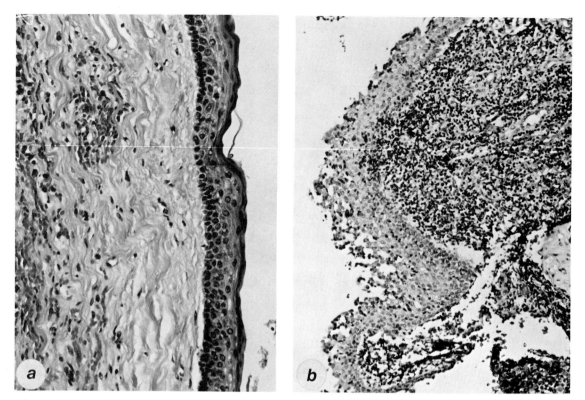

Figure 29-2. *a.* Keratocyst showing regular border along underlying connective tissue, no inflammatory component, and a thin epithelial-cell layer with keratinization at its surface. (×250) *b.* Ordinary squamous epithelial-lined cyst of jaw with inflammatory component and no definite keratinization. (×160)

Benign fibro-osseous lesions of the jaws are relatively common. They encompass such a wide spectrum concerning the amount of osseous component that they defy strict classification. But pathologically they fit into the general category of fibrous (fibro-osseous) dysplasias. Benign, densely collagenous, fibroblastic tissue contains a variable amount of bone, which typically arises as a metaplastic change in the former. Occasional lesions are large, expansile masses that may bulge into and distort the sinuses, and for which the term "fibrous osteoma" or "osteofibroma" is preferred by some. Most are centrally originating lesions that vary greatly in size and radiopacity. They may be incidental roentgenographic findings or produce pronounced distortion of the bone. A minority are a part of the polyostotic fibrous dysplasia complex. Even cherubism, with its fibrous expansion of the jaws of children that is characteristically familial, bilateral, and tends toward spontaneous resolution, is usually called "fibrous dysplasia." The least conspicuous end of the spectrum is the periapical fibrous dysplasia. All of these fibro-osseous lesions, although they may recur, are benign. Conservative surgical management is indicated. Unless exposed to radiation therapy, they have practically no tendency to malignant change. Some osteosarcomas of the jaws are so lacking in overt anaplasia that they pose a problem in differentiation from fibrous dysplasia.

"Fibrous dysplasia" and "fibro-osseous lesion" are the terms applied to the various members of this group by Waldron and Giansanti, who concluded that although similarities exist, they can be separated into these two families of diseases much of the time.

The WHO classification advocated in 1972, although relatively elaborate, is reproduced here because it is reliable and valid and because most of the lesions encountered can be fitted into an appropriate niche.

Histologic Typing of Odontogenic Tumors, Jaw Cysts, and Allied Lesions

I. Neoplasms and other tumors related to the odontogenic apparatus
  A. Benign
    1. Ameloblastoma
    2. Calcifying epithelial odontogenic tumor
    3. Ameloblastic fibroma
    4. Adenomatoid odontogenic tumor (adenoameloblastoma)
    5. Calcifying odontogenic cyst
    6. Dentinoma
    7. Ameloblastic fibro-odontoma
    8. Odontoameloblastoma
    9. Complex odontoma
    10. Compound odontoma
    11. Fibroma (odontogenic fibroma)
    12. Myxoma (myxofibroma)
    13. Cementomas
      a. Benign cementoblastoma (true cementoma)
      b. Cementifying fibroma
      c. Periapical cemental dysplasia (periapical fibrous dysplasia)
      d. Gigantiform cementoma (familial multiple cementomas)
    14. Melanotic neuroectodermal tumor of infancy (melanotic progonoma, melanoameloblastoma)
  B. Malignant
    1. Odontogenic carcinomas
      a. Malignant ameloblastoma
      b. Primary intraosseous carcinoma
      c. Other carcinomas arising from odontogenic epithelium, including those arising from odontogenic cysts
    2. Odontogenic sarcomas
      a. Ameloblastic fibrosarcoma (ameloblastic sarcoma)
      b. Ameloblastic odontosarcoma
II. Neoplasms and other tumors related to bone
  A. Osteogenic neoplasms
    1. Ossifying fibroma (fibro-osteoma)
  B. Non-neoplastic bone lesions
    1. Fibrous dysplasia
    2. Cherubism

3. Central giant cell granuloma (giant cell reparative granuloma)
4. Aneurysmal bone cyst
5. Simple bone cyst (traumatic, hemorrhagic bone cyst)

III. Epithelial cysts
   A. Developmental
      1. Odontogenic
         a. Primordial cyst (keratocyst)
         b. Gingival cyst
         c. Eruption cyst
         d. Dentigerous (follicular) cyst
      2. Non-odontogenic
         a. Nasopalatine duct (incisive canal) cyst
         b. Globulomaxillary cyst
         c. Nasolabial (nasoalveolar) cyst
   B. Inflammatory
      1. Radicular cyst
IV. Unclassified lesions

This chapter is not meant to supplant standard texts on this complex subject. Some of the lesions are rare. For instance, we have recognized only one melanotic progonoma.

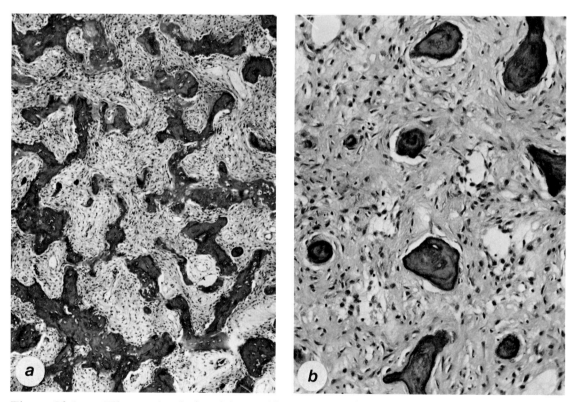

Figure 29-3. *a.* Fibrous dysplasia of jaw. This characteristic pattern may occur in lesions of the jaw of patients with polyostotic involvement, even in Albright's syndrome. (×160) *b.* Fibro-osseous "lesion." Such tumors may resemble those of fibrous dysplasia, making roentgenologic and surgical findings essential to their interpretation. (×160)

Ameloblastoma

There are about 125 ameloblastomas in the Mayo Clinic's total series of oral lesions, which includes 50 osteosarcomas of the jaws. Ameloblastoma is the most common of the odontogenic tumors in our surgical series, and yet it comprises only about 1 percent of the cysts and tumors seen in the area of the maxilla and mandible (Gorlin and coworkers, 1961). There is no notable sex predilection, and the tumor occurs throughout adulthood and old age. It is distinctly rare in young children. More than three fourths of the lesions arise in the mandible, most commonly in the molar-angle region. Slowly growing, the tumor is usually painless. Swelling is the usual symptom. The roentgenogram shows a cystlike radiolucent expansion, which may be multilocular or unilocular and is simulated by various lesions. The tumor often contains cysts and may be so predominantly cystic that squamous epithelium-lined cyst with incidental non-neoplastic ameloblastic elements in its wall becomes a differential consideration.

The proliferating epithelial elements belie their derivation from ameloblasts. The outer layer in the cellular islands is usually of cells of columnar type, with nuclei tending to be away from the basement membrane. The cells often become stellate and loosely arranged in the centers of the islands. Although follicular and plexiform patterns are described, these merge in many tumors. A variable amount of non-neoplastic collagen may separate the epithelial islands. Sometimes, large zones of spindle-shaped epithelial cells are suggestive of sarcoma. Squamous metaplasia is relatively frequent and may be so extensive as to suggest that the tumor is squamous cell carcinoma. Rare ameloblastomas contain cells that are granular; such cells may comprise the entire tumor. Some ameloblastomas are so vascular that they have been called "ameloblastohemangiomas." The histogenesis of melanoameloblastoma (melanotic progonoma, retinal anlage tumor) is obscure, but this rare tumor of infancy is nearly always found in the jaws, especially the maxilla. By definition, ameloblastomas produce no recognizable mature dental substances. The extremely rare but distinctive calcifying epithelial odontogenic tumor described by Pindborg (1958) may be a variant of ameloblastoma; it behaves like one. It contains characteristic spherical calcific masses. Some of these peculiar ameloblastic tumors contain a substance that looks and stains like amyloid. It is important to recognize this primary tumor of the jaws partly because it may be confused with metastatic carcinoma. One of our tumors occurred in the basal cell nevus syndrome.

Treatment principles for ameloblastoma are still controversial, but it seems reasonable to adopt a relatively conservative attitude since metastasis practically never occurs. The tumor does have marked capacity to recur unless widely excised.

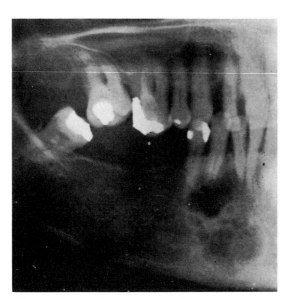

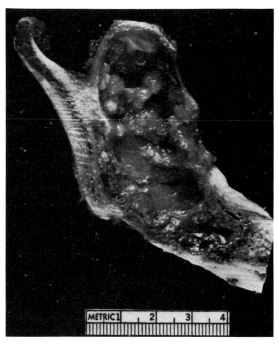

Figure 29-4. Recurrent multilocular ameloblastoma of anterior part of mandible.

Figure 29-5. Partially cystic ameloblastoma bulging from region of angle of mandible.

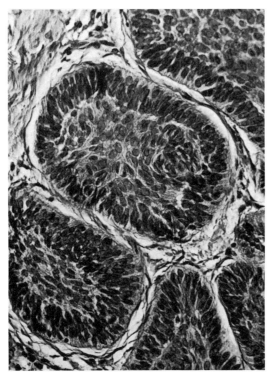

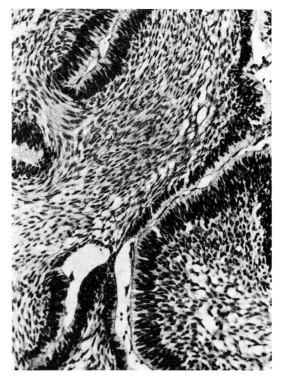

Figure 29-6. *Left.* Solidly packed islands of cells show typical peripheral palisading of ameloblasts. (×325) *Right.* In this tumor, cells of centers of anastomosing clusters show prominent spindling quality. (×200)

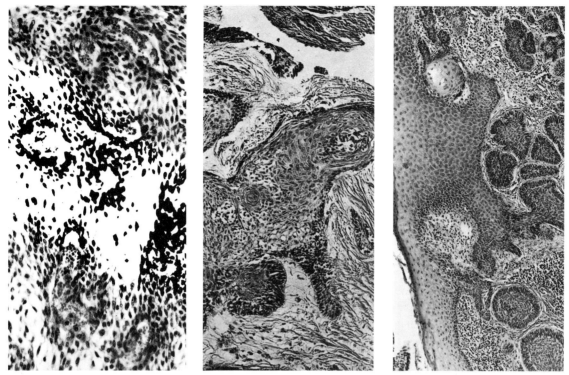

Figure 29-7. Patterns of ameloblasts. *Left.* Prominent vascularity such as seen here has prompted some to consider this lesion hemangioameloblastoma. (×200) *Middle.* Squamous metaplasia, which is not an extremely unusual finding. (×125) *Right.* Ameloblastoma eroding to and fusing with gingival epithelium. (×70)

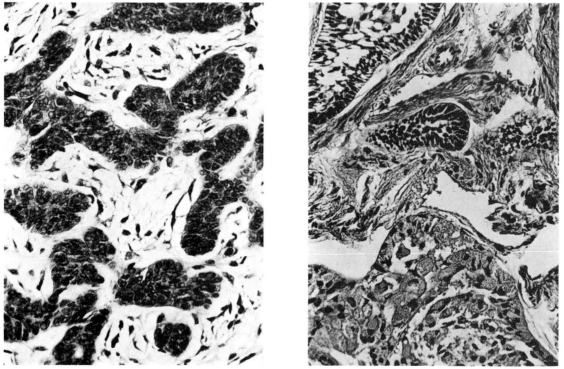

Figure 29-8. *Left.* Trabecular pattern sometimes seen in ameloblastomas mimics histologic appearance of ameloblastic fibroma somewhat. Characteristic fibrous component of latter lesion is lacking. (×250) *Right.* Granular cells such as these comprise part or all of an ameloblastoma in rare instances. (×250)

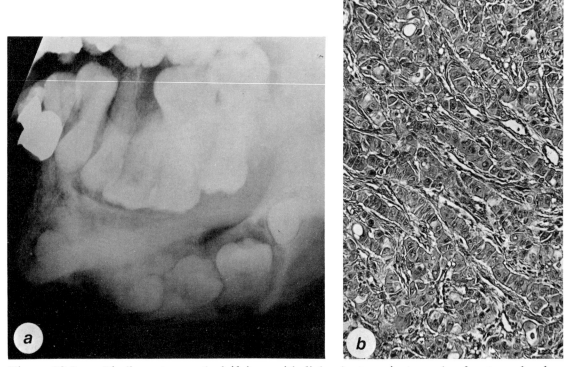

Figure 29-9. *a.* Pindborg tumor (calcifying epithelial odontogenic tumor) of extremely slow growth. *b.* Strands of epithelial cells in unmineralized area of Pindborg tumor. (×175) (Reproduced with permission from: Vap, D. R., Dahlin, D. C., and Turlington, E. G.: *Cancer,* *25:*629-636, 1970.)

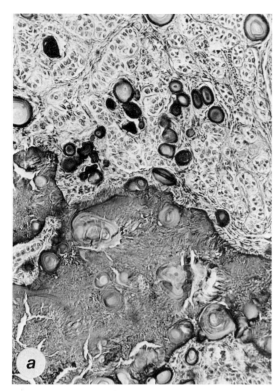 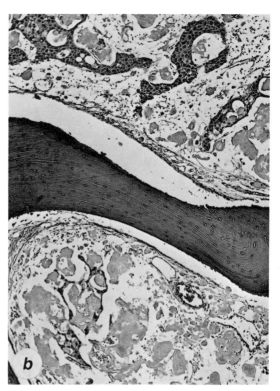

Figure 29-10. *a.* Mineralized portion of Pindborg tumor showing association with epithelial cells. (×150) *b.* Epithelial cells and amyloid deposits in Pindborg tumor that is invading bone at its periphery. (×50) (Reproduced with permission from: Vap, D. R., Dahlin, D. C., and Turlington, E. G.: *Cancer, 25:*629-636, 1970.)

Adenomatoid Odontogenic Tumor (Ameloblastic Adenomatoid Tumor)

This tumor, also called "adenoameloblastoma," should be distinguished from ameloblastoma because it responds to conservative surgical removal, having little tendency to recur. It is much less common than ameloblastoma. The Mayo Clinic files to January 1, 1976, contained only ten examples. Most of approximately forty reported tumors have been in patients whose ages have ranged from eleven to twenty-six years; there has been a slight predominance of females. Approximately two thirds of the tumors have involved the maxilla, and nearly all of them have been located anterior to the first premolars. Tumefaction is the common symptom. Roentgenologically, the tumor produces a cystlike zone, which may display calcific material in a stippled pattern. The "cyst" often contains an unerupted tooth and resembles a dentigerous cyst. Grossly, the lesion is often actually cystic, and the solid tissue may fill only a fraction of the cavity. A few extraosseous tumors of this type have been recognized. The expanding process is well demarcated from surrounding tissue. Microscopically, the tumor is characterized by tubular, ductlike structures lined with columnar or cuboidal epithelium. The central spaces in some of these ductlike structures are empty, others are filled with acidophilic material, and still others are lined by a layer of pink hyaline material. Small calcified spherules or even larger mineralized masses may be found, sometimes within the tubular spaces.

Masses of cells that produce whorllike structures are found among the glandular-appearing elements. These epithelial cells sometimes resemble the stellate reticulum of ameloblastomas, but they are usually distinctly spindle-shaped. These nests of cells lie outside the glandular component, which is in striking contrast to their location within the palisade of columnar cells in ameloblastoma. Although the cells are closely packed, they are regular in size and shape and do not appear to be anaplastic. The prognosis is excellent, local curettage being curative.

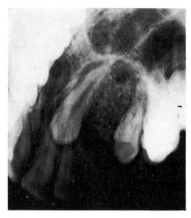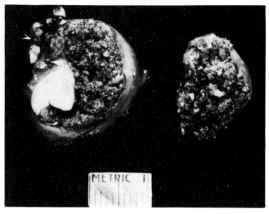

Figure 29-11. *Left*. Ameloblastic adenomatoid tumor presenting as cystlike lesion containing upper right premolar tooth. *Right*. Surgical specimen. Most of premolar tooth was within well-circumscribed tumor, but part of root projected from it. (Reproduced with permission from: Stafne, E. C.: *Oral Surg, 1*:887-894, 1948.)

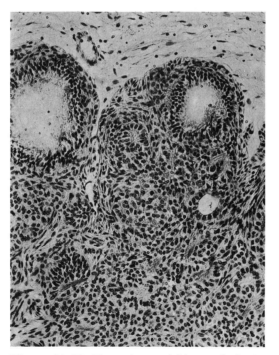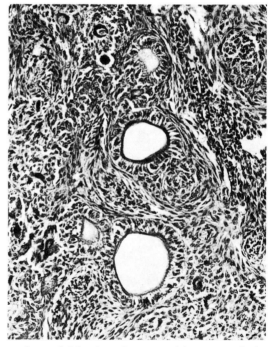

Figure 29-12. Two views of histopathologic pattern of ameloblastic adenomatoid tumor. *Left*. Periphery of mass showing ductular structures of varying size and slightly fusiform cells among them. (×140) *Right*. Central portion of tumor, which has same basic pattern. Small mineralized (darkly staining) masses are present. (×140) (Reproduced with permission from: Stafne, E. C.: *Oral Surg, 1*:887-894, 1948.)

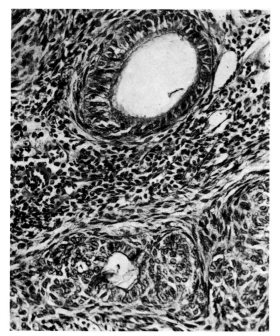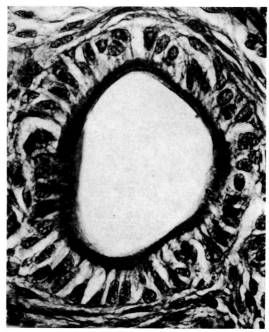

Figure 29-13. *Left.* Another ameloblastic adenomatoid tumor illustrating pronounced similarity to one in Figure 29-12. (×210) All tumors of this type are remarkably alike histologically. *Right.* Higher magnification emphasizes ameloblastic quality of cells lining tubular structures. This one has thin hyalin-appearing lining. (Reproduced with permission from: Stafne, E. C.: *Oral Surg, 1:*887-894, 1948.)

Ameloblastic Fibroma

This lesion, also called "soft mixed odontoma," is rare. Six examples were found in our files. Proliferation of mesenchymal and epithelial odontogenic elements characterize this tumor. In contrast to ameloblastoma, in which the connective tissue is not part of the neoplastic process, ameloblastic fibroma contains an actively proliferating fibroblastic component. There is apparently no sex predilection. It is seen throughout childhood and adolescence but is rare in patients more than twenty-one years of age. Most of these tumors affect the mandible, especially the bicuspid-molar region. Generally, there is painless swelling, and the lesion may be found incidentally on roentgenograms, where it produces a well-circumscribed cyst-like radiolucent zone. Occasionally, an unerupted tooth is associated with the tumor. Grossly, the tissue is a soft fibrous mass. Histologically, the proliferating fibroblasts have plump nuclei that show little variation in size and shape. There are buds, cords, and islands of epithelial cells that are usually only a few cell layers thick. Peripheral cells tend to become columnar, as in ameloblastoma. If one studies many sections in an ameloblastic fibroma, one may find evidence of hard dental structures such as dentin and enamel or preenamel. Hence, this tumor overlaps histologically with ameloblastic odontoma, and both lesions probably should be regarded as hamartomas of a more primitive type than are the composite and compound odontomas.

Nearly all ameloblastic fibromas are easily cured by conservative surgical means, but a malignant counterpart in which fibrosarcoma arises in the stroma occurs. Two such cases were present in our series, and several others have been documented.

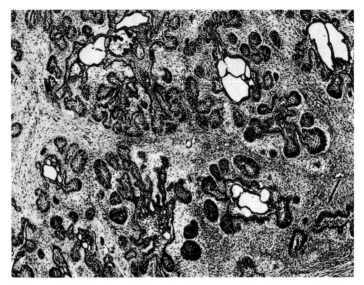

Figure 29-14. Ameloblastic fibroma showing ramifying and branching cords of ameloblastic cells and associated fibroblastic proliferation. (×48)

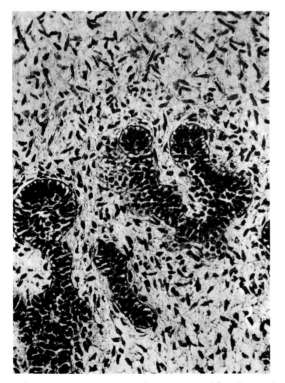

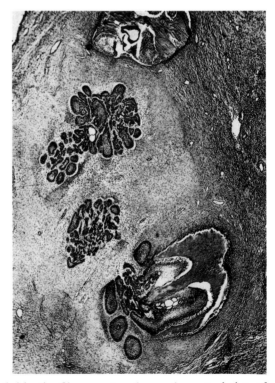

Figure 29-15. *Left.* Higher magnification of ameloblastic fibroma to show characteristics of epithelial component and plump uniform nuclei of fibroblastic portion. (×250) *Right.* Except for small foci of hard dental structure formation, shown here as homogeneous masses, this tumor was typical of ameloblastic fibroma throughout. Tumors like this emphasize kinship of these various hamartomalike tumors that reproduce dental structures or their precursors. (×29)

Ameloblastic Odontoma

This tumor occupies a place between ameloblastic fibroma and the compound and composite odontomas. It contains foci of proliferating ameloblastic cells, which introduce the hazard of mistaking the lesion for ameloblastoma. Dentin and enamel, which are present in a poorly organized state, differentiate it from ameloblastoma and indicate its basically hamartomatous nature. Parts of ameloblastic odontoma may resemble ameloblastic fibroma. Our files yielded only seven cases of this rare tumor, which is usually found in children. Any part of either jaw may be affected, but Gorlin and coworkers (1961) found a predilection for the premolar and molar areas. Delayed eruption or irregular position of teeth and swelling of the alveolar process may result from this tumor. The cystlike zone in the roentgenogram may contain small or large radiopaque bodies. Nearly all of these well-circumscribed tumors are readily cured by conservative surgical means, but sarcomatous change in the connective tissue has been observed on very rare occasions.

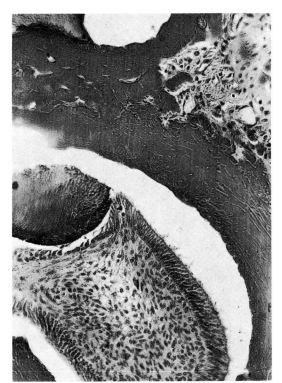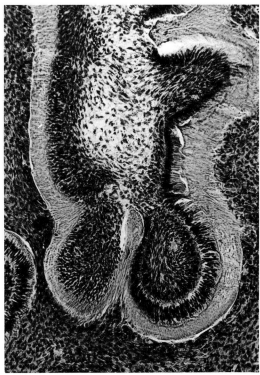

Figure 29-16. Ameloblastic odontoma. *Left.* Variable amounts of hard dental structures are produced by this tumor. Dentin dominates this area, but dark mass at left center is early enamel matrix. (×250) *Right.* Here ameloblastic proliferation is even more prominent. (×125)

Complex Odontoma

This tumor lacks ameloblastic tissue, corresponding to a later stage of development of teeth than does ameloblastic odontoma. A disorderly mixture of hard dental elements characterizes the lesion. It is considered to be somewhat more common in females, and six of the eleven tumors affected this sex. It is found most often in older children and in young adults. It has a predilection for the molar portion of the lower jaw. The lesion is usually an incidental roentgenographic finding and is readily cured by simple removal.

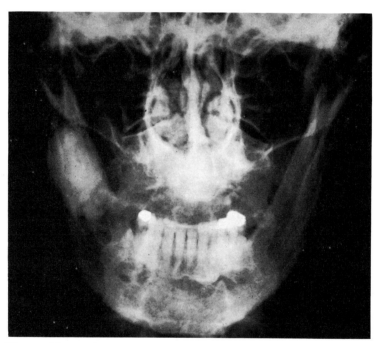

Figure 29-17. Complex odontoma with its poorly formed but recognizable dental structures. *Above.* Well-circumscribed and heavily mineralized tumor in ramus of mandible.

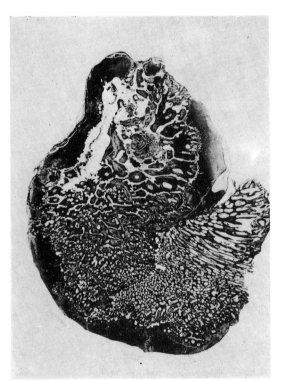 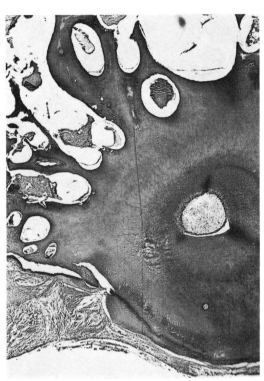

Figure 29-17 *continued. Left.* An entire complex odontoma. (×3) *Right.* Higher magnification showing ramifying dentin in background of fibrous tissue. (×30)

Compound Odontomas

These tumors are composed of grossly recognizable teeth, although they tend to be small and deformed. The number of teeth varies from three or four to many hundred. Complex and compound odontomas merge with one another, being arbitrarily separated on the basis of the degree of morphodifferentiation of the teeth. Both tumors are completely benign. Compound odontoma tends to occur in the incisor-cuspid region.

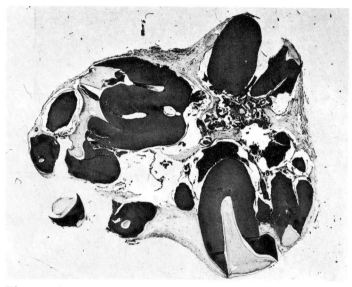

Figure 29-18. Compound odontoma. Here, differentiation toward teeth is definite. (×6) (Reproduced with permission from: Cina, M. T., Dahlin, D. C., and Gores, R. J.: *Proc Staff Meet Mayo Clin, 36:*664-678, 1961.)

Myxoma (Fibromyxoma)

Myxomas of bone practically always occur in the jaws, which suggests that they are probably of odontogenic origin. This suggestion is supported by the resemblance of these tumors to the mesenchymal portion of the tooth germ. Some chondrosarcomas and even fibrosarcomas of the remainder of the skeleton show such prominent myxomatous alteration, probably as a result of degeneration, that they have been classified erroneously among the myxomas and myxosarcomas. In our experience, myxoma of the jaws is approximately one-sixth as common as ameloblastoma. No sex predilection has been noted. Although almost any age may be affected, most of the lesions are discovered during the second and third decades of life. The upper and lower jaws are about equally affected. This slowly growing lesion is usually painless but causes slowly progressive swelling; sometimes severe facial deformity results. Roentgenographically, the tumors may appear to be multilocular or unilocular. They cannot be distinguished from other cystlike rarefying expansile lesions of the jaws. Grossly, the tumor is soft and semitranslucent and may have a bosselated surface. Loose stellate cells dominate the histologic pattern. They have long anastomosing cytoplasmic processes. The intercellular substance may be somewhat granular and basophilic. Some myxomas are hypocellular and obviously benign. Others contain relatively large and bizarre nuclei, suggesting that they are more active, but follow-up studies indicate no correlation between cytologic abnormalities and ability of the tumor to recur. Sometimes zones within myxomas show considerable fibromatous quality, but this does not appear to affect their clinical behavior.

The available evidence suggests that myxoma of the jaws has a capacity to recur similar to that of ameloblastoma, but that it does not metastasize. The therapeutic goal should be total local removal of the lesion. Chondrosarcomas, osseosarcomas, and even fibrosarcomas with myxoid features can simulate myxoma and must be carefully differentiated from the latter.

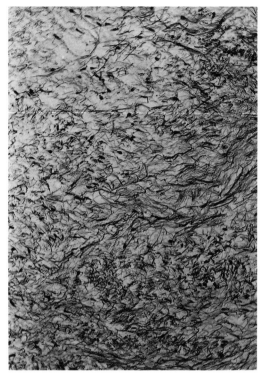

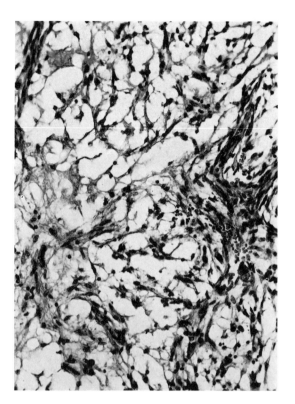

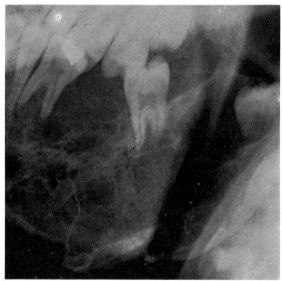

Figure 29-19. *Top left.* Myxoma with scanty, small cells and characteristic slightly fibrillar and almost transparent matrix. (×140) *Top right.* More cellular myxomas such as this have not been associated with poorer prognosis in our material. (×200) *Bottom right.* Expanding "multicystic" myxoma that extended from second bicuspid to coronoid process of right mandible.

Bibliography

1953   Berger, A., and Jaffe, H. L.: Fibrous (Fibro-osseous) Dysplasia of Jaw Bones. *J Oral Surg, 11:*3-17.

1953   Jaffe, H. L.: Giant Cell Reparative Granuloma, Traumatic Bone Cyst, and Fibrous (Fibro-osseous) Dysplasia of the Jaw Bones. *Oral Surg, 6:*159-175.

1958   Chaudhry, A. P., Spink, J. H., and Gorlin, R. J.: Periapical Fibrous Dysplasia (Cementoma). *J Oral Surg, 16:*483-488.

1958   Pindborg, J. J.: A Calcifying Epithelial Odontogenic Tumor. *Cancer, 11:*838-843.

1958   Zimmerman, D. C., and Dahlin, D. C.: Myxomatous Tumors of the Jaws. *Oral Surg, 11:*1069-1080.

1961 Chaudhry, A. P., Robinovitch, M. R., Mitchell, D. F., and Vickers, R. A.: Chondrogenic Tumors of the Jaws. *Am J Surg, 102:*403-411 (September).

1961 Cina, M. T., Dahlin, D. C., and Gores, R. J.: Odontogenic Mixed Tumors: A Review of the Mayo Clinic Series. *Proc Staff Meet Mayo Clin, 36:*664-678.

1961 Gorlin, R. J., Chaudhry, A. P., and Pindborg, J. J.: Odontogenic Tumors. Classification, Histopathology, and Clinical Behavior in Man and Domesticated Animals. *Cancer, 14:*73-101.

1962 Anderson, D. E., McClendon, J. L., and Cornelius, E. A.: Cherubism-Hereditary Fibrous Dysplasia of the Jaws. I. Genetic Considerations. II. Pathologic Considerations. *Oral Surg, 15 (Supplement 2):* 5-16, 17-42.

1962 Cina, M. T., Dahlin, D. C., and Gores, R. J.: Ameloblastic Sarcoma. Report of Two Cases. *Oral Surg, 15:*696-700.

1963 Cina, M. T., Dahlin, D. C., and Gores, R. J.: Ameloblastic Adenomatoid Tumors. A Report of Four New Cases. *Am J Clin Pathol, 39:*59-65

1965 Gorlin, R. J., Vickers, R. A., Kelln, E., and Williamson, J. J.: The Multiple Basal-Cell Nevi Syndrome: An Analysis of a Syndrome Consisting of Multiple Nevoid Basal Cell Carcinoma, Jaw Cysts, Skeletal Anomalies, Medulloblastoma, and Hyporesponsiveness to Parathormone. *Cancer, 18:*89-104 (January).

1965 Shear, M.: The Unity of Tumours of Odontogenic Epithelium. *Br J Oral Surg, 2:*212-221.

1965 Vickers, R. A., Dahlin, D. C., and Gorlin, R. J.: Amyloid Containing Odontogenic Tumors. *Oral Surg, 20:*476-480.

1966 Webb, H. E., Devine, K. D., and Harrison, E. G., Jr.: Solitary Myeloma of the Mandible. *Oral Surg, 22:*1-6 (July).

1967 Garrington, G. E., Scofield, H. H., Cornyn, J., and Hooker, S. P.: Osteosarcoma of the Jaws: Analysis of 56 Cases. *Cancer, 20:*377-391 (March).

1968 Abrams, A. M., Melrose, R. J., and Howell, F. V.: Adenoameloblastoma: A Clinical Pathologic Study of Ten New Cases. *Cancer, 22:*175-185 (July).

1968 Smith, R. L., Dahlin, D. C., and Waite, D. E.: Mucoepidermoid Carcinomas of the Jawbones. *J Oral Surg, 26:*387-393 (June).

1969 Allen, M. S., Jr., Harrison, W., and Jahrsdoerfer, R. A.: "Retinal Anlage" Tumors: Melanotic Progonoma, Melanotic Adamantinoma, Pigmented Epulis, Melanotic Neuroectodermal Tumor of Infancy, Benign Melanotic Tumor of Infancy. *Am J Clin Pathol, 51:*309-314 (March).

1969 Shear, M.: Primary Intra-alveolar Epidermoid Carcinoma of the Jaw. *J Pathol, 97:*645-651 (April).

1970 Cabrini, R. L., Barros, R. E., and Albano, H.: Cysts of the Jaws: A Statistical Analysis. *J Oral Surg, 28:*485-489 (July).

1970 Dhawan, I. K., Bhargava, S., Nayak, N. C., and Gupta, R. K.: Central Salivary Gland Tumors of Jaws. *Cancer, 26:*211-217 (July).

1970 Gorlin, R. J., and Goldman, H. M.: *Thoma's Oral Pathology,* ed. 6, vols. 1 and 2. Saint Louis, Mosby, 1139 pp.

1970 Khosla, V. M., and Korobkin, M.: Cherubism. *Am J Dis Child, 120:*458-461 (November).

1970 Vap, D. R., Dahlin, D. C., and Turlington, E. G.: Pindborg Tumor: The So-Called Calcifying Epithelial Odontogenic Tumor. *Cancer, 25:*629-636 (March).

1971 Huebner, G. R., and Turlington, E. G.: So-Called Traumatic (Hemorrhagic) Bone Cysts of the Jaws: Review of the Literature and Report of Two Unusual Cases. *Oral Surg, 31:*345-365 (March).

1971 Pindborg, J. J., and Kramer, I. R. H.: Histological Typing of Odontogenic Tumours, Jaw Cysts, and Allied Lesions. In *International Histological Classification of Tumours,* no. 5. Geneva, World Health Organization, 43 pp.

1971 Van Blarcom, C. W., Masson, J. K., and Dahlin, D. C.: Fibrosarcoma of the Mandible: A Clinicopathologic Study. *Oral Surg, 32:*428-439 (September).

1972 Brady, C. L., and Browne, R. M.: Benign Osteoblastoma of the Mandible. *Cancer, 30:*329-333 (August).

1972 Browne, R. M., and Gough, N. G.: Malignant Change in the Epithelium Lining Odontogenic Cysts. *Cancer, 29:*1199-1207 (May).

1972 Leider, A. S., Nelson, J. F., and Trodahl, J. N.: Ameloblastic Fibrosarcoma of the Jaws. *Oral Surg, 33:*559-569 (April).

1972 Mehlisch, D. R., Dahlin, D. C., and Masson, J. K.: Ameloblastoma: A Clinicopathologic Report. *J Oral Surg, 30:*9-22 (January).

1972 Payne, T. F.: An Analysis of the Clinical and Histopathologic Parameters of the Odontogenic Keratocyst. *Oral Surg, 33:*538-546 (April).

1972 Trodahl, J. N.: Ameloblastic Fibroma: A Survey of Cases From the Armed Forces Institute of Pathology. *Oral Surg, 33:*547-558 (April).

1973 Anderson, L., Fejerskov, O., and Philipsen, H. P.: Calcifying Fibroblastic Granuloma. *J Oral Surg, 31:*196-200 (March).

1973 Eversole, L. R., Sabes, W. R., and Dauchess, V. G.: Benign Cementoblastoma. *Oral Surg, 36:*824-830 (December).

1973 Ghosh, B. C., Huvos, A. G., Gerold, F. P., and Miller, T. R.: Myxoma of the Jaw Bones. *Cancer, 31:*237-240 (January).

1973 Waldron, C. A., and Giansanti, J. S.: Benign Fibro-osseous Lesions of the Jaws: A Clinical-Radiologic-Histologic Review of Sixty-Five Cases. I. Fibrous Dysplasia of the Jaws. *Oral Surg, 35:*190-201 (February).

1973 Waldron, C. A., and Giansanti, J. S.: Benign Fibro-osseous Lesions of the Jaws: A Clinical-Radiologic-Histologic Review of Sixty-Five Cases. II. Benign Fibro-osseous Lesions of Periodontal Ligament Origin. *Oral Surg, 35:*340-350 (March).

1974 Shafer, W. G., Hine, M. K., and Levy, B. M.: *A Textbook of Oral Pathology,* ed. 3. Philadelphia, Saunders, 853 pp.

1974 van der Kwast, W. A. M., and ven der Waal, I.: Jaw Metastases. *Oral Surg, 37:*850-857 (June).

1975 Altini, M., and Farman, A. G.: The Calcifying Odontogenic Cyst: Eight New Cases and a Review of the Literature. *Oral Surg, 40:*751-759 (December).

1975 Courtney, R. M., and Kerr, D. A.: The Odontogenic Adenomatoid Tumor: A Comprehensive Study of Twenty New Cases. *Oral Surg, 39:*424-435 (March).

1975 Pullon, P. A., Shafer, W. G., Elzay, R. P., Kerr, D. A., and Corio, R. L.: Squamous Odontogenic Tumor: Report of Six Cases of a Previously Undescribed Lesion. *Oral Surg, 40:*616-630 (November).

1975 Waldron, C. A., Giansanti, J. S., and Browand, B. C.: Sclerotic Cemental Masses of the Jaws (So-called Chronic Sclerosing Osteomyelitis, Sclerosing Osteitis, Multiple Enostosis, and Gigantiform Cementoma). *Oral Surg, 39:*590-604 (April).

1976 Budnick, S. D.: Compound and Complex Odontomas. *Oral Surg, 42:*501-506 (October).

1976 Lucas, R. B.: *Pathology of Tumours of the Oral Tissues,* ed. 3. New York, Churchill Livingston.

Index